TABLE OF CONTENTS

D1337936

ACKNOWLEDGEMENTS

The WHO Centre for Health Development, Kobe, Japan, is grateful to the following contributors for their active participation and collaboration at various stages in the preparation and publication of the WHO Global Atlas of Traditional, Complementary and Alternative Medicine.

WHO AFRICAN REGION

Cameroon: Daniel N. Lantum, Martin Ekeke Monono; *Ghana:* Francis Kwabena Oppong-Boachie; *Kenya:* Jack Githae; *Mozambique:* Adelaide Bela Agostinho; *Nigeria:* Tolu Fakeye, Karniyus S. Gamaniel, Abayomi Sofowora; *Swaziland:* D. Nhlavana Maseko; *Uganda:* Joseph Tenywa; *United Republic of Tanzania:* Andrew Y. Kitua, Rogasian Lemmy Anselm Mahunnah, Zacharia H. Mbwambo, Paul Mhame, Sabina Mnaliwa, Mainen J. Moshi, Febronia C. Uiso.

WHO REGION OF THE AMERICAS

Argentina: Silvia Debenedetti, Maria A. Rossella, Susana Zacchino; *Bolivia:* Alberto Gimenez, José Antonio Pagés; *Brazil:* Elaine Elisabetsky; *Canada:* Michael John Smith, Tracey Spack; *Chile:* Ana Christina Nogueira; *Costa Rica:* Philippe Lamy, Gerardo Alberto Mora; *Cuba:* Franscisco Moron; *Dominican Republic:* Dalia Castillo, Carlos Roersch; *Ecuador:* Ximena Chiriboga, Fernando Ortega; *Guatemala:* Armando Caceres, Hilda Leal de Molina; *Honduras:* Jorge A. Mendoza, Cristina Mercedes Montoya, Regina Moncada; *Nicaragua:* Franscisco Beteta; *Panama:* Mahabir Prashad Gupta, Jose De Gracia, Rosaura Jimenez, Ana Isabel Santana, Pablo Solis; *Suriname:* Hanny L. van de Lande, Lucien Kloof; *United States of America:* Joseph Bastien, Rowan J. D. Brixey, Nancy A. Hazleton, Jack Killen, Karen E. Kun.

WHO SOUTH-EAST ASIA REGION

Bangladesh: Mahbub Ara Ummeh Zohra; *Bhutan:* Dorji Wangchuk; *India:* B.B. Gaitonde, P.N.V. Kurup, G.S. Lavekar, Sheyphali B. Sharan, S.K. Sharma; *Indonesia:* M Hayatie Amal, Rachmaniar Brahim, Hardaningsih, Sri Harsodjo, Kustiani, Agnes M. Loupatty, Soetomo, Nani Sukasediati, Imam Waluyo; *Sri Lanka:* Niletthi Nimal Siripala De Silva; *Thailand:* Tipsukon Bamrungwong, Anchalee Chuthaputti, Kunchana Deewised, Pennapa Subcharoen.

WHO EUROPEAN REGION

Denmark: Erling Høg, Karen Worm, *Georgia:* Lali Dateshidze, *Germany:* Gudrun Bornhöft, Thomas Hofmann, Peter F. Matthiessen, Susanne Moebus, *Russian Federation:* Andrey V. Goryunov, Alexey A. Karpeev, Vladimir V. Tonkov, Pavel P. Vetrenko, Andrey S. Zakharevich; *Sweden:* Torkel Falkenberg; *United Kingdom:* Henrietta Bidwell, Gerard Bodeker, Gordon Brown, Gemma Burford, Alison Daykin, Chris Grundy, Penny Ireland, Michael McIntyre, Cora Neumann, Chi-Keong Ong, Kerrie Raggatt, Mushi Rahman, Terence Ryan, Judith Thompson, Diana Walford.

WHO EASTERN MEDITERRANEAN REGION

Egypt: Aly Bayoumi Hammad; *Islamic Republic of Iran:* Majid Cheraghali, Ali Haeri, Mahmoud Mosaddegh, Farzaneh Naghibi; *Kuwait:* Abdul Rahman Abdulla Al-Awadi, Ahmed Regai El-Gendy, Mohammad Sabir; *Pakistan:* Athar Saeed Dil, Anwar-ul-Hassan Gilani, Hakeem Abdul Hannan, Shahzad Hussain, Farnaz Malik; *Saudi Arabia:* Tawfeq A. Al-Howiriny, Abdullah M. N. Al-Bedah; *United Arab Emirates:* Sassan Behjat.

WHO WESTERN PACIFIC REGION

Australia: Alan Bensoussan, David Chapman-Smith, Stephen Myers; *China:* Dequan Ren, Ping Yan Lam, Baoyan Liu, Zhi Xiang Shen, Jarme Sin, Xiaopin Wang, Zhendou Wu, Jiaqing Zhu; *Fiji:* Nacanieli Goneyali; *Japan:* Norio Aimi, Kazuhiko Atsumi, Yukihiro Goda, Ken Hara, Masao Hattori, Munekazu Iinuma, Takeatsu Kimura, Hiroaki Kiyohara, Chiaki Nagase, Shinya Sakai, Ushio Sankawa, Motoyoshi Satake, Setsuko Sekita, Shohachi Tanzawa, Katsutoshi Terasawa, Kazuo

Toriizuka, Kiichiro Tsutani, Haruki Yamada, Takahiro Yamada, Kaisuke Yoneda, Yoshitoku Yoshida; *Lao People's Democratic Republic:* Boun Hoong Sourthavong; *Malaysia:* Abdul Aziz Mahmood; *Mongolia:* Zina, Batchmeg; *Papua New Guinea:* Umadevi Ambihaipahar; *Philippines:* Alfonso T. Lagaya, *Republic of Korea:* Jae-kyu An, Chung-Whan Byun, Il-Moo Chang, Hyun-Woo Han, Seonsam Na, Pyong-Ui Roh, Yoonsook Yoo; *Singapore:* Chris Cheah; *Viet Nam:* Tran Luu Van Hien, Le Van Truyen, Chu Quoc Truong.

WORLD HEALTH ORGANIZATION

WHO Centre for Health Development: Yuji Kawaguchi*, Kin Shein, Yuki Maehira

WHO Headquarters: Xiaorui Zhang, Steeve Ebener, Yaniss Guigoz.

WHO Regional Office for Africa: Rufaro Chatora, Ossy M.J. Kasilo, Marianne Ngoulla, Edoh Soumbey-Alley, Charles Wambebe.

WHO Regional Office for the Americas/Pan American Sanitary Bureau: Sandra Land, Rosario D'Alessio.

WHO Regional Office for South-East Asia: Krisantha Weerasuriya.

WHO Regional Office for Europe: Kees de Joncheere.

WHO Regional Office for the Eastern Mediterranean: Mohamed Bin Shahna, Peter Graaff.

WHO Regional Office for the Western Pacific: Seung-hoon Choi, Ken Chen.

Contributions to the publication of this Global Atlas by Rosamund Williams (WHO style editing), June Morrison (indexing), are also gratefully acknowledged. The WHO Centre for Health Development is also grateful to all the other contributors in the preparation and publication of the Global Atlas.

---

* Dr Yuji Kawaguchi, former Director of WHO Centre for Health Development, is acknowledged for his conceptualization, initiation, and support to the Global Atlas work.

FOREWORD

The International Conference on Primary Health Care, held in 1978 in Alma-Ata in the former Soviet Union, launched "Health for All", a global movement that has shaped the dynamics of public health ever since. Yet, despite indisputable advances made, the situation remains as "health for some". Issues such as disparity in health-care coverage; lack of equitable, accessible and affordable health care for all; and problems with availability of realistic financial resources for health services and medicines are daily realities for the indigent, the marginalized and the underprivileged.

The World Health Organization (WHO) estimates that one-third of the world's population has no regular access to essential modern medicines; in some parts of Africa, Asia, and Latin America, as much as half of the population faces these persistent shortages. However, in these same situations, the rich resources of traditional remedies and practitioners are available and accessible.

Traditional medicines play a primary role in people's health, as they have for thousands of years. The range of therapies and practices is wide, varying greatly from country to country and from region to region. The most well-known are the Ayurveda of India and traditional Chinese medicine and these systems of medicine have now spread to other countries.

The use of herbal medicines, and complementary and alternative medicine, is increasing in industrialized countries, in connection with disease prevention and the maintenance of health. There is an emphasis on self-empowerment and a more holistic approach, in which life is understood as being a union of body, senses, mind and soul; and health as being the combination of physical, mental, social and spiritual well-being. This approach is consistent with WHO's definition of health. The practices of traditional, complementary and alternative medicine focus on the holistic approach and include medicinal plants. Herbal medicines are perceived as "safe", although in reality there are potential risks, such as side-effects, in the use of all medicines. The relatively low cost of traditional remedies and their greater accessibility contrasts with the rising cost and limited availability of a number of even the most essential modern medicines.

The WHO Global Atlas of Traditional, Complementary and Alternative Medicine relates well to one of WHO's overall strategic directions in traditional medicine for 2002–2005; that of tackling excess mortality and morbidity especially among poor and marginalized populations. Traditional medicine's accessibility and affordability are key values for populations struggling against communicable and noncommunicable diseases, especially in their chronic forms.

We have seen a global resurgence of interest in the use of traditional, complementary and alternative medicine over the last decade. The Fifty-sixth World Health Assembly formally acknowledged this in May 2003; Member States discussed the WHO Traditional Medicine Strategy 2002–2005 and adopted resolution WHA56.31. These documents set out squarely the major challenges: the lack of organized networks of traditional practitioners; the lack of sound evidence of the safety, efficacy and quality of traditional medicines; the need for measures to ensure proper use of traditional medicines and to protect and preserve traditional and natural resources necessary for their sustainable application; and measures for training and licensing of traditional practitioners.

The Traditional Medicine Strategy reflects both the value placed on traditional medicine as a resource, and the challenges ahead. It details four directions for our work with countries in this field: in the areas of policy (where we aim to broaden recognition of traditional medicine, supporting its integration into national health systems as appropriate, and protecting indigenous knowledge); safety, efficacy and quality (where our work is to expand the knowledge base on traditional medicine and raise its credibility); access (where we must work to increase availability and affordability, especially for poor populations); and rational use (where the task is to ensure appropriate and sustainable use of these medicines by consumers and providers, preserving and protecting medicinal plant resources and knowledge of traditional medicine).

Mapping the issues through this Atlas gives them fresh impact, illustrating graphically the "gaps", and therefore the needs. In this way it directly supports the implementation of WHO's strategic plans. For example, a map that shows only 25 countries as having a national policy for traditional medicine should stimulate enquiry and remedial action on regulation.

The Atlas is an advocacy tool to show the global community where our efforts are most required and to stimulate joint responsibility for solving the problems. It is also part of the solution. The actual process of its compilation has, in itself, been a useful means of raising the profile of traditional medicine globally. In asking the questions and articulating the issues, constructive progress has already been made in underlining the importance of traditional medicine in the field of public health and highlighting to all Member States where work still needs to be done.

The Atlas provides reliable, evidence-based information on the use and practice of traditional medicine in the world today, to stimulate decision-making in health sector development and reform. It provides a reference and research tool for all those who are working to increase availability and accessibility to cost-effective remedies and methods of treatment; and to promote proper use and to improve training and education of providers of traditional medicines, and complementary and alternative therapies. I believe that the success of these efforts will eventually lead to a more comprehensive health-care delivery which will, in turn, bring us closer to realizing "Health for All" in the 21st century.

Dr Wilfried Kreisel
Director
WHO Centre for Health Development
Kobe, Japan

July 2004

PREFACE

Traditional medicine (TM) has always maintained its popularity worldwide. In addition, for more than a decade, there has been an increasing use of complementary and alternative medicine (CAM) in many developed and developing countries. In line with increased international demand, the safety, efficacy and quality of the products and practices used in TM/CAM have become important concerns for both health authorities and the public. Therefore, WHO Member States are seeking to establish policy frameworks and deciding in what ways these products and practices should be regulated to ensure their safety, efficacy and quality. In this context, it would be beneficial for Member States to share experiences in order to assist each other as they begin to develop their own policies and regulations. The compilation of the WHO Global Atlas of Traditional, Complementary and Alternative Medicine has provided a mechanism for sharing evidence-based information on the current state of TM/CAM.

BACKGROUND TO THE DATA COLLECTION AND WORKING PROCESS

The Global Atlas was designed to record and map the current status of TM/CAM around the world, in terms of policy, regulation, education, research, practices and use. To this end WHO through its Centre for Health Development (WHO Kobe Centre) organized two meetings, in September 2001 and in June 2003. All together, 73 participants, including national health authorities, experts, and representatives of NGOs, from 45 countries in the six WHO regions, engaged in an international collaborative effort to prepare the Global Atlas.

The meeting in 2001 reviewed and discussed the primary data available on the prevalence and utilization of TM/CAM, as well as the development of a working procedure to compile national information and data for the Atlas. Since TM/CAM is not been legally recognized in many countries and there is a lack of data for most countries, the participants decided that the Global Atlas would be based on data from secondary sources. Due to the lack of an effective and generally-accepted tool for the purposes of secondary data collection, three types of indicator were proposed; background, structural (including a survey quality assessment indicator), and process indicators (see Annexes in the map volume). These indicators were employed to gather the demographic information, infrastructural development of TM/CAM at the national level, and its utilization and popularity.

Before launching the global collection of information, the feasibility of using the indicators was field-tested in Indonesia, Panama, Thailand, and Viet Nam in cooperation with national authorities relating to TM. In order to gather these data, the WHO Kobe Centre together with the Traditional Medicine Team at WHO Headquarters and the six WHO regional offices set up a working group in each region. The WHO European Region coordinators working at Global Initiative for Traditional Systems (GIFTS) of Health at Oxford University, United Kingdom, were commissioned by the WHO Kobe Centre to collate the information received from the six regional working groups. Each working group contacted national focal points and/or working partners in the countries of their respective region to collect information and data. After global data collection, analysis and collation by the regional working groups had been completed, a meeting was convened in June 2003, at which it was agreed that the Global Atlas would consist of a map volume and a text volume. After the meeting, the WHO Kobe Centre sent the final draft of each country chapter to the respective national health authorities for their review and comments.

UTILIZATION OF THE GLOBAL ATLAS

The Global Atlas facilitates an easy review of many aspects of the situation regarding the use of TM/CAM in different countries, which therapies are most popular worldwide, how many countries have already established policy and regulation of TM/CAM, etc. It provides a rich source of information to assist Member States seeking to develop their national policies on TM/CAM. However, it should be noted that the Global Atlas was prepared on the basis of information and data from secondary sources and references are included at the appropriate points.

One of the four objectives of the WHO Traditional Medicines Strategy 2002–2005 is to assist Member States to integrate TM/CAM with national health-care systems, as appropriate, by developing and implementing national TM/CAM policies and programmes. From the information gathered in an ongoing WHO global survey of national policy and regulation of TM/CAM and herbal medicines, it is clear that the situation is evolving rapidly and that many countries are currently engaged in establishing national policies and regulations.

Thus, in order to capture this changing scenario, the Global Atlas will need to be updated regularly. Meanwhile, it provides an excellent overview of the situation of TM/CAM in the world today.

Dr Xiaorui Zhang
Coordinator, Traditional Medicine
Department of Essential Drugs and Medicines Policy
World Health Organization, Geneva, Switzerland

July 2004

INTRODUCTION

Kin Shein[1] and Yuki Maehira[2]

[1] Coordinator, Traditional Medicine Programme, WHO Centre for Health Development,
Kobe 651-0073, Japan.
Email: sheink@who.or.jp

[2] Technical Officer, Traditional Medicine Programme, WHO Centre for Health Development,
Kobe 651-0073, Japan.
Email: maehiray@who.or.jp

The developments and achievements in biomedical disciplines and advances in modern medical sciences in general, in the prevention, control and treatment of various diseases and other medical conditions is unprecedented in the history of medicine. However, the benefits derived from these developments are not necessarily available, accessible and affordable to a significant proportion of the people in many developing countries. Under such circumstances, traditional medicine (TM) continues to play an important role in the provision of primary health care in many countries. For example, in Africa, up to 80%, and in India, 70% of the population depend on traditional medicine to help meet their health-care needs (1).

In the last two decades, many developed countries have also been interested in traditional medicine. It is being referred to as complementary and alternative medicine (CAM) and therapies. As many as 42% of the people in the USA, 48% in Australia, 70% in Canada and 77% in Germany used CAM at least once in the 1990s (1).

Various systems of traditional medicine are used in different parts of the world today; yet there is no reference information on their utilization. A need has been expressed to bring together such information, especially on the popularly-used TM, for better understanding of the various systems of medicine contributing to the people's health. The various modalities of therapies and practices employed in TM/CAM, insofar as they are beneficial and not harmful to peoples' health and well-being, are potential resources for health care. They need to be explored for their possible contributions to health. It is crucial to understand their role because it is important to systematize the contributions of all systems of medicine in the development of "Health for All" in the 21st century. Therefore sharing the countries' information and experiences is necessary. This Global Atlas aims to provide a range of information relating to the use of TM/CAM, including the national policy and regulation, popularly-used therapies, research and education, among others.

The Development of WHO Global Atlas on Traditional/Complementary and Alternative Medicine

Since 1999, the WHO Centre for Health Development (WHO Kobe Centre/WKC) has been working in the area of TM to examine its valid contributions to health system development in the 21st century (2). It is envisaged that modalities of treatment in various systems of medicine—whether conventional, traditional, complementary or alternative, that have been proven to be effective and not harmful to peoples' health and well-being when used properly, might contribute to improve access to preferred methods of health care in national health and welfare systems.

There is lack of information and documentation on a number of different systems of TM/CAM. Hence, the WHO Kobe Centre convened an international consultative meeting in September 2001 (3) as the first step in the collection of global information on practices and utilization of TM/CAM. The indicators for the collection of information were selected and field-tested in Indonesia, Panama, Thailand and Viet Nam. Thereafter, the collection of information was carried out globally.

In June 2003, the Centre organized another international meeting to review the data (4). This was attended by 48 experts and national health authorities from 33 countries. The participants reviewed the information collected and developed the structure of the Global Atlas, a brief description of which is given below.

Purpose of the WHO Global Atlas

The purpose of the WHO Global Atlas is to:

- Provide the latest information on the status of development of TM/CAM in the world to the Member States, academia, researchers, the industry, NGOs and other interested parties; and,

- Provide information on commonly-used TM/CAM in different countries, as well as documenting their global prevalence.

The Global Atlas consists of two volumes, i.e. the map volume and the text volume (4). They are arranged to provide a more complete picture regarding peoples' reliance and dependence on different traditional health systems.

The map volume presents information on the current status of TM/CAM around the world by means of maps, figures and tables, on the following aspects:

- National legislation and policy;

- Availability of public financing;

- Status of education and professional regulation;

- National legal recognition of TM/CAM practitioners by therapy,

- Conventional health-care professionals entitled to provide TM/CAM;

- Popularity, or use of different systems of TM/CAM around the world.

The text volume includes six regional overview chapters and 23 selected country chapters on practices and utilization of TRM/CAM, with a view to provide country-specific information from developing as well as developed countries.

Conclusion

The availability of more complete information on the health systems prevalent in a country could facilitate a more comprehensive national health-system development and/or health sector reform where this is necessary and desirable. These developments are important to the endeavours of nations around the world in their quest to improve the health-care coverage and provision to their citizens safe, effective, affordable, and culturally-accepted therapies and practices.

Glossary of selected terms

In order to read easily and use the information included, definitions of the terms commonly used in this Global Atlas are given below. The following definitions of key terms are quoted from other WHO publications for consistency and have already been used in the Member States.

Traditional Medicine (TM)

Traditional medicine has a long history. It is the sum total of the knowledge, skills and practices based on the theories, beliefs and experiences indigenous to different cultures, whether explicable or not, used in the maintenance of health, as well as in the prevention, diagnosis, improvement or treatment of physical and mental illnesses (5).

Complementary and Alternative Medicine (CAM)

The terms complementary/alternative/non-conventional medicine are used interchangeably with traditional medicine in some countries. The term complementary and alternative medicine is used in some countries to refer to a broad set of health care practices that are not part of the country's own tradition and are not integrated into the dominant health care system (5).

Herbal Medicines

Herbal medicines (5) include herbs, herbal materials, herbal preparations and finished herbal products.

Herbs

Herbs include crude plant material such as leaves, flowers, fruit, seed, stems, wood, bark, roots, rhizomes or other plant parts, which may be entire, fragmented or powdered.

Herbal materials

Herbal materials include, in addition to herbs, fresh juices, gums, fixed oils, essential oils, resins and dry powders of herbs. In some countries, these materials may be processed by various local procedures, such as steaming, roasting, or stir-baking with honey, alcoholic beverages or other materials.

Herbal preparations

Herbal preparations are the basis for finished herbal products and may include comminuted or powdered herbal materials, or extracts, tinctures and fatty oils of herbal materials. They are produced by extraction, fractionation, purification, concentration, or other physical or biological processes. They also include preparations made by steeping or heating herbal materials in alcoholic beverages and/or honey, or in other materials.

Finished herbal products

Finished herbal products consist of herbal preparations made from one or more herbs. If more than one herb is used, the term mixture herbal product can also be used. Finished herbal products and mixture herbal products may contain excipients in addition to the active ingredients. However, finished products or mixture products to which chemically defined active substances have been added, including synthetic compounds and/or isolated constituents from herbal materials, are not considered to be herbal.

Ayurveda

Ayurveda (6) originated in the 10th century BC, but its current form took shape between the 5th century BC and the 5th century AD. In Sanskrit, Ayurveda means "science of life". Ayurvedic philosophy is attached to sacred texts, the Vedas, and based on the theory of Panchmahabhutas—all objects and living bodies are composed of the five basic elements: earth, water, fire, air, and sky. Similarly, there is a fundamental harmony between the environment and individuals, which is perceived as a macrocosm and microcosm relationship. As such, acting on one influences the other. Ayurveda is not only a system of medicine, but also a way of living. It is used to both prevent and cure diseases. Ayurvedic medicine includes herbal medicines and medicinal baths. It is widely practised in South Asia, especially in Bangladesh, India, Nepal, Pakistan, and Sri Lanka.

Chiropractic

Chiropractic was founded at the end of the 19th century by Daniel David Palmer, a magnetic therapist practising in Iowa, USA. Chiropractic is based on an association between the spine and the nervous system and on the self-healing properties of the human body. It is practised in every region of the world. Chiropractic training programmes are recognized by the World Federation of Chiropractic if they adopt international standards of education and require a minimum of four years of full-time university-level education following entrance requirements.

Homeopathy

Homeopathy was first mentioned by Hippocrates (462-377BC), but it was a German physician, Hahnemann (1755-1843), who established homeopathy's basic principles: law of similarity, direction of cure, principle of single remedy, the theory of minimum diluted dose, and the therapy of chronic diseases (6). In homeopathy, diseases are treated with remedies that in a healthy person would produce symptoms similar to those of the disease. Rather than fighting the disease directly, medicines are intended to stimulate the body to fight the disease. By the latter half of the 19th century, homeopathy was practised throughout Europe as well as in Asia and North America. Homeopathy has been integrated into the national health care systems of many countries, including India, Mexico, Pakistan, Sri Lanka and the United Kingdom.

Traditional Chinese medicine

The earliest records of traditional Chinese medicine (6) date back to the 8th century BC. Diagnosis and treatment are based on a holistic view of the patient and the patient's symptoms, expressed in terms of the balance of yin and yang. Yin represents the earth, cold, and femininity. Yang represents the sky, heat, and masculinity. The actions of yin and yang influence the interactions of the five elements composing the universe: metal, wood, water, fire, and earth. Practitioners of traditional Chinese medicine seek to control the levels of yin and yang through 12 meridians, which bring energy to the body. Traditional Chinese medicine can be used for promoting health as well as preventing and curing diseases. It encompasses a range of practices, including acupuncture, moxibustion, herbal medicines, manual therapies, exercises, breathing techniques, and diets. Surgery is rarely used. Chinese medicine, particularly acupuncture, is the most widely-used traditional medicine. It is practised in every region of the world.

Unani Medicine

Unani (6) is based on Hippocrates' (462–377 BC) theory of the four bodily humours: blood, phlegm, yellow bile, and black bile. Galen (131–210 AD), Rhazes (850–925 AD), and Avicenna (980–1037 AD) heavily influenced Unani's foundation and formed its structure. Unani draws from the traditional systems of medicine of China, Egypt, India, Iraq, Persia (Islamic Republic of Iran), and the Syrian Arab Republic. It is also called Arabic medicine.

Medication therapies

Therapies employing medications include African medicine, Ayurveda, traditional Chinese medicine, herbal medicine, homeopathy, Siddha medicine, Unani medicine and other traditional medicines which are popularly used worldwide (3).

Non-medication therapies

These therapies are also called "traditional procedure-based therapies" in some countries. Therapies that do not use medicines internally are acupuncture, chiropractic, osteopathy traditional exercises (e.g. Qigong, Yoga), manual therapy (e.g. Shiatsu), and others (3, 7).

References

1. *WHO Traditional Medicine Strategy 2002-2005.* Geneva, World Health Organization, 2002 (WHO/EDM/TRM2002.1).

2. *Traditional Medicine – its contributions to human health development in the new century. Report of an International Symposium, Kobe, Japan, 9 November 1999.* Kobe, WHO Centre for Health Development, World Health Organization, 2000.

3. *Global Information on Traditional Medicine/Complementary and Alternative Medicine Practices and Utilization. Proceedings of an International Consultative Meeting, Kobe, Japan, 19–21 September 2001.* Kobe, WHO Centre for Health Development, World Health Organization, 2001.

4. *Global Atlas of Traditional Medicine. Proceedings of an International Meeting, Kobe, Japan, 17–19 June 2003.* Kobe, WHO Centre for Health Development, World Health Organization, 2004.

5. *Traditional Medicine – Growing Needs and Potential.* WHO Policy Perspectives on Medicines, Geneva, World Health Organization, 2002 (WHO/EDM/2002.4).

6. *General guidelines for methodologies on research and evaluation of traditional medicine.* Geneva, World Health Organization, 2000 (WHO/EDM/TRM/2000.1).

7. *Legal Status of Traditional Medicine and Complementary/Alternative Medicine – A Worldwide Review.* Geneva, World Health Organization, 2001 (WHO/EDM/TRM/2001.2).

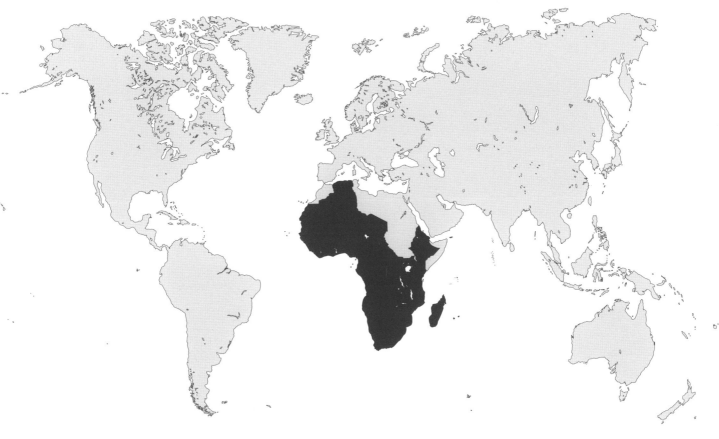

WHO AFRICAN REGION

REGIONAL OVERVIEW AND
SELECTED COUNTRY CHAPTERS

CHAPTER 1

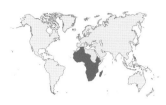

REGIONAL OVERVIEW: AFRICAN REGION

Ossy MJ Kasilo[1],
Edoh Soumbey-Alley[2],
Charles Wambebe[3]
and Rufaro Chatora[4]

[1] Regional Adviser for Traditional Medicine, Division of Health Systems and Service Development, World Health Organization Regional Office for Africa, P.O. Box 6, Brazzaville, the Republic of the Congo. E-mail: kasiloo@afro.who.int

[2] Regional Adviser for Health Information Systems, Division of Health Systems and Service Development, World Health Organization Regional Office for Africa, P.O. Box 6, Brazzaville, the Republic of the Congo. E-mail: soumbeye@afro.who.int

[3] Short-Term Professional in the Traditional Medicine Programme, Division of Health Systems and Service Development, World Health Organization Regional Office for Africa, P.O. Box 6, Brazzaville, the Republic of the Congo. E-mail: wambebec@afro.who.int

[4] Director, Division of Health Systems and Services Development, World Health Organization Regional Office for Africa, P.O. Box 6, Brazzaville, the Republic of the Congo. E-mail: chatorar@afro.who.int

1.1. INTRODUCTION

African Traditional Medicine (ATRM) is embedded in the culture of the population. In some communities, it is the only form of health care that is available, affordable and accessible. Only about 50% of the population in the WHO African Region (AFR) has regular access to essential pharmaceuticals, whereas more than 80% use ATRM (*1*). Africa is endowed with a rich biodiversity estimated at 40 000 plant species (*2*) and ATRM is 90% plant-based. About 6377 plant species are used in tropical Africa, of which more than 4000 species are used medicinally (*3*). Traditional knowledge is transmitted mostly by oral tradition, while some specific recipes are disclosed only to family members who can be trusted to keep such heritage.

In recognition of the role that traditional medicine (TRM) and its practitioners play in the development of health systems and services and the achievement of 'Health for All', WHO governing bodies at global and regional levels have adopted several resolutions on TRM. These include Resolution AFR/RC50/R3 on Promoting the Role of Traditional Medicine in Health Systems: A Strategy for the African Region adopted at the fiftieth session of the WHO Regional Committee for Africa, held in Ouagadougou, Burkina Faso, in 2000 (*4*); and Resolution WHA56.31 on traditional medicine at the World Health Assembly in May 2003 (*5*).

More recently, there has been a renewed political commitment to TRM at both country and WHO levels, as evidenced by the institution, with effect from August 2003, of the ATRM Day for Advocacy – on 31 August each year – in Member States. The first such Day was launched in Pretoria, South Africa in 2003 with the theme Traditional Medicine: Our Culture, Our Future. The African Summit of Heads of State and Government declared in Abuja, Nigeria, in April 2001 that TRM research was a priority, and in Lusaka, Zambia, in July 2001 it designated the period 2001–2010 as the Decade for the Development of ATRM. A plan of action, which received WHO support, was adopted in Tripoli, Libyan Arab Jamahiriya, in April 2003 and endorsed in Maputo, Mozambique, by the African Summit of Heads of State and Government in July 2003. The strategy for its implementation has been developed by WHO and was submitted to the African Union in December 2003. Furthermore, the African Summit of Heads of State and Government, held in Maputo in July 2003, declared that it would continue to support the implementation of the plan of action for the Decade for ATRM, especially research in the area of treatment for HIV/AIDS, tuberculosis, malaria and other infectious diseases in Africa (*6*).

Countries will need time to capitalize on this renewed political commitment to enhance ATRM in AFR. Currently, about half of the countries in the Region have formulated TRM policies and developed functional structures for the practice of TRM.

1.2. BACKGROUND INDICATORS

1.2.1. Morbidity and mortality

The estimated total population in AFR in 2002 was about 672 238 000. The average annual growth rate of the population is estimated at 2.2%. The average life expectancy at birth, both sexes combined, is 48.9 years. The per capita total expenditure on health, in international dollars, ranged from $12 in the Democratic Republic of the Congo to $770 in the Seychelles in 2001, with an average across AFR of $109.30. Infant mortality rates in 2001 ranged from 13 per 1000 live births in Seychelles to 182 per 1000 live births in Sierra Leone, while maternal mortality rates ranged from 0 per 100 000 live births in Seychelles to 1837 per 100 000 live births in the Democratic Republic of the Congo in 2001 (7).

The ten most common causes of morbidity in AFR are HIV/AIDS, malaria, lower respiratory tract infections, childhood diseases, diarrhoeal diseases, perinatal conditions, neuropsychiatric disorders, road traffic accidents and other unintentional injuries, maternal conditions, and violence (8). The ten most common causes of mortality are HIV/AIDS, malaria, lower respiratory tract infections, childhood diseases, diarrhoeal diseases, perinatal conditions, unintentional injuries, malignant neoplasm, cerebrovascular disease and ischaemic disease.

1.2.2. Numbers of prescribers and TCAM providers

The total number of prescribers in AFR estimated during 1995–2003 was 822 374, composed of: physicians – 106 685; midwives – 48 044; nurses – 485 705; pharmacists – 32 801; dentists – 17 675 and other health workers – 131 464. In 2003, Nigeria had 25 000 physicians, 10 000 pharmacists and 8386 nurses, whereas in 1996, South Africa had 23 855 physicians, no midwives, 200 000 nurses, 15 794 pharmacists and 7544 dentists (8).

The total number of traditional, complementary and alternative medicine (TCAM) providers within and outside the conventional health system varies from one country to another. Most of them are traditional health practitioners (THPs). Surveys conducted by WHO and other organizations show that in many parts of Africa, THPs greatly outnumber medical doctors. For example, in 1982, Hedberg and colleagues (9) reported that there were about 30 000–40 000 THPs and 600 medical doctors in the United Republic of Tanzania. A similar situation is observed in other countries. In Ghana for example, the ratio of medical doctors to the population is 1:20,000 and that of THPs to the population 1:200 whereas in Mozambique the ratio of medical doctors to the population is 1:50 000 and that of THPs to the population 1:200 (10).

1.2.3. Total Expenditure on Health

The total expenditure in the conventional health-care sector is illustrated in Table 1.1, Table 1.2 and Figure 1.1. Table 1.1 shows the expenditure by type of provider, including nongovernmental organizations (NGOs) and for-profit private sectors, in selected Eastern and Southern Africa (ESA) countries. Table 1.2 shows the health expenditure by level of care in the public sector of ESA countries. Figure 1.1 shows the breakdown of direct care delivery expenditure by level of care across the region as a whole (8).

There has always been doubt expressed internationally that hospital expenditure is too high in relation to expenditure on primary health care in developing countries. The evidence presented in this comparative analysis of the national health accounts in ESA countries does not, however, tend to support this concern. Table 1.1 shows that the proportion of total expenditure devoted to hospital care tends to decrease in most countries with the addition of the private sector. This is, however, largely due to expenditure in pharmaceutical outlets in the private sector, which is difficult to classify into primary care or otherwise. In the case of the United Republic of Tanzania, the high proportion of expenditure on hospitals can be explained by the fact that many hospitals are run by religious organizations which receive only subsidies from the Government.

Table 1.1. Total health expenditure in Eastern and Southern Africa (ESA) countries by type of provider, including NGOs and for-profit private sectors (*11*).

Provider type	Percentage of total health expenditure by provider in countries:						
	ETH	*KEN*	*MAL*	*RWA*	*SAF*	*UGA*	*URT*
Hospitals	18.53	27.07	11.54	33.44	39.31	10.14	53.25
Outpatient care centres	33.15	21.46	24.41	12.29	5.44	6.83	18.57
Hospitals and clinics (not separated)	NA	NA	12.28	NA	NA	22.81	NA
Private medical practitioners	NA	NA	NA	NA	16.12	NA	NA
Public health programmes	NA	NA	12.27	NA	2.65	21.79	16.28
Producers of pharmaceuticals & medical supplies	33.07	23.46	2.87	24.66	14.13	14.12	NA
Administration	7.15	2.53	11.18	23.92	6.11	4.75	11.90
Research	0.66	1.09	NA	NA	0.25	0.12	NA
Training	1.89	1.17	NA	NA	1.97	1.79	NA
Treatment abroad	NA	NA	NA	1.21	NA	NA	NA
THPs/healers	4.90	NA	2.19	4.31	NA	1.46	NA
Others	NA	NA	0.16	NA	10.88	NA	NA
Not classified	0.66	23.23	23.11	0.17	3.14	16.19	NA
Total	**100**	**100**	**100**	**100**	**100**	**100**	**100**

ETH, Ethiopia; KEN, Kenya; MAL, Malawi; RWA, Rwanda; SAF, South Africa; UGA, Uganda; URT, United Republic of Tanzania.

NA, not available (this does not mean that there was no expenditure on these provider types, but rather that it was not separated from the other providers shown in the table).

Table 1.2 and Figure 1.1 show that mid-level care has the highest proportion of expenditure allocated to it by the public sector. This may impede the achievement of the goals contained in the health policies of the countries concerned, where primary care is suggested to be a priority.

Table 1.2. Health expenditure in selected Eastern and Southern Africa (ESA) countries, by level of care in the public sector only (*8*).

Level of care	Percentage of total health expenditure by level of care in countries:						
	ETH	*MAL*	*MOZ*	*RWA*	*SAF*	*UGA*	*AFR*
Tertiary	11	11	38	25	23	11	23
Mid level (1st and 2nd)	33	24	36	53	53	37	52
Primary care (non-hospital)	56	65	26	22	24	52	25
Total	100	100	100	100	100	100	100

ETH, Ethiopia; MAL, Malawi; MOZ, Mozambique; RWA, Rwanda; SAF, South Africa; UGA, Uganda; AFR, WHO African Region.

1.2.4. Expenditure in the Traditional Health Sector

Information on total expenditure in the traditional health sector is scanty, so it is difficult to make meaningful comparisons between the formal and traditional sectors, but a few examples can be cited. Figure 1.2 combines the results of a study on affordability (*12*) and a comparison of health expenditures (*13*) in KwaZulu-Natal Province in South Africa, which showed that the estimated annual cost of treatment per individual, paid by patients using herbal products and consulting traditional health practitioners, was less than the provincial per capita annual health expenditure on public health care not paid by patients.

Figure 1.1. Breakdown of direct care delivery expenditure by level of care across the WHO African Region as a whole (public sector only) in 2001 (*11*).

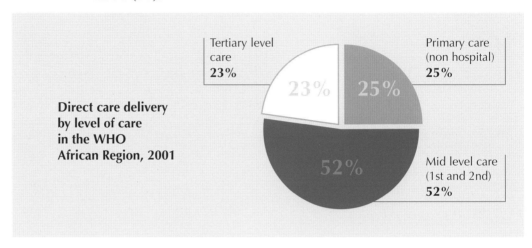

Similarly, Figure 1.3 shows results of a study on comparative cost of malaria treatments in Dangme West District, Ghana, where self-treatment using herbs and over-the-counter medications was less expensive for patients than the cost of malaria treatment at a clinic (*14*).

1.3.1. Official National TCAM Policies

Government reports and surveys undertaken by WHO and other partners indicate that at least 20 (56%) countries in AFR have an official national policy on TCAM, (including policy whose endorsement by Cabinet is pending). Those with policies are mostly in western, southern and eastern Africa. Those without policies include a number of countries in central and north-western Africa, together with some of the smaller countries in the south and east (e.g. Lesotho, Malawi, Seychelles and Swaziland).

Figure 1.2. Health expenditures (in US$) in KwaZulu-Natal Province, South Africa (12, 13).

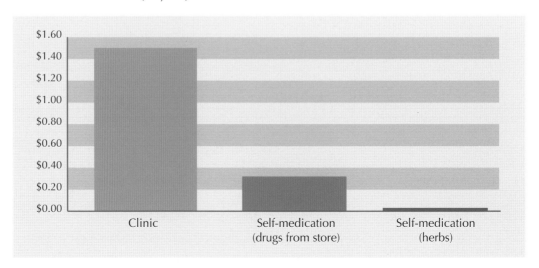

Figure 1.3. Out-of-pocket expenditure (in US$) for malaria treatments in Dangme - West District, Ghana (14).

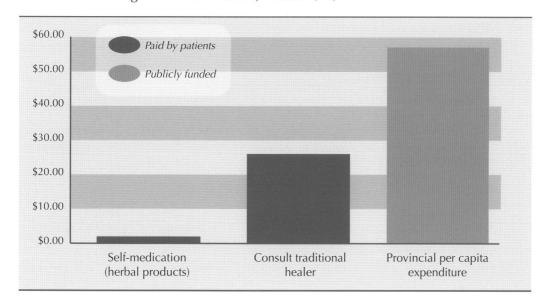

1.3. STRUCTURAL INDICATORS

Selected structural indicators are summarized in Table 1.3 and discussed in further detail below.

1.3.2. TCAM Legislation

A national law or regulation of TRM exists in the following countries: Burundi, Côte d'Ivoire, the Democratic Republic of the Congo, Equatorial Guinea, Ethiopia, the Gambia, Ghana, Guinea, Lesotho, Liberia, Madagascar, Malawi, Mali, Mauritius, Namibia, Nigeria, Senegal, Sierra Leone, Swaziland, Togo and Zimbabwe. Certain forms of TRM are regulated in Botswana, Ethiopia, Ghana, Lesotho, Madagascar, Mauritius, Nigeria, Sierra Leone, South Africa, Swaziland, Togo, the United Republic of Tanzania, and Zimbabwe. TCAM providers are legally recognized in Botswana, Burkina Faso, Cameroon, the Congo, Ethiopia, Gambia, Ghana, Guinea, Kenya, Lesotho, Mali, Mauritius, Namibia, Niger, Nigeria, Senegal, Sierra Leone, South Africa, Swaziland, Togo, the United Republic of Tanzania, and Zimbabwe (1).

Currently, THPs are the most common professional category entitled to provide TCAM in most countries in AFR. There are others however; in Nigeria, for example, chiropractors and osteopaths are recognized within the conventional health system. In Mauritius, there are no provisions for ATRM, but registered practitioners of Ayurveda, homeopathy and traditional Chinese medicine are legally recognized. In Mali, chartered THPs, all medical staff, and retired paramedical staff may open private TCAM consultation clinics. Chartered medicinal plant sellers, graduates from the Katibougou Rural Polytechnic Institute or equivalent, and graduates from the Superior Normal School or its equivalent are allowed to open medicinal herb stores (1). Similarly, in South Africa, allopathic doctors retain the right to practise homeopathy, regardless of their level of homeopathic education, since these professionals are legally recognized TCAM providers.

1.3.3. Existence of a Ministry, Institution or National Expert Committee

Sixteen (44%) countries indicated that a national expert committee on TCAM has been established whose mandate includes, among others, TCAM control, education, information and/or research (Table 1.5). Furthermore, 14 (39%) countries have established a national programme on TCAM. Thirty-one countries (86%) indicated that a National Office of TCAM has been established within the Ministry of Health, whereas 28 (78%) indicated that TRM research is being carried out.

1.3.4. National Voluntary Self-regulatory Bodies for TCAM

National voluntary self-regulatory bodies for TCAM, mostly THPs' associations, exist in Benin, Burkina Faso, Congo, Ethiopia, Ghana, Kenya, Mali, Mozambique, Nigeria, Senegal, South Africa,

Uganda, the United Republic of Tanzania, Zambia and Zimbabwe. It is interesting to note that in Mali there are over 32 THP associations, and a Federation of THPs has been established. In most countries, however, the number of associations ranges from one in small countries to five in larger ones. They are mostly concentrated in urban areas.

Table 1.3. **Summary of selected structural indicators in the WHO African Region**

Structural indicator	No. (%) of countries with indicator	Reference
National Office of Traditional Medicine in the Ministry of Health	31 (86)	(15)
Conducting research related to traditional medicine	28 (78)	(1,16)
National policies on traditional medicine	22 (61)	(1,15)
National traditional medicine programmes	12 (33)	(15)
National law or regulation on traditional medicines	21 (58)	(1,15)
National expert committee	16 (44)	(15)
Registration system	7 (19)	(15)
GMP requirements for manufacturing of herbal medicines	7 (19)	(15)
Associations of traditional health practitioners	22 (73)	(16)
Conservation of medicinal plants	17 (59)	(16)
Management bodies for coordinating traditional medicine activities	17 (57)	(16)
Training programmes for traditional birth attendants	17 (57)	(16)
Legal framework for the practice of traditional medicine	16 (53)	(16)
Local production of traditional medicines	15 (50)	(16)

1.3.5. Public Sector Financing Mechanisms for TCAM

In most countries of AFR, the free provision of health care in the public sector does not include TCAM therapies (1). Both herbalists and private practitioners of TCAM charge user fees (17). For example, in South Africa, Zambia and Zimbabwe, TCAM treatments are not covered by insurance. In the Congo, an attempt has been made to standardize fees for TCAM treatment, but no patient reimbursement exists for such fees. Even in Niger, where a health insurance programme was introduced for government health-care services, it does not cover any traditional treatments (17). The World Health Report 2003 indicates that in 2001 social security expenditure as a percentage of general government expenditure on health accounted for 0.8% in Ethiopia, 0.1% in Guinea-Bissau, 8.1% in Mauritius and 0.6% in Rwanda (8).

1.3.6. Education, Information and Advisory Services Relating to TCAM

Regarding education and training, some countries have initiated training programmes to improve the skills and public health-care knowledge of THPs, including traditional birth attendants. Some others provide training in TRM for pharmacists, doctors and nurses and THPs (Burkina Faso, Cameroon, the Congo, Equatorial Guinea, Gambia, Ghana, Guinea, Kenya, Lesotho, Liberia, Madagascar, Malawi, Mali, Rwanda, Senegal, Sierra Leone, South Africa, Uganda and the United Republic of Tanzania). For example, the Kwame Nkrumah University in Ghana offers a bachelor's degree in herbal medicines; Kenya has established a Karati Rural Service and School of Alternative Medicine and Technology; Zimbabwe has a School of Traditional Medicine and a Bachelor of Science degree in Natural Medicine; and Nigeria has established diploma courses for traditional herbalists.

Information and advisory services are available in Benin, the Central African Republic, Congo, Ghana, Guinea, Kenya, Mali, Mauritania, Mozambique, Senegal, South Africa, Togo, Uganda and the United Republic of Tanzania. In west Africa, Benin is developing a guide for the rational use of traditional pharmacopoeia and researchers at the University of Benin carry out research on medicinal plants. In Ghana, Volume 1 of the Ghana Herbal Pharmacopoeia contains scientific information on 50 medicinal plants (*18*), and a second volume is currently in preparation. The International Development Centre in Conakry, Guinea, has conducted regional workshops for THPs of francophone Africa and in Senegal, NGOs such as ENDA (Environnement pour le Développement) and PROMETRA (Promotion des Médicines Traditionnelles) provide information on medicinal plant horticulture and self-medication, and on all aspects of TRM, including training of THPs. The Ministry of Health and Social Action in Senegal has produced a publication on medicinal plants sold across the world (*19*). In central Africa, the National Centre of Traditional Medicine in the Congo promotes information exchange between institutions.

Table 1.5. National expert committees for TCAM in the WHO African Region

Countries with national expert committees for TCAM	No expert committee, or no information supplied on this indicator	
Botswana	Algeria	Angola
Burkina Faso	Benin	Cameroon
Burundi	Cape Verde	Chad
Central African Republic	Comoros	Congo
Côte d'Ivoire	Equatorial Guinea	Eritrea
Democratic Republic of the Congo	Gabon	Guinea-Bissau
Ethiopia	Lesotho	Kenya
Gambia	Madagascar	Malawi
Ghana	Mali	Mauritania
Guinea	Niger	Rwanda
Liberia	Senegal	Seychelles
Mauritius	South Africa	Swaziland
Mozambique	Togo	Uganda
Namibia	United Republic of Tanzania	Zambia
Nigeria	Zimbabwe	
Sierra Leone		

In eastern and southern Africa, Mozambique has a number of programmes sponsored by NGOs in collaboration with district or provincial health authorities, one of which aims to coordinate research in TRM and to establish a research-derived information base about traditional beliefs and practices. In South Africa, the Traditional Medicine Programme at the University of Cape Town was established to carry out research and provide appropriate information to THPs and other health professionals (*1*). In Uganda, a NGO called Traditional and Modern Health Practitioners Together Against AIDS (THETA) has established a resource and training centre to facilitate the collection and dissemination of information on TRM (*20*). The Kenyan Society of Ethnoecology, founded in 2000, promotes research, field trips and information exchange on herbal medicine and other subjects related to the traditional use of plants, and holds an annual conference. There is also a Kenyan Resource Centre for Indigenous Knowledge. Similarly, the Tanzanian Society of Ethnoscience, based at Sokoine University in Morogoro, United Republic of Tanzania, was established in 2002 with UNESCO funding to promote research and information-sharing in all branches of ethnoscience, including TRM. The Maasailand Resource Centre for Indigenous Knowledge (MARECIK) is based in Arusha, United Republic of Tanzania, as are the NGOs Aang Serian and Terrawatu, which have a joint library on medicinal plant use and traditional health care (G. Burford, personal communication, 2003).

1.3.7. TCAM User Surveys

TCAM user surveys conducted in some of the countries of AFR in the past 20 years indicate that TCAM is used by approximately 90% of the population in Burundi and Ethiopia (*21*), 80% in Burkina Faso, the Democratic Republic of Congo and South Africa, 70% in Benin, Côte d'Ivoire, Ghana, Mali and Rwanda; and 60% in the Congo, the United Republic of Tanzania, and Uganda (*1*).

1.4. PROCESS INDICATORS

1.4.1. Estimated Prevalence of TCAM Use

Within AFR as a whole, over 80% of the population uses traditional medicines for primary health-care needs. Of the five most popular individual therapies at a regional level, the estimated % of the population using each is as follows: herbal medicines 80% (ranges from 60% in some countries to 95% in others (*4*); spiritual therapies 13%; manual therapies 5%; homeopathy and chiropractic less than 1%.

1.4.2. Medical Determinants for TCAM Use

In most countries, the patients seeking treatment with TRM often present with conditions related to morbidity, including: malaria; HIV/AIDS and opportunistic infections; diarrhoeal diseases; childhood illnesses; illnesses related to reproductive health; asthma; gastro-intestinal disorders; diabetes; hypertension; sickle-cell anaemia; mental illness and epilepsy.

1.4.3. Patient Satisfaction and Perceived Outcomes of TCAM Treatment

Patients are normally very satisfied with traditional therapy and the services that they obtain from THPs as these health care providers listen to their problems, counsel them and treat their physical, social and psychological illnesses in a holistic manner. Traditional medicines are affordable and accessible. Therefore, patients continue to resort to THPs for consultation and treatment. The outcome of the treatment is usually good as they get relief from the signs and symptoms of their illnesses, except in very few cases when adverse reactions or interactions, poisoning, or some immunological reactions occur. Some of these adverse reactions may be related to inappropriate use or overdose of traditional medicines.

1.4.4. Sociodemographic Characteristics of Consumers

The use of TRM is a part of the African cultural belief system. Therefore, all types of consumers with different sociodemographic characteristics including rural and urban dwellers, very poor, low-, middle- and high-income earners, educated (including religious leaders, administrators and politicians) and uneducated people use TRM. Some of the elite tend to use TRM secretly, consulting THPs at night.

1.4.5. Out-of-pocket Payments and Total National Expenditure

Precise data on out-of-pocket payments and total national expenditure on TCAM are not available, as no specific survey on this issue has been carried out. However, consumers and patients who use TRM pay 100% of their medical bill out-of-pocket. At present most Member States in AFR do not have National Health Insurance Plans. In cases where such plans exist, they normally exclude, for purposes of reimbursement, expenses related to the use of TRM. Total national expenditures for TRM utilization are difficult to estimate, bearing in mind that few countries have a national budget for the practice, or for patients and consumers who get treated in hospitals due to occasional adverse reactions, interactions and poisoning. The cost of medicines, time and salaries paid to hospital personnel during hospitalization of patients affected by these adverse reactions is also not budgeted.

It is not possible to make a meaningful comparison between traditional health sector and conventional health sector expenditures because the former costs are not readily available. Furthermore, payment is not always in monetary terms; in some cases it depends on the ability to pay, or on what the consumer thinks he or she should pay, or appreciation can be demonstrated in kind. On the other hand, hospital expenditure in AFR in relation to primary health care is not as high as initially thought. Information on primary health care expenditure is central to policy monitoring and evaluation. This is very difficult when so much of the primary care level expenditure is captured by financial systems at higher levels, such as district hospitals that supervise and implement public health programmes or clinics, or even central-level departments. The challenge remains for governments in the Region to improve their accounting systems to reflect resource use at the various levels in the health-care system. This will yield better estimates of national health accounts to inform, monitor and evaluate policy decisions and facilitate regional comparison.

1.5. DISCUSSION

There are important differences between the countries in AFR, with regard to their degree of development of national policy and organizational structures for the practice of TRM. There are some countries in which few or no structures are in place, whereas in others considerable organizational structures exist.

A number of countries are moving towards licensing traditional medicines, which are being locally produced on a small scale. To this end, about 21 (58%) countries in AFR have national laws or regulations for herbal medicines (1, 14). In order to promote the registration and marketing of safe, effective and good quality traditional medicines (TRMs) in its Member States, the WHO Regional Office for Africa has organized two Regional Workshops on Regulation of Traditional Medicines. These took place in Johannesburg, South Africa from 1 to 3 April 2003, and in Madrid, Spain in conjunction with the International Conference on Drug Regulatory Authorities from 13 to 14 February 2004, respectively. Participants at the first workshop reviewed and adopted guidelines on registration of TRMs in AFR; these guidelines were then used for training the participants from national regulatory authorities in the second Regional Workshop.

In order to support countries in institutionalizing TRM within their national health systems and establishing functional structures for the practice of TRM within the framework of the African Regional Strategy on Promoting the Role of Traditional Medicine in Health Systems, the WHO Regional Office for Africa has also developed a number of documents. These can be used as tools for the following: policy formulation and national master plans for the development of TRM; legal frameworks for the practice of TRM; codes of ethics for THPs; and registration of traditional medicines. In addition, tools for continuing education of THPs in primary health care and for allopathic health care providers in TRM, and research methodologies have been developed to support countries in documenting safety, efficacy and quality of traditional medicines used for the treatment of priority diseases. A tool for documenting ATRM and a regional intellectual property framework for the protection of traditional medical knowledge have also been developed. These documents are at various stages of the publication process.

There are diverse forces that influence the integration of services and professionalization of THPs. For example, due to the cultural acceptance of TRM, the majority of the population in AFR uses TRM for primary health care needs. However, in some communities TRM is the only form of health care available to the population. For diseases such as HIV/AIDS that have no known cure, the majority of patients resort to extensive use of TRM, as it is accessible and affordable to them. Experience in some African countries, such as Burkina Faso, Ghana, Kenya, Nigeria, Senegal, South Africa, Uganda, the United Republic of Tanzania and Zimbabwe, shows that allopathic health care providers have been collaborating with THPs in the use of TRM in research as well as in HIV/AIDS prevention activities. Researchers have observed a reduction in the viral load and increase in the CD4:CD8 ratio; improvement of the clinical condition of patients; and in some cases (such as Burkina Faso), a weight increase of up to 20 kg. Similar experiences have been reported by the NGOs THETA in Uganda and PROMETRA in Senegal. Experience from Chinese and Ayurveda systems of medicine suggests that TRM is apparently more effective than allopathic medicines in the management of chronic disorders.

1.6. CONCLUSIONS

The renewed political interest in the development of TRM by African leaders as well as WHO cannot be underestimated. This political momentum has been made evident by the declarations of the various African Summits of Heads of State and Government. These include the announcement of the period 2001–2010 as the Decade for African Traditional Medicine, and the institution, by WHO, of African Traditional Medicine Day for Advocacy. Countries need to capitalize and build on the renewed political and economic momentum, resulting from the recent global resurgence in the use of natural medicines, in order to enhance TRM in the Region.

References

1. *Legal status of traditional medicine and complementary/alternative medicine: a worldwide review.* Geneva, World Health Organization, 2001 (WHO/EDM/TRM/2001.2).

2. Mahunnah RLA. Ethnobotany and conservation of medicine plants in Africa: the way forward in the next decade, 2001–2010. In: *OAU Decade for African Traditional Medicine. Proceedings of the fifteenth meeting of the Inter-African Expert Committee on African Traditional Medicine and Medicinal Plants, Arusha, Tanzania, 15–17 January 2002,* Scientific Technical Research Commission of the African Union, Lagos, 2002.

3. Bosch CH et al. *Plant resources of tropical Africa. Basic list of species and commodity grouping.* Wageningen, Plant Resources of Tropical Africa (PROTA) Program, 2002.

4. *Promoting the role of traditional medicine in health systems: a strategy for the African Region.* Harare, World Health Organization Regional Office for Africa, 2001 (AFR/RC50/9) and resolution (AFR/RC50/R5).

5. Resolution WHA56.31. Traditional medicine. In: *Fifty-sixth World Health Assembly, Geneva, 19–28 May 2003.* Geneva, World Health Organization, 2003.

6. Heads of State and Government of the African Union: Second ordinary session, Maputo, Mozambique, 10-12 July 2003. Maputo declaration on HIV/AIDS, Tuberculosis, Malaria and Other Related Infectious Diseases The full text of this and other declarations can be found at: www.africa-union.org

7. Regional Health for All Policy for the 21st Century in the African Region: Agenda 2020. World Health Organization Regional Office for Africa, (document AFR/RC50/8 Rev: 1 and resolution AFR/RC50/R1), 2002.

8. *The World Health Report 2003: shaping the future.* Geneva, World Health Organization, 2003.

9. Hedberg I et al. Inventory of plants used in traditional medicine in Tanzania. I. Plants of the families Acanthaceae–Cucurbitaceae. *Journal of Ethnopharmacology,* 1982, 6:29–60.

10. Chatora R. Situation analysis of traditional medicine in the WHO African Region. In: World Health Organization Regional Office for Africa, ed. *Traditional medicine: our culture, our future. African Health Monitor.* Brazzaville, World Health Organization Regional Office for Africa, (January-June), 2003, 4(1):4-7.

11. Nabyonga J et al. *National health accounts in Eastern and Southern Africa.* Country reports, AFRO, 2002.

12. Mander M. *Marketing of indigenous medicinal plants in South Africa. A case study in KwaZulu-Natal.* Roma, Food and Agriculture Organization of the United Nations, 1999.

13. McIntyre D et al. (eds). Marketing of indigenous medicinal plants in South Africa. In: *Equity in public sector health care financing and expenditure in South Africa. Technical report: South African Health Review 1999.* Durban, Health Systems Trust, 1999.

14. Ahorlu CK et al. Malaria-related beliefs and behaviour in southern Ghana: implications for treatment, prevention and control. *Tropical Medicine and International Health,* 1997, 2:488–499.

15. Summary of situation of herbal medicines and regulations in the WHO African Region based on results of global survey. In: *Report of the Second Regional Workshop on Regulation of Traditional Medicines in the WHO African Region. Madrid, Spain, 13-14 February 2004,* WHO Regional Office for Africa, Brazzaville (AFRO/EDM/AFRO/2004.2) (in press).

16. Green, EC. The WHO Forum on Traditional Medicine in Health Systems. *Journal of Alternative and Complementary Medicine.* 2000, 6(5):379-382.

17. D'Avanzo CE, Geissler EM. *Cultural health assessment,* 3rd ed. Philadelphia, Mosby, 2003.

18. Ghana Herbal Pharmacopoeia. Accra, Ghana: Policy Research and Strategic Planning Institute, 1992.

19. Burford G et al. Traditional medicine and HIV/AIDS in Africa: a report from the International Conference on Medicinal Plants, Traditional Medicine and Local Communities in Africa. *Journal of Alternative and Complementary Medicine,* 2000, 6:457–472.

20. Kyeyune P et al. The role of traditional health practitioners in increasing access to HIV/AIDS prevention and care: The Ugandan Experience. In: World Health Organization Regional Office for Africa, ed. *Traditional medicine: our culture, our future. African Health Monitor,* 2003, 4(1):31–32.

21. Bishaw M. Promoting traditional medicine in Ethiopia: a brief historical review of government policy. *Social Science and Medicine,* 1991, 33:193–200.

CHAPTER 2

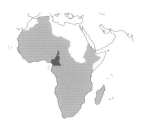

REPUBLIC
OF CAMEROON

Daniel N. Lantum[1]
and Martin Ekeke Monono[2]

[1] Medical Doctor, Professor of Public Health, Consultant, P.O. Box 4285, Nlongkak Yaounde, Cameroon. E-mail: dlantum@camnet.cm

[2] Medical Doctor, Director, Health Care Organization and Health Technology, Ministry of Health, Yaounde, Cameroon.

2.1. INTRODUCTION

The Republic of Cameroon has a land area of 475 000 km2 and over 250 ethnic groups (*1*) in a total population of 15 472 557 inhabitants.

Cameroonian Traditional Medicine has existed from time immemorial as an important component of social and cultural development. It seeks to prevent illness, promote general well being and carry out diagnosis and treatment. Traditional medicine (TRM) of Africa in general and that of Cameroon in particular is the medicine of particular peoples or ethnic groups, and thus varies in its particularities from people to people and with different ecological zones (forest, savanna, scrubland, coastal and riverine – Cameroon being Africa in miniature). It is part and parcel of the peoples' culture (*2*). However, in urbanizing cosmopolitan communities, TRM providers (medicine men) have migrated from the countryside to live in new cities, although they still depend on their places of origin for replenishment of supplies (*3*).

The training of practitioners of traditional medicine (tradi-practitioners) is still largely informal but it is continuous and well established to ensure a constant number in society. Interested and motivated individuals move into the field and work full time, but due to economic pressures, some learn other skills and accept more lucrative job opportunities (*3*).

A number of studies of Cameroonian medicinal plants and traditional medicine are recorded. They are summarized in Table 2.1 and have been reported in the draft document of the National Strategic Plan (*4*). The objective of the Cameroon National Strategic Plan for the development of TRM is to integrate this medicine into the national health-care delivery system.

In 1979, a unit for TRM was created within the Department of Health and in 1981 a Traditional Medicine Unit was set up in Central Hospital, Yaoundé. This was followed in 1989 by the creation of a Community Health and Traditional Medicine Service with a Unit in charge of TRM. In 1990 the Law on Freedom of Association was passed by the National Assembly, which led to the creation of many Traditional Healers' Associations in the country and was followed a year later by a note issued by the Ministry of Health requesting the collaboration between the traditional healers and the public health sector. In 2002, the Service for Traditional Medicine was established including two units; one for ethics and deontology and another for legislation and control. Besides these, there is a scientific network sub-department to help promote medicinal plants in the Ministry of Public Health. At the same time as these official units were established, there were decrees establishing formal institutions for research (see section 2.5).

In addition to this national commitment, the Republic of Cameroon also subscribed to the Lusaka Declaration of the African Union Heads of State held in July 2001, on the designation of the period 2001–2010 as the Decade for African Traditional Medicine and to its plan of action for implementation adopted by the Ministers of Health Conference held in Tripoli, Libyan Arab Jamahiriya, in April 2003 (*5*). The plan of action and mechanisms for its implementation were endorsed by the African Union Summit of Heads of State and Government, which took place in July 2003 in Maputo, Mozambique (*6*) (see also Chapter 1).

Table 2.1. Some historical studies of TRM in the Cameroon (4)

Year	Study
1889	Georges Zenker, botanist from the botanic garden in Naples, Italy, visited Cameroon
1900	The Sultan of Bamun, Ibrahim Njoya recorded in his language some traditional medicine used by his people
1913	Milbread, in a study conducted in the Central part of Cameroon, noticed the use of 100 plants among which some were of medicinal benefit
1926	Santesson, in an ethnobotanic study conducted around Mount Cameroon, collected 42 species and in 1935 he listed their local names and their medicinal usage
1941	Canabis in the northern part of Cameroon noticed some traditional phytotherapy acting on psychiatric disorders. (cited by Saivet in 1975)
1950	Malzy (cited by Saivet in 1975) recorded the usage of 300 plants of the northern part of Cameroon with their local and scientific names
1955	Surville made studies of some medicinal plants in the southern Cameroon
1961	Couteix studied the art and the pharmacopoeia of the Ewondos traditional healers around Yaoundé. He published a collection of treatments given for psychiatric and psychosomatic disorders. He also gave the local and scientific names of certain plants and their usage
1970	Mallard, a researcher of ORSTOM (Office de la Recherche Scientifique et Technique d'Outre-Mer) studied for more than a year the "Evouzock therapeutic in Ebolowa area"
1975	Saive, within the framework of a doctorate thesis in pharmacy, began an ethno-pharmacological study in Cameroon

2.2. STATE OF DEVELOPMENT OF TRADITIONAL, COMPLEMENTARY AND ALTERNATIVE MEDICINE IN THE CAMEROON

Cameroonian traditional, complementary and alternative medicine (TCAM) has kept its popularity but side-by-side with its new competitors (7). From the patients' viewpoint, when in need, they first use what is accessible at home. If not successful, they consult the nearest healer. If still not successful, they then go to more reputed health centres or hospitals and pharmacies to seek aid. Their aim is to get well by any means known, reputable and affordable, and especially provided by someone who can explain the nature of their illness, get rid of it, and advise on how to avoid it (8). This indigenous medicine, which is very much a way of life and practised by all, is spearheaded by its masters who are called tradi-practitioners, medicine men, or traditional healers (9, 10). In the urbanizing communities, these masters are found in large numbers alongside others who carry foreign certificates in homeopathy, naturopathy, nutrition medicine, palmistry and other systems including Chinese medicine (7). They are popular in spite of public or state hospitals, health centres, maternity centres, pharmaceutical dispensaries and mobile health education and mass vaccination campaigns which propagate allopathic medicine (11). The tradi-practitioners of Oku and the Pygmies of the Congo basin are the most reputed (12).

Although a government policy to identify and count tradi-practitioners and other alternative healers has existed in Cameroon since 1976, the structure for implementation was never properly put in place (DN Lantum, unpublished, 2003). However statistics for allopathic medicine are well kept in Annual Reports of Activities of the Health Ministry for review, periodic planning and budgeting of health care delivery services (2).

2.3. Background Indicators

For purposes of communication, morbidity and mortality data must be reported in the language of allopathic medicine, though TCAM has some equivalent terms and many more besides (*13, 14*). Furthermore, for the most part TCAM treats symptoms and symptom-complexes and vague illness entities (*15*). Occasionally, practitioners depend for specific diagnosis on allopathic medicine, but often associate a social dimension since there is a social cause to every disease (*16*). In general, diagnosis among tradi-practitioners is largely symptomatic.

2.3.1. Causes of Morbidity

The most common causes of morbidity vary from clinic to clinic, hospital to hospital and by geographic region of the country; also by the specific age groups of the patients, by gender and by season (*17*). However, malaria was recorded to top the list in medical and paediatric wards in all the hospitals, regions and age groups. This was followed, in internal medicine wards, by bronchopneumonia, high blood pressure, gastroenteritis, peptic ulcers, HIV/AIDS, diabetes mellitus, typhoid fever, asthma, hepatitis, coma and tuberculosis. The surgical wards reported burns, snakebites, fractures, splenic rupture, accidental wounds, inguinal hernia, appendicitis and peritonitis as common causes of morbidity.

In the paediatric services, common causes of morbidity often included, in descending order of frequency, malaria, bronchopneumonia, cerebral malaria, gastroenteritis, meningitis, severe anaemia, malnutrition, neonatal infection, measles, and sickle cell disease (*18*).

In the maternity services, the causes of morbidity included, normal delivery, malaria, abortion, postpartum haemorrhage, threatened abortion, foetal suffering, ovarian cysts, extrauterine pregnancy and pelvic inflammatory disease. According to gynaecology/obstetric records, the top ten causes of illness for the North Region were: pelvic infections, threatened abortions, malaria in pregnancy, urethritis, uterine fibroids, secondary sterility, ovarian cysts, extrauterine pregnancies and primary infertility.

In all the regions of the Cameroon, the following disease entities and symptoms figured among the most common in traditional healers' records: malaria, dysentery, chronic urethritis, jaundice, witchcraft, fractures, poison, ulcers, gastritis, protection, chance/misfortune, spells, bottom belly, sterility, arthritis, haemorrhoids, body pains, common infections, diseases of the lung (*2, 19*).

The above trends are only for severe cases who are hospitalized. The most common causes of morbidity described in ambulant health-care services include: malaria, common cold, wounds, common infections, buccal problems, conjunctivitis, pain and fevers, urethritis, skin rashes, intestinal worms, burns, and diseases of the lung (*18*). Among tradi-practitioners, the most common presenting symptoms include lumbago, malaria/fever, diarrhoea, sub-fertility, anaemia, male impotence, jaundice, constipation, asthenia, and witchcraft or sorcery (*2*).

2.3.2. Causes of Mortality

As for morbidity, the causes of mortality vary with hospital, region, age group, service unit and type of medicine (allopathic versus TCAM). Gastroenteritis, severe anaemia, meningitis, measles, cerebral malaria, leukaemia, malnutrition, tetanus, intoxications or acute poisoning and bronchopneumonia were all recorded as common causes of mortality in paediatric services (*18*). In general medicine wards, malaria, typhoid, HIV/AIDS, hypertension, tuberculosis, bronchopneumonia, meningitis, cardiopathies, hepatoma and tetanus are common, while in surgical services, septicaemia, gangrene, amputations, extra-dural haematoma, multiple injuries, severe anaemia, and cancer, are the most common causes of death.

Records of traditional healers and complementary medicine scarcely showed any causes of death since moribund cases are invariably referred to public hospitals or managed in their own homes by visiting tradi-practitioners and family members (*2*).

2.3.3. Total Number of TCAM Providers

A partial census of traditional healers has been carried out from which the total number may be estimated to about 10 000 in Cameroon. This is equivalent to 1 per 700 inhabitants but the proportion is greater in towns. However, those recognized and recorded by community are no more than 6000 (1/2333 inhabitants). For census purposes, a tradi-practitioner is a native healer recognised by his/her community, since they do not carry any formal certificate or diploma awarded by the State. In comparison in 2001, Cameroon had at her disposal, 1 medical doctor to 10 083 inhabitants and 1 qualified nurse to 2249 inhabitants with a significant difference from one province to another.

2.3.4. *Total Health Expenditure*

Whereas money is the means of payment in the formal public and private allopathic medical sectors, the system of compensation in TRM is radically different, permitting for payments in kind (goats, chickens, palm wine, services, specially-valued token gifts, values of prestige and precedence, etc.) (*11*). As every citizen is a member of a community, the community is committed to protect his or her life and welfare by all reasonable means. It is not possible to quantify the cost of this social commitment and care. However a lot of medicinal plant elements are now sold in popular markets (*3*). Thus, an annual expenditure of CFA 10 billion for TRM is a reasonable estimate (*20*).

In the native communities, TRM is largely gratuitous as a communal responsibility (*9*).

2.4. Structural and Process Information

In Cameroon, TRM structures are part of the ethnic and cultural organization for survival. Hence it is easier to visualise the system from the social and cultural anthropological context (*9, 21*). All chiefs of clans and lineages are medicine men by dint of office and medicine is mixed with their religious authority to strengthen their leadership positions and power of command. Hence all professional tradi-practitioners or medicine men are specialized arms of their chiefs who must periodically bless the medicines of the clan. Although professionals have been identified and recognized, almost every citizen knows some TRM as part of his practical vocabulary and skill. Hence all attempts to abolish TRM have failed.

Although the training of the younger generation tends to be by parents to their children, gifted masters of TRM are well-known established trainers, and their dwellings constitute informal schools for inculcation by apprenticeship or participant-observation. Initiation is often done by these trainers or by parents and community leaders. A traditional healer is first recognised by his or her community before venturing out (*22*). If trained in another ethnic entity, he or she must be formally received and recognized by the native community before settling down to practise with confidence.

In fact, there are several traditional healers' associations at district and regional levels. However, they are not well organized and seem to fight for leadership in the field. These different associations have a lot of activities, including the training of other traditional healers.

Many traditional healers apply to the Ministry of Health for eventual official authorization. Others set up some traditional techniques to improve presentation of their preparations for patients. Some traditional healers are overzealous and sometimes use modern diagnosis inappropriately, merely for advertisement purposes.

Legislation to promote TRM as a system is scanty, and indeed it is thanks to external pressures, particularly those of the World Health Organization, that TRM has come to enjoy official respectability in spite of its ubiquitous presence and utility (*7*). Cameroon may be classified in the Inclusive System of WHO where TRM is recognized, but not completely integrated in all aspects of the health system.

2.5. Research and Development of traditional medicine in Cameroon

In 1979, a decree organizing the General Delegation of Technical and Scientific Research, created a Research Institute of Medicine and the Study of Medicinal Plants, and in 1989 the first Seminar Workshop on Traditional Medicine and Cameroonian Pharmacopoeia was organized.

In 1993, a Centre for Research on Medicinal Plants and Traditional Medicine was created and today contains a number of traditional medicines pending ratification by the Ministry of Public Health. A census and identification of almost 200 species of plants has been done, with the determination of the composition of certain plants and their therapeutic properties (*23*).

In State Universities during the last 20 years, several scientific studies are done every year and have permitted the discovery of antiseptic, antimycotic, anti-inflammatory and insect-killing properties of medicinal plants in Cameroon (*12*).

Moreover, an ethnobotanic survey, conducted by the Organization for African Unity, Scientific and Technical Commission, and published in 1996, made it possible to collect interesting information concerning more than 600 Cameroonian plants (*24*). Since the colonial period, the scientific study of medicinal plants by ethnobotanists is widely known, and reports are abundant (*25*) and a national herbarium exists. However, these studies were not carried out with the intention of promoting traditional medicine and its practitioners (*26*). The limited effort in the study of TCAM has been generally for purposes of exploitation of medicinal plants rather than helping the growth and development of TCAM (*27*). It is not, therefore, surprising that the study of TCAM has been a meeting ground for researchers of several scientific disciplines, including foresters, botanists, phytochemists, pharmacologists, physicians, theologians, wonder-workers, conservationists, anthropologists, ecologists, social geographers, pathologists and others (*24*).

2.6. CONCLUSIONS AND SUMMARY

The TRM of Cameroon is very much alive as part of people's culture. It is unfortunate that it was driven into clandestine practice during the long colonial period. However, a number of favourable policies are beginning to emerge which augur well for the future. There is a political will to create the legislation necessary to give official recognition, as well as lay down guidance for its operation. This will give opportunities for TRM to flourish even more.

The Alma–Ata declaration of 1978 created opportunities for integrating TRM into conventional health-care systems. In Cameroon, this process has been slow but steady and has gathered momentum in the last few years. A number of major government actions have been undertaken:

- Encouragement of a census of tradi-practitioners;

- Provision for tradi-practitioners to be members of dialogue committees at Health Area and District jurisdiction of health care services;

- Authorization for setting up Chinese medicine hospitals in Cameroon e.g. Guider and Mbalmayo (since 1970s);

- Creation of a service of Traditional Medicine in the Health Ministry in 1995 (2);

- Acknowledgement that TCAM can contribute to fighting against the HIV/AIDS epidemic (15);

- Invitation to tradi-practitioners to the national medical conference and organization of special sessions on TCAM in 2002 – 2003;

- Official implementation of First Annual Celebration of Traditional Medicine Day on 31 August 2003 (2).

The preparation of the National Strategic Plan of Traditional Medicine is well underway.

References

1. *Enquête Camerounaise des Ménages [Inquiry into Cameroonian households]*, 2001.

2. Lantum DN. *Traditional medicine-men of Cameroon: the case of bui: trad med report series No.1*, P.H.Unit CUSS, University of Yaounde, Trad. Med. Occasional Paper No. 2, 188, 1985.

3. Betti, Jean Lagarde, "Medicinal Plants Sold in Yaounde Markets, Cameroon" in *African Study Monographs*, 23(2): 47-64, 2002.

4. *Draft Document de Plan National Stratégique de Développement de la Médecine Traditionnelle au Cameroun [Draft document of strategic national plan of development of traditional medicine in Cameroon]*, 2003.

5. Sambo LG. Integration of traditional medicine into health systems in the African Region – The journey so far. *African Health Monitor*. WHO Regional Office for Africa, 2003, 4:8-11.

6. Heads of State and Government of the African Union: Second ordinary session, Maputo, Mozambique, 10-12 July 2003. Maputo declaration on HIV/AIDS, Tuberculosis, Malaria and Other Related Infectious Diseases The full text of this and other declarations can be found at: www.africa-union.org

7. *WHO Traditional Medicine Strategy 2000–2005.* Geneva, World Health Organization, 2002 (WHO/ EDM/TRM/2002.1).

8. Tegha SM. *Traditional health beliefs, concept of health and traditional medical practice in Mezam Division, Cameroon* [thesis]. Sociology, University of Ibadan, 1983.

9. Cora du Bois. *The people of Alor.* Harper Torchbooks, The Academy Library, University of Minnesota, 1960.

10. Leiderer Rosemaire. *La medecine traditionnelle chez les bekpak (bafia) du Cameroun [Traditional medicine at the bekpak (bafia) of Cameroon], Vol I, II,* Collectanea Instituti Anthropos, Haus Volker and Kulturen, D – 5205 Sankt Augustin, 1982.

11. Lantum DN. *The pros and cons of traditional medicine in Cameroon / pour ou contre la medicine traditionnelle au Cameroun,* abbia Cameroon Cultural Review, No. 35-36-37, pp79-, 1978.

12. Betti, Jean Lagarde. *An Ethnopharmacological Study of Medicinal Plants Among the Baka Pygmies in the Dja Biosphere Reserve.* Cameroon Dept. of Forestry, University of Dschang, Cameroon, 2001.

13. Eric de Rosny. Ndimsi – *ceux qui soignent dans la nuit [Ndimsi - those who look after in the night].* Etudes et Documents Africains, Editions Cle Yaounde, 1974.

14. Eric de Rosny. *Les yeux de ma chevre [Eyes of my goat],* (A film on witchcraft in Douala Cameroon), 1993.

15. Lantum DN. "Role of Traditional Medicine-men in the prevention and control of HIV/AIDS pandemic in Africa" in *Biodiagnostics and Therapy,* No. 19, December 2002:5-10.

16. Gebauer P. *Spider divination,* Milwaukee Public Museum Publications in Anthropology, No. 10, 1964.

17. Dommaul Fankam P. *Rapport de Stage de Médicine Intégrée a l'Hôpital Central d'Enongal [Report of training course of integrated medicine at the Central Hospital of Enongal]* 1/10/1997 au 7/2/1998.

18. Kongnyuy Eugene Justin Kongnyuy. *Report of Integrated Medicine Posting in Banso Baptist Hospital,* 6 October 1997 to February 1998.

19. Lantum DN. *Traditional medicine men of centre province* (Mfoundi, Mefou and Nyong et Soo): Traditional medicine census report series No. 2. P.H.Unit, UCHS/CUSS, University of Yaounde, May 1989.

20. Etude sur l'accessibilité et les déterminants de recours aux soins (Study on accessibility and determinants of recourse to the care), MINSANTE, 2002.

21. Malinowski B. *Magic, science and religion and other essays,* A Doubleday Anchor Book, 1948.

22. Gelfand M. *Medicine and custom in Africa,* E and S Livingstone Ltd., Edinburgh and London, 1964.

23. *Rapport d'Activités Institut des Recherches Médicales et d'Etude des Plantes Médicinales [Report of medical research and study for institutional management of medicinal plants],* 2000.

24. OAU/Scientific Tech. And Research Commission, *Traditional medicine and pharmacopoeia: contribution to ethnobotanical and floristic studies in Cameroon, Impression,* CNPMS BP 135 Porto Novo BENIN, 1996:641.

25. Cipcre, *Connaissez-vous les plantes médicinales ?* Cipcre – Yoirp Cameroun, Projet de promotion des Plantes médicinales *[Do you know the medicinal plants? – Project for promotion of medicinal plants],* BP 1256, Bafoussam, 2000.

26. Minrest. *Flore du Cameroun,* Serie No. 34, minrest, Yaoundé, 1998.

27. Ankoud Angele R. *Rapport de Stage de Médicine Intégrée a l'Hôpital Provincial de Bertoua [Report of training course of Integrated Medicine at the Provincial Hospital of Bertoua],* 7 Octobre 1996 – 06 Février 1997.

CHAPTER 3

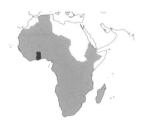

REPUBLIC
OF GHANA

F. K. Oppong-Boachie

Immediate Past Director of the Centre for Scientific Research into Plant Medicine,
P.O. Box 73, Mampong-Akuapem, E/R, Ghana.
E-mail: oppongboachie@yahoo.com

3.1. INTRODUCTION

The Republic of Ghana is located on West Africa's Gulf of Guinea just a few degrees north of the equator. It borders the North Atlantic Ocean to the south, Burkina Faso to the north, Côte d'Ivoire to the west and Togo to the east. It has a total area of 238 540 km² of which 230 020 km² is land and the rest is covered by rivers. A tropical rain forest belt, split by heavily forested hills, extends northward from the shore near the Côte d'Ivoire border. This area produces most of the country's cocoa, minerals and timber. Low bush, park-like savanna and grassy plains, where many medicinal plants and herbs can be found, cover the area north of this belt.

The country is divided administratively into 10 regions and 110 local districts and has a population of some 18.8 million people (1). In 2001, the average annual growth rate was 3%, with a per capita gross domestic product of US$ 390 and an average life expectancy of 60 years (2).

Traditional, complementary and alternative medicine (TCAM) knowledge and practices in Ghana stem from some of the area's oldest traditions. In recognition of this heritage, successive post-independence governments have sought to develop TCAM services as viable and necessary alternatives to allopathic health care. The first attempt to organize the TCAM sector was in 1961 when the first President of Ghana, Osagyefo Dr Kwame Nkrumah, encouraged the formation of the Ghana Psychic and Traditional Healers Association. The Ghana Federation of Traditional Medical Practitioners' Associations (GHAFTRAM) was established in 1999, and since then it has greatly advanced the cause and development of TCAM in Ghana.

3.2. BACKGROUND INDICATORS

3.2.1. Leading Causes of Mortality

Various institutional data have revealed malaria, anaemia, stroke, pneumonia, tuberculosis (TB), injury, liver disease, HIV/AIDS, hypertension, diarrhoea, sickle cell and neonatal injury as the leading causes of death in Ghana. Malaria and anaemia together account for up to 40% of reported deaths in children aged 15 years and below, while pneumonia and diarrhoea cause a significant number of deaths in all age groups. Liver disease, HIV/AIDS and TB are major causes of death in the adult population over 15 years old, while stroke, hypertension and type 2 diabetes mellitus are the predominant causes of death of both men and women over the age of 45 years (3). Injury and liver disease exact a higher burden on men than women, in contrast to HIV/AIDS-related deaths, which are higher in women (2).

In Ghana, children under five years of age constitute less than 20% of the population and yet account for more than 50% of the estimated 192 000 deaths each year (2). The under-five mortality rate is therefore generally considered as a good overall indicator of the health of the Ghanaian population. Ghana's under-five mortality rate fell from 154 in 1988 to 110 per 1000 births in 1998 (4), a decline of 27%. Generally, children in rural areas are 1.6 times more likely to die before their fifth birthday than those in urban areas.

Maternal mortality rates vary from 214 per 100 000 live births in urban centres to 740 per 100 000 live births in rural communities. Leading causes of death are haemorrhage, hypertensive diseases in pregnancy, abortions, sickle cell disease, genital tract infections, anaemia and obstructed labour (5).

It is projected that improvements in education and health technology will improve childhood and adult mortality statistics over the next 5–10 years.

3.2.2. Leading Causes of Morbidity

Morbidity statistics from hospital data indicate that the number of attendance per person per year at outpatient departments have increased from 0.32 in 1996 to 0.42 in 2000. Malaria, upper respiratory tract infection (URTI), diarrhoea, skin diseases, eye infections and injury are the leading causes of visits to outpatient departments. Malaria (42%) and URTI (8%) account for half of the total visits for both sexes and all age groups (3).

Admissions to public health facilities were about 24 per 1000 persons in 1999 with differences across the regions of the country. For example, regional admissions in the Ashanti Region were 4 per 1000 persons, as compared to 48 per 1000 persons in the Central Region. At Korle-Bu Teaching Hospital in the Greater Accra Region, perinatal conditions account for 66.6% of infant admissions (6), which may be attributed to the fact that this hospital is a tertiary referral facility. Injury represents 20% of admissions for both sexes in the 5–14-year age group. Maternal and gynaecological disorders accounted for 78% of admissions of women aged 15–44 years. Stroke, injuries and heart failure are the leading causes for admission of the elderly of both sexes.

3.2.3. Epidemic and Other Causes of Mortality and Morbidity

Environmentally-related diseases, epidemics and HIV/AIDS also contribute to mortality and morbidity. At various times in its history, Ghana has experienced major epidemics of cholera, cerebrospinal meningitis, yellow fever, rabies and HIV/AIDS. Major cholera epidemics occur every 9–11 years. The latest cholera epidemic was in 1999 when 9463 cases resulted in 259 deaths (7). The last epidemic of cerebrospinal meningitis was in 1997 when 18 703 cases and 1356 deaths occurred (8). In 2000, two regions reported rabies outbreaks with ten deaths reported in the Central Region (9).

Guinea worm disease declined by 96% from 179 556 cases in 1989 to 7402 in 2000 (2). Reported cases of HIV/AIDS increased from 42 in 1986 to 6289 in 1999 (10). In 2000, the cumulative number of reported AIDS cases reached 43 587.

3.2.4. Providers of Conventional Health Care

A 1999 annual report of the Ministry of Health (MOH) in Ghana indicates the number and type of health facilities as shown in Table 3.1 (2). The total number of medical personnel recruited by MOH to work in the public health sector is 30 612. Of this number, the distribution of medical and paramedical staff by profession and region is indicated in Table 3.2 (2).

The two teaching hospitals (Korle-Bu Teaching Hospital in the Greater Accra Region and Komfo Anokye Teaching Hospital in the Ashanti Region) alone employ 469 or 42.1% of all qualified doctors and MOH headquarters employs 40 or 3.6% of the national total, leaving very few doctors to meet the needs of the rest of the country. The three northern regions have only 68 doctors, or 6.1% of the national total. It has been recommended that public health facilities employ another 268 doctors, 5694 nurses, 293 dentists, 871 pharmacists, 36 physiotherapists, 1206 clinical laboratory assistants, 160 radiologists and 8705 other staff to reach the estimated optimum operational standards (2).

Table 3.1. Number and type of health facilities in Ghana

Facility type	Number
Teaching hospitals	2
Regional hospitals	9
District hospitals	91
Clinics	1085
Other hospitals	124
Health centres	558
Maternity homes	320
Pharmacy shops	800
Chemists' shops	4000

3.2.5. TCAM Providers

The two main types of TCAM in Ghana are traditional medicine and alternative medicine. A traditional medicine practitioner is defined as a person who possesses the knowledge and skills of holistic health care, and who is recognized and accepted for health care based on indigenous theories, beliefs and experiences handed down through generations. In Ghana, as in other parts of Africa, traditional medical practitioners include herbal healers, bone-setters, traditional birth attendants, spiritualists, shrine operators, eye specialists, throat specialists, animal bite healers, veterinary healers and surgeons (e.g. incisors of tribal and disease prevention marks on the body).

Table 3.2. Numbers of MOH staff in Ghana for 1999

Region	Doctors	Dentists	Medical Assistants	Nurses	Others*	Total
MOH Headquarters	40	1	1	0	34	76
Ashanti	256	2	47	2118	905	3323
Greater Accra	435	12	55	3894	408	4804
Eastern	84	5	43	2019	2388	4647
Northern	29	1	29	942	1559	2442
Western	69	3	40	1056	1588	2747
Brong-Ahafo	59	0	32	1048	2079	3218
Volta	57	0	29	1560	2341	4087
Central	47	2	31	1134	1352	2566
Upper East	25	1	14	706	800	1546
Upper West	14	1	12	495	710	1232
Total	**1115**	**28**	**333**	**14972**	**14164**	**30688**

* Others include village health workers and community-based distributors.

Alternative medicine practices are those practices and therapies outside allopathic and traditional medicine. Alternative medicine involves cooperation with natural forces and the natural defence mechanisms of the body and includes homeopathy, chiropractic, hydrotherapy, acupuncture, naturopathy, radionics and reflexology. These therapies are recent additions to health care in Ghana and are mainly practised in urban areas such as Accra, Kumasi, Takoradi and Tema.

In November 2002 and March 2003, the Traditional and Alternative Medicine Directorate of MOH produced a draft census report of registered TCAM practitioners for the Ashanti, Central, Greater Accra, Northern, Upper East, Upper West and Western Regions respectively (*11*). The overall objective of the census was to initiate effective planning and human resource management within the traditional medicine sector for eventual integration into the national health-care delivery system. Although the draft report of the remaining three regions, namely Brong-Ahafo, Eastern and Volta, is yet to be published, results from the seven regions show similar trends. Table 3.3 summarizes some of the trends and shows that in the seven regions, registered TCAM practitioners are thirty-fold more numerous than allopathic physicians (*11*). This figure could rise with the inclusion of TCAM practitioner totals from the remaining Eastern and Volta Regions. It must be emphasized that there could be thousands of TCAM practitioners who are not registered.

In the Ashanti, Central, Greater Accra and Western Regions, of the enumerated TCAM practitioners (7999), 7633 or 95.4% considered indigenous medicine as their primary or secondary profession, while 366 or 4.6% practiced alternative medicine. TCAM practitioners who practice plant or herbal indigenous medicine were by far the largest group at 65.5%. This was followed in descending order by traditional birth attendants (16.6%), psychic practitioners (13.4%), bone-setters (3.5%) and all others (1.1%). Similar trends were observed from the three northern regions where of the 3292 enumerated: 41.9% or 1379 practice herbalism, 15.3% are traditional birth attendants, 11.4% are psychic healers, and 5.8% presented as bone-setters. Acupuncture, naturopathy and chiropractic accounted for 0.03%, while "not stated" and "others" (e.g. practitioners of scarification) constituted the remaining 25.6%. The sociodemographic distribution of TCAM practitioners with respect to sex, age, education and religion was similar in the seven regions.

Table 3.3. Population statistics of registered TCAM practitioners (TCAMP) in Ghana

Region	Total No. of TCAMP	No. (%) TCAMP in urban areas	No. (%) TCAMP in rural areas	TCAMP as % of population	Allopathic physicians as % of population
Ashanti	2995	740 (24.7)	2255 (75.3)	0.094	0.0008
Greater Accra	1207	645 (53.4)	562 (46.6)	0.004	0.0015
Western	1708	620 (36.3)	1088 (63.7)	0.093	0.0003
Northern	1704	506 (29.7)	1198 (70.3)	0.092	0.0002
Central	2089	690 (33.0)	1399 (67.0)	0.013	0.0003
Upper East	822	69 (8.4)	753 (91.6)	0.009	0.0003
Upper West	766	416 (54.3)	350 (45.7)	0.013	0.0002
Total	**11 291**	**3686**	**7605**	**0.009**	**0.0003**

3.2.6. Health Expenditure

Total health expenditure from 1997 to 2000 is shown in Table 3.4. Contributors are the Government of Ghana, internally-generated funds from health facilities, donors, and creditors. The percentage of the total contributions made by the Government was 42.8, 54.8, 50.4 and 60.5 in the years 1997–2000, respectively. Total investment and recurrent expenditure (including wages and salaries) from 1997 to 1999 are also shown in Table 3.4 (2).

Table 3.4. Total health expenditure (1997–2000)

Year	Total health expenditure (US$ million)	Total investments (US$ million)	Recurrent expenditure (US$ million)
1997	159	70	89
1998	155	47	108
1999	129	23	106
2000	114	NA	NA

The capital expenditure was distributed to the various levels of health care namely; MOH Headquarters, the teaching hospitals (tertiary), the regions (secondary), and the districts (primary) from 1997 to September 1999 as indicated in Table 3.5 (2). The distribution is based mainly on the number of health personnel at each level of health care and special needs e.g. control of an epidemic at a particular level.

3.3. TRADITIONAL MEDICINE POLICY AND OUTCOMES

3.3.1. Mission, Vision and Goals of TCAM

The mission of the 2000 medium-term strategy document for TCAM aims to make traditional health care a well-defined and recognized system, complementary to other health systems throughout Ghana. This strategy seeks to establish a health-care system, based on Ghanaian traditions, that provides acceptable quality of care. The end goal is to improve the health status of all people living in Ghana through the use of traditional health care.

The strategy highlights that the regulation and control of TCAM practice is, in part, the responsibility of the Traditional and Alternative Medicine Council (TAMC), which is to oversee the practice and the practitioners through registration, licensing and prescription of appropriate codes of ethics, in consultation with the recognized TCAM associations. The TAMC is also mandated to institute a national expert committee on control, education, research and promotion of TCAM in Ghana. The TAMC, in collaboration with the Food and Drugs Board, regulates the manufacturing, sale and registration of scientifically assessed traditional products for commercial purposes. The MOH, through its Traditional and Alternative Medicine Directorate, has a duty to develop policy guidelines that allow for growth of the traditional medicine sector.

Table 3.5. Capital health expenditure by levels of health care

Year	Expenditure (US$ million) by level of health care				
	HQ	*Tertiary*	*Secondary*	*Primary*	*Total*
1997	14.0	11.5	24.8	15.8	66.1
1998	1.4	5.0	27.8	13.8	48.0
1999 (Jan–Sep)	0.8	0.5	0.1	0.4	1.8
Total	16.2 (13.9%)	17.0 (14.7%)	52.7 (45.5%)	30.0 (25.9%)	115.9 (100%)

3.3.2. Achievements

A chronological summary of the institutional, policy and regulatory structures that have worked to advance TCAM in Ghana includes:

- establishment of the Centre for Scientific Research into Plant Medicine in 1973, which was given statutory recognition in 1975 (*13*);

- institution of the Directorate for Herbal Medicine at MOH in 1991;

- formation of the Food and Drugs Board in 1997 (*14*);

- establishment of the Traditional and Alternative Medicine Directorate at MOH in 1999;

- formation of GHAFTRAM in 1999;

- development of a strategic plan for traditional health care in Ghana in 2000 (*15*);

- introduction of the Traditional Medicine Practice Act, 2000 (*16*);

- institutionalization of an annual "traditional medicine week" for awareness and advocacy;

- development of a training manual for traditional health practitioners, including traditional birth attendants in primary health care, nutrition, diagnosis, prevention of diseases and proper record-keeping in 2002 (*17*);

- drafting of the Alternative Medicine Practice Bill of 2002, presently before Parliament (*18*);

- publication of a manual on procedures for assessing the safety, efficacy and quality of plant medicines in Ghana (*19*); and

- institution of a Bachelor of Science Degree in Herbal Medicine at the Kwame Nkrumah University of Science and Technology (KNUST).

3.3.3. Research

Institutions such as the Nogouchi Memorial Institute of Medical Research, Departments in the Universities of Ghana, Cape Coast, KNUST, and a few private entrepreneurs are furthering the field of traditional Ghanaian medicine through research on herbal medicine.

3.4. USES OF TCAM

3.4.1. Medical determinants of use

The 2002–2003 census report on the three northern regions and Accra, Ashanti, Central and Western Regions (*11*) revealed that TCAM practitioners manage and treat multiple conditions or diseases in their primary, secondary or tertiary stages of development. The type and frequency of condition or diseases seen in patients seeking TCAM (as a % of total visits) is assessed as infertility (12.9%), malaria (9.2%), convulsion (8.5%), boils (4.0%), stroke (3.7%), abdominal pains (3.6%), hernia (3.0%), asthma (2.9%), skin diseases (2.7%), waist pains (2.5%), measles (2.5%), snake bites (2.0%), diabetes mellitus (1.5%), cough (1.2%), eye problems (1.1%), diarrhoea (1.0%), worms (0.8%) and chest pains (0.7%) (*11*). The total (63.8%), added to which are the unreported cases, supports common estimates that 80% of the Ghanaian population relies on TCAM.

The outpatient department of the Centre for Scientific Research into Plant Medicine sees on average 50 patients per day presenting with, in order of frequency, malaria, typhoid fever, sexually transmitted diseases, impotence, hypertension, diabetes mellitus, stroke, various types of cancer, anaemia, skin diseases and sickle cell conditions (K. Oppong-Boachie, unpublished data, 2003).

3.4.2. Out-of-pocket payments

The largest single source of health expenditure, including formal and informal providers, governments, health facilities and pharmacists, comes from patient out-of-pocket spending. This contributes about 50% of total spending and has created a potential access barrier for the poor in Ghana. It is hoped that the establishment of a national health insurance scheme will greatly aid the poor and improve overall health in Ghana.

Although the practice of TCAM is widely tolerated and regulated, it is not considered a mainstream health service. Because of this, government financing for TCAM is largely neglected. This anomaly must be addressed.

3.5. CONCLUSIONS AND SUMMARY

Regulations on practice of TCAM in Ghana have been developed by the national government. Statistics indicate that TCAM providers in Ghana far outnumber allopathic physicians. Irrespective of these data, TCAM is yet to be formally recognized, regulated and controlled. It is hoped that the laudable recommendations put forth in Ghana's strategic plan for the development and eventual integration of TCAM into the Ghana Health Service will be achieved. Through this, it is believed that the people of Ghana would benefit more fully from TCAM practices.

References

1. Ghana Home Page (http://www.ghanaweb.com, accessed 22 April 2004).

2. *The health of the nation: reflections on the First Five Year Health Sector Programme of Work, 1997–2001.* Accra, Ministry of Health, Government of Ghana, 2001.

3. *Report of Health and Disease Analysis Task Team.* Accra, Ministry of Health, Government of Ghana, 2001.

4. *Ghana Demographic and Health Survey.* Claverton, Maryland, Ghana Statistical Service and Macro International Inc., 1999.

5. Wagstaff A. Socioeconomic inequalities in child mortality: comparisons across nine developing countries. *Bulletin of the World Health Organization.* 2000, 78:19–29.

6. Biritwum RB, Gulaid J, Amaning AO. Pattern of diseases or conditions leading to hospitalization at Korle-Bu Teaching Hospital, Ghana in 1996. *Ghana Medical Journal.* 2000, 34:197–205.

7. *Annual Report.* Accra, Public Health Division, Ministry of Health, Government of Ghana, 1999.

8. Woods CW, et al. Emergency vaccination against epidemic meningitis in Ghana: implications for the control of meningococcal disease in West Africa. *Lancet,* 2000, 355:30–33.

9. *Annual Report, Central Regional Health Report, 2000.* Accra, Ministry of Health, Government of Ghana, 2000.

10. *AIDS Surveillance Report.* Accra, National AIDS Commission Programme, Ministry of Health, Government of Ghana, 1999.

11. *Draft census report on the three northern regions and Accra, Western, Central and Ashanti regions.* Accra, Traditional and Alternative Medicine Directorate, Ministry of Health, Government of Ghana, November 2002 and March 2003.

12. Foster M, et al. In: *1999 Health sector review: supplementary report on health sector finance.* Accra, Ministry of Health, Government of Ghana, 2000.

13. *NRC Decree 344.* National Redemption Council, Ghana, 1975.

14. *PNDC Law 305B.* Provisional National Defence Council, Ghana, 1992.

15. *A Strategic Plan for Traditional Health Care in Ghana (2000-2004).* Accra, Traditional and Alternative Medicine Directorate, Ministry of Health, Government of Ghana, 1999.

16. *Traditional Medicine Practice Act 575.* Parliament of Ghana, 2000.

17. *Draft training manual for traditional health practitioners.* Accra, Traditional and Alternative Medicine Directorate, Ministry of Health, Government of Ghana, 2000.

18. *Draft Alternative Medicine Practice Bill.* Accra, Traditional and Alternative Medicine Directorate, Ministry of Health, Government of Ghana, 2000.

19. *A manual of harmonized procedures for assessing the safety, efficacy and quality of plant medicines in Ghana.* Accra, Traditional and Alternative Medicine Directorate, Ministry of Health, Government of Ghana, 2003.

CHAPTER 4

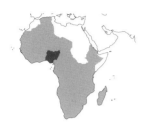

FEDERAL REPUBLIC OF NIGERIA

Karniyus S. Gamaniel[1],
Tolu Fakeye[2]
and Abayomi Sofowora[3]

[1] Director, Department of Pharmacology and Toxicology, National Institute for Pharmaceutical Research and Development (NIPRD), P.M.B. 21, Abuja, Nigeria. E-mail: ksgama@yahoo.com

[2] Coordinator, National Traditional Medicine Development Programme, Federal Ministry of Health, Shehu Shagari Way, P.M.B.083, Garki, Abuja, Nigeria. E-mail: tfakeye@hotmail.com

[3] Professor of Pharmacognosy, Department of Pharmacognosy, Faculty of Pharmacy, Obafemi Awolowo University, Ile-Ife, Nigeria. E-mail: abayomisofowora@yahoo.com

4.1. BACKGROUND

The Federal Republic of Nigeria is situated along the Gulf of Guinea, in the eastern part of the West African subcontinent. It extends over an area of 923 768 km², making it the tenth largest country in the world. The country has a wide diversity of habitats, ranging from arid areas, through many types of forests, to swamps. Associated with the varied zones is an array of plant and animal species. The major vegetation formations are the mangrove forest and coastal swamps, freshwater swamps, lowland rain forest, derived savanna, Northern Guinea savanna, Sudan savanna, Sahel, montane, sub-montane forest and grassland. A country report published in 2002 by the Federal Environmental Protection Agency (*1*) indicates that Nigeria possesses more than 5000 recorded species of plants; 22 090 species of animals, including insects; 889 species of birds; and 1489 species of microorganisms.

Traditional medicine plays a significant role in meeting the health-care needs of the majority of Nigerians. It also provides a livelihood for a significant number of people who depend on it as their main source of income. A National Investigative Committee on Traditional and Alternative Medicine carried out a nationwide survey of traditional medicine in 1985 under the aegis of the Federal Ministry of Science and Technology. In the report presented by the committee (*2*), it was stated that 75% to 80% of the Nigerian population use the services of traditional healers.

Medicinal plants are the primary source of medicines used by traditional healers in Nigeria. Several medicinal plants of global importance originate in the country. For example, Calabar bean (*Physostigma venenosum*) was traditionally used in Nigeria as an "ordeal poison" in trials of wrong-doers. From it, the major component physostigmine (eserine) and its derivatives have been discovered, and are now used against intraocular pressure (glaucoma) (*3*). Nigeria has been ranked eleventh in Africa for plant diversity. Out of the estimated 5000 plant species that exist in the country, 205 are considered endemic, making the country the ninth highest among the 42 African countries in the level of endemic species (*4*). With an estimated population of over 120 million people, distributed among over 250 distinct ethnic groups or tribes, the country is unique in having high cultural diversity and a significant share of the global biological diversity.

The Federal Government of Nigeria, through the Federal Ministry of Health (FMH), declared its intention to incorporate traditional medicine into the national health-care system as far back as 1992, and took immediate steps to actualize this intention. Since then, the Government of Nigeria has put in place a number of measures to support traditional medicine development and control. The questions that remain are, firstly, how much impact these measures have had on the integration of traditional medicine into the official health sector of the Nigerian economy; and secondly, whether there are specific bottlenecks that must be addressed in order to harness the full benefits of traditional medicine. This chapter aims to give a brief overview of the current situation in Nigeria, and to recommend steps that will boost the contribution of traditional medicines to national health care.

4.2. BACKGROUND INDICATORS

Information about some selected background indicators is shown in Table 4.1.

Table 4.1. Selected background indicators for Nigeria.

Background indicator (year)	Value
Total population (2002)	120 911 000
Average annual growth of the population (1992–2002)	2.8%
Life expectancy at birth, total population (2002)	48.8 years
Per capita expenditure on health (2001)	Int$ 31.00
Infant mortality rate (per 1000 live births) (2001)	110
Maternal mortality rate (per 100 000 live births) (2001)	800

4.2.1. Infant Mortality and Maternal Mortality Rates

Trends show that mortality is high compared to more advanced countries, but it has declined over the years, due to improved standards of living and public health. According to the FMH (4) the infant mortality rate was 187 per 1000 live births in the 1960s, compared with 110 in 2001, while the reported maternal mortality rate per 100 000 live births for the same year was 800.

4.2.2. Causes of Morbidity and Mortality

National health records of the FMH (7) indicate that malaria, simple diarrhoea, diarrhoea with blood (dysentery), pneumonia, typhoid and paratyphoid fevers, measles, gonorrhoea, other sexually-transmitted diseases, pertussis and food poisoning were the ten most common causes of morbidity in Nigeria in 2002. Lassa fever, neonatal tetanus, cerebrospinal meningitis, snake bite, HIV/AIDS, tetanus, cholera, tuberculosis, food poisoning and measles were the ten leading causes of mortality in the same year.

4.2.3. Health Sector Personnel

According to the Health Manpower Registration Councils/Boards, in the year 2000 the numbers of prescribers included registered medical practitioners (30 885), registered pharmacists (8642) registered dental practitioners (2221) and registered nurses (10 673) (7).

4.2.4. Number of TCAM Providers

There is no proper record of the total number of TCAM providers in Nigeria. All of them operate outside the conventional health system, and the practices vary from one locality to another. There is a traditional healer in almost every village and it is estimated that there are over 200 000 traditional healers spread all over the country (8). This means that a very significant number of Nigerians, especially those living in the countryside, still receive their medical care through the traditional system. The term 'traditional healers' includes herbalists (general practitioners), herb sellers, bone-setters, psychic healers and traditional birth attendants. Some faith healers – diviners and spiritualists – also use medicinal plants, but not as the primary source of healing.

4.2.5. National Health Expenditure

Out of an estimated total annual health expenditure of 65 billion Naira (US$ 500 million) in the conventional health-care sector, about 50 billion Naira (US$ 385 million), 5 billion Naira (US$ 38.5 million) and 10 billion Naira (US$ 77 million) are allocated to the tertiary, secondary and primary health care levels respectively (8).

There is no information on traditional health sector expenditures. There is very little literature on traditional health practitioners (THPs) although there is plenty on the herbs that they use. The discipline also derives little or no benefit from the formal system. There is hardly any proper documentation of the diseases cured by THPs.

4.3. Structural Indicators

4.3.1. Traditional Medicine Development Programme

The Nigerian National Drug Policy has incorporated a full chapter on traditional medicines (9). Similarly, the draft Nigerian National Pharmacopoeia has a section devoted solely to traditional medicines (10). In taking these steps, the desire of the Government was to maintain and encourage the growth and development of traditional medical practice through coordination and control. To this end, the Government has established a Traditional Medicine Development Unit under the FMH, to coordinate the programme. The unit has prepared documents on the regulation and control of traditional medical practice in Nigeria, and is pursuing appropriate legislation.

The National Agency for Food and Drugs Administration and Control (NAFDAC) is mandated to regulate and guide the use and distribution of herbal medicines to ensure safe use, efficacy and quality. The Agency has completed its work on the criteria for evaluating the quality, safety and efficacy of herbal products used in traditional medicine and their registration, in line with WHO guidelines (11). NAFDAC has already developed guidelines for the registration and listing of herbal medicines and related products (12).

4.3.2. Research and Development

The National Institute for Pharmaceutical Research and Development (NIPRD) was established by the National Science and Technology Act CAP 276 (13) to promote research on traditional remedies so that they can serve as alternatives to modern medicines. NIPRD provides scientific validation and standardization of medicinal plant products used in traditional medicine. A 52-hectare ($520\,000$ m^2) plot was allocated by the federal government to NIPRD for the cultivation and preservation of selected medicinal and aromatic plants. The institute has been involved in the bulk processing and standardization of phytomedicines, as well as maintenance of a full herbarium and ethnobotanical data.

UNDP approved, in 1993, a pilot plant project entitled "Techno-Economic Development of Nigeria's Medicinal and Aromatic Plants for Industrial Utilization". The project, which was funded by UNDP and executed by NIPRD with UNIDO assistance, was aimed at promoting sustainable development and industrial use of medicinal and aromatic plants in Nigeria. The NIPRD Pilot Plant now produces NIPRISAN and NIPRD AM1, which are phyto-drugs developed for the management of sickle cell anaemia and malaria respectively.

Most universities and research institutes involved in the investigation of medicinal plants collaborate with traditional healers in the collection of the plants which they investigate. Many universities are involved, e.g. Obafemi Awolowo University (OAU) Ile-Ife, Ahmadu Bello University, Zaria, the University of Nigeria, Nsukka, and Abubakar Tafawa Balewa University, Bauchi. Work at OAU Ile-Ife on the use of "Fagara" in managing sickle cell anaemia has included characterization of the active ingredients after demonstrating the anti-sickling activity in vivo of the root extracts of *Zanthoxylum zanthoxyloides* (14). Research findings, including standardization work, were published and lead to the listing of the plant in the African Pharmacopoeia (15).

In 1991, the Organization for African Unity's Scientific, Technical and Research Commission (OAU/STRC now AU/STRC) published a report entitled Traditional Medicine and Pharmacopoeia: Contributions to Ethnobotanical and Floristic Studies of South-Western Nigeria (16). This report contains an analysis of medicinal plant use in the Yoruba-speaking parts of Southern Nigeria.

4.3.3. Conservation and Sustainable Use

The National Policy on the Environment (17) is also supportive of the conservation and sustainable use of traditional medicine resources. The Federal Ministry of Environment has undertaken ethnobotanical and ethnomedical studies of parts of Nigeria in conjunction with NIPRD and other agencies. The Ministry developed the first annotated checklist of Nigerian flora (18), and has established and managed national parks, wildlife sanctuaries and other protected areas. Most of the endangered species of medicinal plants are today found in these national parks and reserves. The Forest Research Institute of Nigeria (FRIN), under the Federal Ministry of Agriculture, also carries out the confirmation of the identity of plants at the forest research herbarium in Ibadan, where about 120 000 species are kept, and in this way assists research and development work on medicinal plants and traditional medicine.

4.3.4. Education and Training

Diploma courses in African traditional medicine were proposed, reviewed and approved by Government at the ministerial level in 1999–2000 (*19*). Currently, some courses in traditional medicine are being taught to undergraduate and graduate students of pharmacy and medicine in Nigeria. These come within the context of ethnopharmacology and history of pharmacy. The Nigerian Natural Medicine Development Agency also provides training courses in traditional medicine, and issues certificates in Lagos (*19*).

From a regulatory perspective, the Federal Government has not yet approved the proposed National Traditional Medicine Council. The Council will be vested with authority to regulate the training and accreditation of traditional health practitioners.

4.4. CURR5PTENT PRACTICES

The mode of practice of traditional medicine in Nigeria varies from one community to another. Almost every practitioner prepares his or her own remedies, without reference to any universal protocol or formulated standards. Despite the developments in education and training noted above (see 4.3.4.), there are virtually no accredited formal training institutions. Due to a high level of poverty, many traditional healers employ a low level of technology in the preparation of their products. The medicaments being produced are largely non-standardized in quantity and uncontrolled in quality. This makes some people reluctant to accept the use of the medicines even where there is proof of efficacy.

The mother in the home constitutes the first level of health care in the rural communities and if the patient does not respond to treatment, the traditional healer is contacted. Midwives provide pre- and post-natal care. Free or inexpensive effective herbal treatments exist for infections, anaemia, skin ailments, minor pain, and nutritional disorders, and many more complaints that are mundane rather than life-threatening. Various skin infections of bacterial and fungal origin are cured by *Terminalia avicennoides* (bark). Neem (*Azadirachta indica*), a widespread exotic tree, is used to treat malaria and is an effective insecticide. These and other high-demand plants of traditional medicine, used to fight the day-to-day burden of diseases, are potential candidates for scientific validation.

Presently there are no adequate structures that enable the efficient use of traditional medicines with the necessary regulation and control. In order to ensure that medicinal plant resources are used rationally and that the requirements for their use are assessed as accurately as possible, much research and development work is needed to standardize the nomenclature, collection, extraction, process, formulation procedures, quality, safety, dosage, indications, contraindications, etc. The National Health Policy and National Health Plan (*20*) emphasize the development and facilitation of the use of traditional medicine in Nigeria, and the establishment of a country-specific institutional framework for the practice of traditional medicine. The Government has also realized that there is a need to conserve the plant resources within the overall framework of its policy on the environment, which advocates biodiversity conservation and sustainable utilization of resources through effective management plans and resources inventories, as well as community participation. For instance, medicinal plants have been recognized as a priority area in conservation and sustainable use of biodiversity in Nigeria. This issue was reiterated in Nigeria's contribution at the Fifth Conference of the Parties to the Convention on Biological Diversity through submissions of the G7 countries and China in Nairobi, Kenya, in 2000 (*21*). Therefore, there is great opportunity to develop traditional medicines and practice in Nigeria today.

4.5. DISCUSSION

In view of the dearth of specialist providers coupled with the non-availability of essential medicines within the allopathic sector, traditional medicine has become an indispensable component of health care in Nigeria. For instance, persons living with AIDS often desperately seek herbal treatments with the hope of obtaining cure or relief of symptoms. Traditional medicines that are used empirically need to be evaluated for safety and efficacy in treatment of AIDS and other priority diseases.

At the Special Health Forum held at the Economic Community of West African States Secretariat in Abuja, Nigeria, in 1999, the President of the Federal Republic of Nigeria, Chief Olusegun Obasanjo, directed that the traditional medicine development programme should be incorporated into the national health-care plan of his Government. Since then however, there has not been any significant boost in the necessary recognition and support. Yet traditional medicine is used by the majority of the population in Nigeria. This calls for an immediate review of the current strategies.

One of the greatest challenges facing the management of medicinal plant diversity and traditional medicines in Nigeria is the dearth of comprehensive, adequate and reliable information to inform precise and rational decision-making with respect to policy and implementation in the country. Although a number of policies exist that seek to support the development of traditional medicine, national efforts to put these into effect have been poorly coordinated between implementing bodies. There is, therefore, a significant gap between policy formulation, policy implementation and activities of the scientific community. Furthermore, the present regulatory system gives prominence to Government authorities, with near-total exclusion of the traditional healers themselves. The direct involvement of all stakeholders in traditional medicine regulation will give it greater legitimacy and acceptance by society as a whole.

The vital role that traditional medicine practice plays in the health sector has often been overlooked by economists and planners, especially in the extent to which its use provides a buffer against poverty and offers opportunities for self-employment in the informal sector. Most of the herbs used in Nigerian traditional medicine are collected from the wild and used unsustainably. High population growth rates and poverty, coupled with dwindling economic resources in the country, lead the people to access these cheap resources for their immediate needs. As the population increases, the demand for traditional medicine will increase, and pressure on the supply will become greater than ever. There is hardly any 'warning system' that will allow introduction of appropriate measures to regulate, protect and restore natural resources. As some of the medicinal plants used in traditional medicine become articles of global commerce, their collection from the wild becomes an intense informal activity, and a major threat to biodiversity and traditional medicine practice in Nigeria.

Traditional medical practice also needs urgent attention in the areas of mass education, training and awareness-building. Practitioners need appropriate information on the sustainable use of medicinal plants and alternative ways of earning their living. There is a need to harmonize national activities around environmental protection, sustainable use and conservation of natural resources, especially of medicinal plants, so as to develop new economic opportunities. The crucial issues to be addressed at the moment are:

- the threat to indigenous knowledge of traditional medicine, which forms an important part of the cultural heritage of local communities, and may be lost;
- the continued loss of medicinal plant species and habitats through deforestation, land conversion and overexploitation;
- the lack of reliable quantitative data on volumes of plant material harvested and used locally and nationally, and their value to national economies;
- the lack of proper coordination and involvement of all stakeholders.

There is an urgent need to sensitize the public, especially rural communities, about the availability and benefits of traditional health therapies and cost-effective means of delivering them. There is also a need to encourage government and donor agencies to support scientific validation of the safety and efficacy of herbal medicines, and promote their rational use; and to caution that the loss of the medicinal plant resource base and biodiversity will have negative long-term impacts for the poor and for humanity as a whole.

4.6. CONCLUSIONS AND SUMMARY

The Government should support and promote professionalism among traditional health practitioners themselves by approving the Council for Traditional Medicine Practitioners, similar to other existing professional regulatory bodies. Once the Council is approved, it will control practice through professional licensing and discipline, and Nigeria is likely to witness a dramatic improvement in traditional medicine and health care, especially at the grass roots.

There is a need to foster effective collaboration between allopathic and traditional health practitioners. There is also a need to strengthen technical expertise and to foster close collaboration between appropriate ministries, research institutes, communities and traditional health practitioners associations. Novel intellectual property rights and benefit-sharing arrangements, need to be developed at national level, bearing in mind the cultural and traditional norms of the local communities, so that the producing communities can benefit from medicinal plants and in this way contribute to their conservation.

There is a need for an information network on traditional medicines, to ensure exchange of information and monitoring of emerging trends through data collection and analysis. This will also assist in information-sharing, education and awareness-building. A national database on traditional medicines should be developed and the on-going Herbal Pharmacopoeia concluded. The Government should be encouraged to support, with adequate funding, actions that validate the safety and efficacy of herbal medicines scientifically and promote their rational use.

References

1. Federal Government of Nigeria. *National biodiversity strategy and action plan*. Abuja, Government Press, 2002:2–7.

2. Federal Ministry of Science and Technology, Federal Republic of Nigeria. *Report of the National Investigative Committee on Traditional and Alternative Medicine*. Abuja, Government Press, 1985.

3. Holmstedt B. The ordeal bean of Old Calabar: *the pageant of Physostigma venenosum in medicine*. In: Swain T, ed. *Plants in the development of modern medicine*. Cambridge, Harvard University Press, 1972:303–360.

4. Federal Government of Nigeria. *National assessment report on sustainable development in Nigeria: ten years after Rio (UNCED) World Summit on Sustainable Development*. Abuja, Government Press, 2002.

5. *The World Health Report 2003: Shaping the future*. Geneva, World Health Organization, 2003.

6. *The official summary of the state of the world's children*. New York, UNICEF, 2003.

7. Federal Ministry of Health, Federal Republic of Nigeria. *Report of the Department of Planning Research and Statistics*. Abuja, Government Press, 2003.

8. Federal Ministry of Health, Federal Republic of Nigeria. *Report of the Traditional Medicine Development Programme Unit, 2003*. Abuja, Government Press, 2003.

9. Federal Ministry of Health, Federal Republic of Nigeria. *Revised National Drug Policy*. Abuja, Government Press, 2003.

10. Federal Ministry of Health, Federal Republic of Nigeria. *Report of the Pharmacopoeia Development Committee*. Abuja, Government Press, 2003.

11. *Guidelines on the quality control of herbal drugs*. Geneva, World Health Organization, 1991.

12. National Agency for Food and Drug Administration and Control (NAFDAC). *Guidelines for the regulation and listing of herbal medicines and related products*. Abuja, Government Press, 2002.

13. Federal Republic of Nigeria. *National Science and Technology Act CAP 276*. Federal Government Press, Lagos, 1987:11059–11062.

14. Sofowora EA, Isaac-Sodeye WA, Ogunkoya LO. Isolation and characterisation of an anti-sickling agent from *Fagara zanthoxyloides*. *Lloydia*. 1971, 34:33.

15. Organization of African Unity, Scientific Technical and Research Commission. *African pharmacopoeia*. Vols. I & II Lagos, 1985.

16. Ajanohoun E., Ahyi MRA, Ake-Assi L, Dramane K, Elewude JA, Fadoju, SO, Gbile ZO, Goudote E, Johnson CLA, Keita A, Morakinyo O, Ojewole JAO, Olatunji OA and Sofowora A. *Contribution to Ethnobotanic and Floristic Studies in Western Nigeria*. OAU/STRC, Lagos, Nigeria, 1991.

17. Federal Ministry of Environment, Federal Republic of Nigeria. *National policy on the environment*. Abuja, Government Press, 2003.

18. Federal Ministry of Environment, Federal Republic of Nigeria. *Annotated checklist of Nigerian flora*. Abuja, Government Press, 1999.

19. Federal Ministry of Science and Technology, Federal Republic of Nigeria. *Report of the Presidential Policy Advisory Committee*. Lagos, Government Press, 1999.

20. Federal Ministry of Health, Federal Republic of Nigeria. *Report of the Traditional Medicine Development Programme Unit, 2000*. Abuja, Government Press, 2000.

21. *Fifth Conference of the Parties to the Convention on Biological Diversity*. Nairobi, WIPO/UNEP, 2000 (UNEP/CBD/COP/5/INF/26).

CHAPTER 5

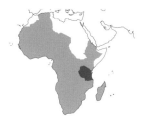

UNITED REPUBLIC OF TANZANIA

R. L. A. Mahunnah[1],
F. C. Uiso[2],
A. Y. Kitua[3],
Z. H. Mbwambo[4],
M. J. Moshi[5],
P. Mhame[6]
and S. Mnaliwa[7]

[1] Associate Research Professor, Institute of Traditional Medicine, Muhimbili University College of Health Sciences, University of Dar es Salaam, P.O. Box 65001, Dar es Salaam, United Republic of Tanzania. E-mail: mahunnah@yahoo.co.uk

[2] Senior Research Fellow, Institute of Traditional Medicine, Muhimbili University College of Health Sciences, University of Dar es Salaam, P.O. Box 65001, Dar es Salaam, United Republic of Tanzania. E-mail: fcuiso@muchs.ac.tz

[3] Director General, National Institute for Medical Research, P.O. Box 9653, Ocean Road, Dar es Salaam, United Republic of Tanzania. E-mail: akitua@nimr.or.tz

[4] Senior Research Fellow, Institute of Traditional Medicine, Muhimbili University College of Health Sciences, University of Dar es Salaam, P.O. Box 65001
Dar es Salaam, United Republic of Tanzania. E-mail: zmbwambo@muchs.ac.tz

[5] Director, Institute of Traditional Medicine, Muhimbili University College of Health Sciences, University of Dar es Salaam, P.O. Box 65001, Dar es Salaam, United Republic of Tanzania. E-mail: mmoshi@muchs.ac.tz

[6] Medical Officer, National Institute for Medical Research, P.O. Box 9653, Ocean Road, Dar es Salaam, United Republic of Tanzania. E-mail: pmhame@yahoo.com

[7] Medical Officer, Traditional Medicine Section, Ministry of Health, P.O. Box 9083, Dar es Salaam, United Republic of Tanzania. E-mail: smnaliwa@moh.go.tz

5.1. INTRODUCTION

The United Republic of Tanzania has a land area of 939 400 km[2] and over 120 ethnic groups (*1*). The history of the practice of traditional medicine (TRM) in the United Republic of Tanzania goes back far beyond the establishment of allopathic health-care systems. In pre-colonial Tanzania (Tanganyika), traditional healers, who are sometimes also referred to as traditional health practitioners or traditional medical or medicine practitioners (*2*), had a wider range of control over the social conditions of health. During the colonial period of the 1890s to 1961, the authority of the pre-colonial healers and the practice of TRM were much suppressed, and in 1929 the restrictive Witchcraft Ordinance was introduced. In the same year, the Medical Practitioners and Dentists Ordinance was introduced, which carried a provision for the practice of TRM by traditional healers in their localities (*3*).

After independence in 1961, there was more tolerance and promotion of TRM practice. The Ministry of Health issued a new Medical Practitioners and Dentists Ordinance in 1968, which recognized the right of traditional healers to exist and operate. In 1996, traditional healers and birth attendants formed a national association known as the Tanzania Traditional Health Practitioners' Association. The Tanzanian Government has demonstrated politically its commitment to TRM, and the Health Policy of the United Republic of Tanzania (*4*) recognizes TRM, together with alternative systems of healing, as a complementary health system to allopathic health care. The political will of the Government has been further demonstrated by the legislation passed by Parliament in 2002 to establish the United Republic of Tanzania Traditional and Alternative Medicine Act (*5*), which includes the practices of traditional birth attendants.

In addition to this national commitment, the United Republic of Tanzania also subscribes to the Lusaka declaration of the African Union Heads of State, on the designation of the period 2001–2010 as the Decade for African Traditional Medicine and to its plan of action for implementation adopted by the Ministers of Health Conference held in Tripoli, Libyan Arab Jamahiriya, in April 2003. The plan of action and mechanisms for its implementation were endorsed by the African Union Summit of Heads of State and Governments, which took place in July 2003 in Maputo, Mozambique (*6*) (see also Chapter 1).

Today, traditional societies in the United Republic of Tanzania, as in many parts of Africa, attach great importance to traditional systems of medicine in spite of the rapid advance of allopathic health care. This is largely because such traditional systems are holistic in approach, and is integrated in the particular socio-cultural and religious views of the people (*7*). Approximately 60% of the urban population and over 80% of the rural population in the United Republic of Tanzania uses TRM for day-to-day health care, most of which (90%) is plant-based (*8, 9*). The United Republic of Tanzania has perhaps the richest flora in tropical Africa, estimated at about 12 667 plant species of which 1122 are endemic (*1*). Current research shows that about 1000 plant species are utilized in traditional medicine practices, representing about 10% of the country's flora (*9*).

5.2. Background Indicators

The total population of the country is 34 569 232 and the annual population growth rate is 2.9% (*10*). The life expectancy at birth of the total population is 46.5 years (*11*). The ten most common causes of morbidity and mortality include malaria (acute febrile illness), HIV/AIDS, tuberculosis, pneumonia, diarrhoeal diseases, cerebrovascular disease (stroke) and hypertension, diabetes, asthma, epilepsy, liver disease and cancer (*12*). Mortality rates, in general, are considered to be lower in urban than in rural areas (*12*). Reasons may include easier access to health services, higher incomes and a more educated population. However, differentials in mortality are also likely to exist within urban areas.

The total number of allopathic physicians is 378 (*13*). There are no TRM providers or complementary/alternative medicine providers within the official health-care system. The practice of traditional and complementary/alternative medicine (TCAM) is still outside the formal health sector, but the recently established legislation (*5*) encourages close collaboration between the two health systems. Today, there are about 75 000 traditional health practitioners in the country (*14*).

5.3. Structural Indicators

5.3.1 Policy and Legislation

Efforts to promote TRM in the provision of primary health care were initiated in 1985 through the WHO Safe Motherhood Programme. This Programme established a system using the services of traditional birth attendants to refer patients to allopathic health care services for complicated deliveries.

The National Health Policy of 1996 recognizes the practice of TRM in the country, but the practice of complementary/alternative medicine is not officially recognized. A Traditional Medicine Unit exists within the Ministry of Health, and this Unit, together with the Institute of Traditional Medicine (ITM) and the National Institute for Medical Research (NIMR), is involved in policy regulation issues. These institutions are the bodies responsible for coordination of TRM research, development and practice, and they act as a national expert team for TCAM. A national voluntary, self-regulatory body for TCAM does not exist formally in the country, but a National Traditional Health Practitioners' Association was established in 1996 (see above) and this regulates registered traditional health practitioners. The country has recently passed legislation on Traditional Medicine and Alternative Medicine Practice (*5*). This legislation establishes a Traditional Health Practitioners' Council which regulates the registration of practitioners and their herbal medicines and TCAM practice through Standing Committees, which include Professional Conduct, Academic and Research and Development Committees. According to the policy and recently enacted legislation, only registered traditional health practitioners and practitioners of alternative systems of healing are allowed to provide TCAM services.

5.3.2. Research

The ITM is the national institution conducting research and development activities on TRM. It was established by the Government in 1974 as a Unit, and elevated to the status of Institute in 1991 (*15*).

Some TRM research is also carried out by the Chemistry Department of the University of Dar es Salaam, and by NIMR. The management and conservation of medicinal plants, both in situ and ex situ, is carried out by ITM in close collaboration with other stakeholders, such as forestry institutions.

5.3.3. Education, Training and Information

There are currently no formal TCAM education programmes or training curricula for medical students. The recent legislation (5) has provisions for such training for both allopathic health-care providers and TCAM practitioners. The training will be introduced when the necessary mechanisms are in place. Short exposure courses for medical, pharmacy, dental and nursing undergraduate students are in place at the Muhimbili University College of Health Sciences, Dar es Salaam (E.J. Kayombo, personal communication, 2003). Also, at the Regional Dermatology Training Centre of the Tumaini University of Health Sciences and Kilimanjaro Christian Medical Centre in Moshi, paramedical students are taught short courses in preparation of traditional medicines and appropriate partnerships with traditional health practitioners (G. Burford, personal communication, 2003). There are no formal information and advisory services relating to TCAM, but these are foreseen in the current legislation.

5.3.4. Financing systems

There is no financing system that contributes to the provision of TCAM, but this is incorporated in the current policy and legislation and is likely to be introduced in the future.

5.3.5 User surveys

A study conducted in two regions of the United Republic of Tanzania on illness patterns and utilization of available health services, including TRM, showed a 73.5% utilization of allopathic health care (3). Otherwise, there has been no TCAM user survey conducted in the country in the past twenty years.

5.4. Process Indicators

TRM is used throughout Tanzania for primary health-care needs including the management and treatment of infectious and degenerative diseases. TRM does not incorporate the use of manual therapy, chiropractic, homeopathy and yoga, although these practices are known to exist in the country.

The diseases and conditions that determine the use of TRM are mostly those with high morbidity and mortality as indicated above (see section 5.2 above). Patients tend to be satisfied with traditional medicine therapy and services because they are natural, affordable and accessible, and grounded in the socio-cultural setting of the society. Traditional health practitioners are trusted by their patients, which have an important psychological effect on the outcome of TCAM treatments. Usually the outcome of the treatment is good, in spite of the fact that in some cases patients resort to TCAM treatment when their disease or condition is quite advanced and difficult to treat. Hence, the legal framework (under preparation) advocates and re-emphasizes the importance of a referral system between TCAM and allopathic health care.

TRM is embedded in culture, and is used by all socio-demographic categories of consumers. Consumers and patients who use TCAM still pay for all treatments out-of-pocket, and there is no national health insurance scheme for the beneficiaries of TCAM. Similarly, national insurance schemes for allopathic health care in the United Republic of Tanzania are in the early stages of development, and medical bills for conventional treatment are also paid out-of-pocket. This is largely because medical care in the country was provided free for a long time after independence, and a cost-sharing programme was introduced only recently. There is no national budget for TCAM, and hence total expenditures on TCAM are not known.

5.5. Discussion

In the United Republic of Tanzania TCAM is in transition, and in the future a shift may be expected from the present tolerant situation to a parallel or dual health-care model (e.g. India; see Chapter 12) where both allopathic health care and TRM are separate components of one national health system or to an integrated model (e.g. China; see Chapter 26) where allopathic health care and TRM are integrated both in medical education and medical practice. The recent law encourages close collaboration between allopathic and TCAM practices. Hence a situation is foreseen whereby TCAM providers will play an active role in the allopathic health-care system, and an even greater role outside this system. The legal framework on TCAM practice currently in preparation will ensure improved standards for traditional health clinics and other workplaces; adherence to codes of ethics; education and training; standardization of medicines and therapies; and the sustainability of materia medica, traditional medical knowledge and intellectual property rights.

There are ongoing efforts to develop a legal framework for a public financing mechanism for the TCAM sector, similar to that of the allopathic sector.

Improved knowledge is potentially of great value for health policy, allocation of resources and formulation of intervention strategies. The number of prescribers is likely to increase with the expansion of medical universities and increased student enrolment at the Muhimbili University College of Health Sciences, where student intake has increased two- to three-fold in the past few years.

5.6. CONCLUSIONS AND SUMMARY

TRM practice in Africa, and in the United Republic of Tanzania in particular, is in transition from the informal to the formal sector. The country is taking positive steps in this direction through the enactment of enabling legislation and the development of appropriate legal frameworks. Organizational arrangements of the Tanzania Traditional and Alternative Medicine Council are in their final stages. This multidisciplinary national body, with relevant committees on academia, professional conduct, and research and development, is spearheading the promotion of TCAM practice in the country. It will be responsive to the key issues in the national policy, including: formulation of a legal framework and the development of norms and standards for the practice of traditional medicine; development of education and training, as well as continuing education programmes; compilation of a code of ethics for traditional healers; development of mechanisms for the official recognition of TCAM; capacity building; research promotion to improve safety, efficacy and quality of medicines; rational use of TCAM; development of local capacity to produce plant-based medicines; cultivation and sustainable conservation of medicinal plants and other materia medica; and protection of traditional medical knowledge and intellectual property rights.

Towards these ends, the WHO Regional Office for Africa has prepared appropriate guidelines on various subjects including policy formulation and plans, legal framework and a code of ethics, education and training, and registration of traditional medicines, protection of traditional medical knowledge and intellectual property rights. It has also produced protocols on research methodologies for evaluation of traditional medicines used for the treatment of priority diseases, aimed at assisting Member States to institutionalize traditional medicine in their national health-care systems (16). The United Republic of Tanzania, as a member of the African Union (formerly the Organization of African Unity), subscribes to the African Union Model Law on the Protection of Local Communities, Farmers and Breeders, and to the Regulation of Access to Biological Resources (17). This relates to the regulation of access to medicinal plant resources, traditional medical knowledge and intellectual property rights and is in harmony with other global bodies like WTO, WIPO and international conventions such as the Convention on Biological Diversity and the Agreement on Trade-Related Aspects of Intellectual Property Rights.

References

1. *Tanzania country study on biological diversity.* Nairobi, United Nations Environment Programme, 1998.

2. *Promoting the role of traditional medicine in health systems: a strategy for the African region.* Brazzaville, World Health Organization Regional Office for Africa, 2001 (AFR/RC50/9).

3. Kilewo JZJ, et al. Traditional medicine practice in Tanzania: history and developments. *Tanzania Medical Journal.* 1987, Special Issue 25:7–10.

4. *National Health Care Policy.* Dar es Salaam, Ministry of Health, United Republic of Tanzania, 1996.

5. *The Traditional and Alternative Medicine Act No. 23 of 2002, United Republic of Tanzania.* Dar es Salaam, Government Printer, 2002.

6. Sambo LG. Integration of traditional medicine into health systems in the African Region – The journey so far. *African Health Monitor.* WHO Regional Office for Africa, 2003, 4: 8–11.

7. Chabra SC. Plants used in traditional medicine in Eastern Tanzania – 1: Pteridophytes and Angiosperms (Acanthaceae to Canellaceae). *Journal of Ethnopharmacology.* 1987, 21:253–277.

8. Mahunnah RLA. Intellectual property rights and biodiversity of medicinal plants and food crops in Tanzania. In: Mshana RN, Ndoye M, Ekpere JA, eds. *Proceedings of the First OAU/STRC/DEPA/KIPO Workshop on Medicinal Plants and Herbal Medicine in Africa: Policy Issues on Ownership, Access and Utilization, Nairobi, Kenya, 14–17 April 1997.* Lagos, Organization of African Unity, 1998:86–92.

9. Mahunnah RLA. Ethnobotany and conservation of medicinal plants in Africa: the way forward in the next decade. In: Adeniji, ed. *Proceedings of the Fifteenth Meeting of the Inter-African Experts Committee on African Traditional Medicine and Medicinal Plants, Arusha, Tanzania, 15–17 January 2002.* Lagos, Organization of African Unity, 2002:70–80.

10. *National Census.* Bureau of Statistics United Republic of Tanzania. Calverton, Maryland, Macro International Inc., 2002.

11. *WHO Strategy on Traditional Medicine 2002–2005.* Geneva, World Health Organization, 2002.

12. *Policy implications of adult morbidity and mortality.* Dar es Salaam, Ministry of Health, United Republic of Tanzania, 1997:324.

13. *Health statistics abstract, Vol. 2: inventory statistics.* Dar es Salaam, Ministry of Health, United Republic of Tanzania, 1999:173.

14. *The history of healthcare in Tanzania: an exhibition on the development of the health sector in more than 100 years.* National Museums of Tanzania. Dar es Salaam, Tanzania Printers Ltd., 2001.

15. *The Muhimbili University College of Health Sciences Act of Parliament No. 9 of 1991.* Dar es Salaam, United Republic of Tanzania, 1991.

16. World Health Organization Regional Office for Africa. Situation analysis of traditional medicine in the WHO African Region. In: *Proceedings of the International Meeting on the Global Atlas of Traditional Medicine,* 17–19 June 2003, World Health Organization Centre for Health Development, Kobe, Japan, 2004.

17. Ekpere JA. *The OAU's Model Law: the protection of the local communities, farmers and breeders, and for the regulation of access to biological resources – An explanatory booklet.* Lagos, Organization of African Unity, Scientific, Technical and Research Commission, 2000.

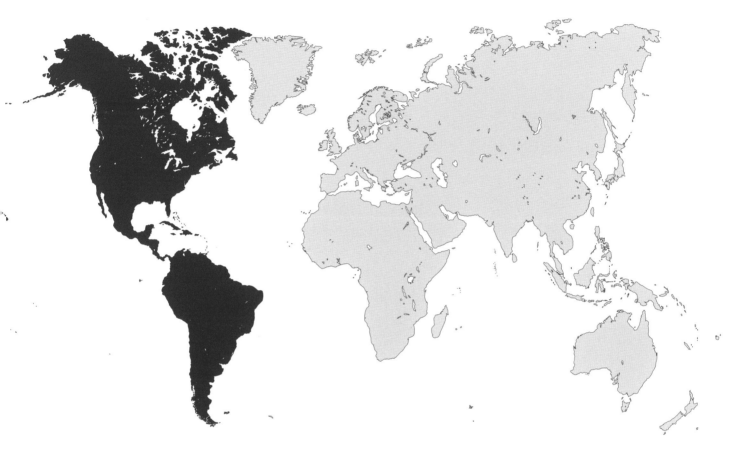

WHO REGION OF THE AMERICAS

REGIONAL OVERVIEW AND
SELECTED COUNTRY CHAPTERS

CHAPTER 6

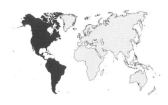

REGIONAL OVERVIEW: REGION OF THE AMERICAS

Mahabir P. Gupta

Research Professor of Pharmacognosy, and International Coordinator, CYTED, Centre of Pharmacognostic Research on Panamanian Flora, College of Pharmacy, University of Panama, Estafeta Universitaria, Apartado 10767 Panama City, Panama.
Email: cytedqff@ancon.up.ac.pa

6.1. INTRODUCTION

There are 48 countries in the Americas, with a total population of over 850 million inhabitants (*1, 2*) of multicultural and multilingual backgrounds. However, this paper reviews only the 35 Member States and one Associate Member (Puerto Rico) of WHO included in the WHO Region of the Americas (AMR). AMR has a high percentage of native indigenous populations, who rely heavily on traditional medicine and a broad range of practices and traditions are found across the Region (*3*). The countries in which over 40% of the total population is indigenous are Bolivia, Ecuador, Guatemala and Peru, and those in which 5–20% of the total population is indigenous are Belize, Chile, El Salvador, Guyana, Honduras, Mexico, Nicaragua, Panama and Suriname. Brazil, the United States of America, Uruguay and Venezuela have less than 5% (*4*).

In Latin America, traditional medicine is practised mainly among Indian tribal groups, rural peoples and lower-income urban groups. Folk healers such as herbalists, masseurs, bonesetters and spiritualists co-exist with, and in many cases replace, allopathic health-care professionals. The services of traditional midwives (partera empirica or comadrona) are mostly used by indigenous peoples of Indian tribal groups throughout Latin American countries. At this time, the overall use of traditional, complementary and alternative medicine (TCAM) in the Americas is steadily increasing.

The Pan American Health Organization (PAHO) has recognized the importance of collecting information on the customs and beliefs of the American peoples regarding illness and traditional therapeutic methods. PAHO has organized a number of regional consultations on the status of TCAM and the health of indigenous peoples of the Americas, and has produced a series of publications.

6.2. SUMMARY OF INFORMATION ON BACKGROUND INDICATORS

A survey of background indicators in AMR reveals that at the conclusion of the "Health for All by 2000" initiative, the countries had, on average, achieved many of the objectives.

The average mortality rate in the Region has fallen from 9.1 per 1000 inhabitants in the 1980s to 6.9 per 1000 at the end of the 1990s. The main causes of mortality in AMR are cardiovascular diseases, communicable diseases, neoplasm, diabetes, respiratory and urinary tract infections, traffic accidents, septicaemia and AIDS. The lowest infant mortality rates are in Cuba and Uruguay. Data on the principal causes of morbidity are not available for all AMR countries. However, in general, the main causes of morbidity are malaria, malnutrition, dengue, diarrhoea, acute respiratory infections, tuberculosis, high-risk pregnancy and AIDS (*1, 2*).

Table 6.1 shows the total number of prescribers in the countries of AMR. The number of doctors per 10 000 inhabitants has shown a significant increase during recent years, from 13.1 in 1980 to 19.8 in 1999. This indicator varies greatly between countries from a minimum of 1.8 in Guyana to a maximum of 58.2 in Cuba.

With the exception of a few countries, no information is available on the total number of TCAM providers within and outside the allopathic health-care system. For example, in Bolivia, the Bolivian Society of Traditional Medicine estimates that there are 1600 TCAM providers; and in Nicaragua, there are an estimated 2500. In the United States, there are more than 12 000 licensed acupuncturists (see Chapter 9). However, various providers of CAM therapies, such as chiropractors, acupuncturists, bonesetters, naturopaths, masseurs, aromatherapists, magnetotherapists, and homeopaths, practise widely throughout AMR. The numbers of other health-care providers are not available.

Table 6.1. Summary of background indicators on health-care providers

Country	Doctors per 10 000 population	Total no. of doctors	Nurses per 10 000 population	Total no. of nurses	Dentists per 10 000 population	Total no. of dentists
Antigua and Barbuda	11.5	75	32.2	209	2.2	14
Argentina	26.8	11 540	5.3	22 387	7.9	29 976
Bahamas	16.3	507	23.4	730	2.9	90
Barbados	13.7	368	51.2	1 377	1.9	51
Belize	7.4	175	13.2	311	1.1	26
Bolivia	3.2	2 786	1.6	1 393	0.4	248
Brazil	14.4	244 588	4.5	78 618	9.4	115 306
Canada	22.9	71 604	89.7	280 474	5.9	18 448
Chile	13.0	20 266	10.0	15 589	4.2	6 547
Colombia	9.3	40 450	4.3	18 703	5.7	24 792
Costa Rica	15.0	6 300	11.3	4 746	4.0	1 680
Cuba	58.2	65 609	17.4	19 615	8.9	10 033
Dominica	4.9	34.3	41.6	291.2	0.6	4.2
Dominican Republic	19	16 414	3.0	2 592	NA	NA
Ecuador	13.2	17 308	4.6	6 031	1.6	2 098
El Salvador	11.8	7 694	4.2	2 788	4.0	2 608
Grenada	8.1	72	19.5	173	1.1	10
Guatemala	9.0	10 795	3.5	4 198	1.6	1 919
Guyana	1.8	138	8.4	643	0.4	31
Haiti	2.5	2 100	1.1	924	0.1	84
Honduras	8.3	5 588	3.3	2 222	2.2	1 481
Jamaica	2.5	655	11.3	2 962	0.2	52
Mexico	15.6	158 873	10.8	109 989	1.0	10 184
Nicaragua	6.2	3 315	3.3	1 764	0.6	321
Panama	12.1	3 560	10.8	3 177	2.6	765
Paraguay	4.9	2 831	1.2	693	0.7	404
Peru	10.3	27 319	6.7	17 770	1.1	2 917
Puerto Rico	17.5	6 979	42.5	16 949	2.5	997
Saint Kitts and Nevis	11.7	46	49.8	194	2.0	8
Saint Lucia	5.8	88	22.6	341	0.9	14
Saint Vincent and the Grenadines	8.8	102	23.9	277	0.5	6
Suriname	5.0	210	22.8	960	0.8	34
Trinidad and Tobago	7.5	979	28.7	3 748	1.1	144
Uruguay	37.0	1 252	7.0	2 369	12.6	1 794
USA	27.9	804 999	97.2	2 804 512	6.0	173 118
Venezuela	19.7	49 433	7.9	19 823	5.3	13 299

The figures for total expenditure for allopathic health care are available but not those by sector (i.e. primary, secondary, tertiary). Table 6.2 shows the total health-care expenditure of each country, both in public and private sectors. There is a great disparity between countries. Public sector expenditure varies from 1.4% of gross national product in Guatemala to 6.9% in Costa Rica. The countries that are in the upper 25% in expenditure are Argentina, Barbados, Canada, Chile, Colombia, Costa Rica, Cuba, Nicaragua, Panama and the United States. The private sector expenditure is highest in the United States (7.1% of gross national product) and lowest in Guyana. No figures are available for the total expenditure on TCAM therapies. However, it is clearly on the increase. In the United States and Canada, it was estimated at US$ 27 billion and US$ 2.4 billion, respectively (see Chapters 8 and 9).

Table 6.2. Summary of background indicators on expenditure

Country	Public expenditure as % of GNP	Total public expenditure (US$ millions)	Private expenditure as % of GNP	Total private expenditure (US$ millions)
Antigua and Barbuda	3.4	24	2.1	14.4
Argentina	4.1	16 914	5.9	24 644.60
Bahamas	3.3	150	1.8	82.4
Barbados	4.4	173	2.2	88.7
Belize	2.5	30	2.3	28.8
Bolivia	3.2	601	1.7	315.8
Brazil	3.4	40 258	5	59 384
Canada	6.6	56 156	2.7	22 936.80
Chile	4.4	5 730	2.4	3 164.40
Colombia	5.1	11 459	4.2	9 433.30
Costa Rica	6.9	2 269	2.2	735.5
Cuba	5.5	2 728	1.2	578.4
Dominica	3.9	14	2	7.3
Dominican Republic	1.9	949	4.6	2 326.40
Ecuador	2	652	2	625.6
El Salvador	3.3	906	4.9	1 342.90
Grenada	3.2	21	2.4	15.6
Guatemala	1.4	601	4	1 673
Guyana	3.7	111	0.9	26.7
Haiti	2.5	296	3.4	410
Honduras	2.7	377	4.5	645.5
Jamaica	2.7	231	2.7	231.6
Mexico	2.5	21 607	2.8	24 181.30
Nicaragua	5.5	610	3.7	413.1
Panama	5.4	857	1.9	299.3
Paraguay	2.6	616	4.5	1 058.20
Peru	2.5	2 918	1.9	2 186.10
Puerto Rico	NA	NA	NA	NA
Saint Kitts and Nevis	3.1	13	2.1	8.7
Saint Lucia	2.6	21	2.2	17.9
Saint Vincent and the Grenadines	4.3	25	1.9	11.6
Suriname	3	49	2.8	43.8
Trinidad and Tobago	2.2	242	2.3	257.1
Uruguay	4.8	1331	5.5	1 532.70
USA	5.9	547 370	7.1	66 020.40
Venezuela	2.4	2915	4.7	5 809.60

GNP, gross national product; NA, not available

6.3. Summary of Information on Structural Indicators

Data on structural and process indicators for countries in AMR are summarized in Tables 6.3 and 6.4. However, no information is available for the following countries: Antigua and Barbuda, Bahamas, Barbados, Belize, Dominica, El Salvador, Grenada, Guyana, Haiti, Paraguay, Puerto Rico, Saint Kitts and Nevis, Saint Lucia, Saint Vincent and the Grenadines, Trinidad and Tobago and Uruguay. In addition, almost no information is available on process indicators.

6.3.1. TCAM Legislation and Regulation

A legal framework for TCAM exists only in Bolivia, Canada, Cuba, Guatemala, Honduras and Peru. Some countries, such as Chile, Dominican Republic, Ecuador, Honduras, Mexico and Nicaragua, are in the process of formulating national policies. Many countries have Ministerial Resolutions that control TCAM therapies such as homeopathy, naturopathy, chiropractic and acupuncture. The practice of acupuncture is legal in the United States. A national management or coordinating body for TCAM exists in each of the following countries: Bolivia, Chile, Costa Rica, Cuba, Guatemala, Honduras, Mexico, Panama, Suriname and the United States.

Fifteen countries have TCAM units or departments within their Ministries of Health, indicating that the majority of the countries give high importance to the topic of TCAM.

The countries of AMR have made great advances towards regulation of herbal medicinal products. Legal documents have been passed in Argentina, Bolivia, Brazil, Chile, Canada, Colombia, Costa Rica, Cuba, Ecuador, Guatemala, Honduras, Mexico, Nicaragua, Peru, Panama, the United States and Venezuela. In addition to the WHO publication (5) on the legal status of TCAM, the Iberoamerican Programme on Science and Technology for Development (Programa Iberoamericano de Ciencia y Tecnologia para el Desarrollo; CYTED) has published an updated book, compiling the existing legislation for the regulation of herbal products in Latin American countries.

6.3.2. Professional Associations

All countries of AMR, except the Dominican Republic and Suriname, have associations of practitioners of homeopathy, acupuncture and herbalists.

6.3.3. Integration into National Health Systems

No reliable information is available on whether TCAM is practised at all levels including public hospitals. Likewise there is no specific information on integration of TCAM into national health systems; general information from Cuba, Canada, Peru, Suriname and the United States, shows that TCAM is practised to some extent in some clinics and/or hospitals.

None of the countries of Latin America have provisions for health insurance coverage for TCAM treatment and products. There is partial health insurance coverage for TCAM products and therapies in Canada and the United States. Only Cuba and the United States (National Center for Complementary and Alternative Medicine, NCCAM; see Chapter 9) allocate a national budget for TCAM.

6.3.4. Education and Research

In relation to formal TCAM courses at national universities, only Argentina (see Chapter 7) and Cuba offer such programmes. In Canada and the United States, some universities offer continuing medical education and elective courses in different TCAM therapies, such as acupuncture and traditional Chinese medicine (see Chapters 8 and 9). Various TCAM associations and societies in many countries offer informal courses.

All countries, except Honduras, have ongoing research programmes on medicinal plants and natural products. Two important regional initiatives are CYTED in Fine Pharmaceutical Chemistry for natural product drug discovery in 21 countries, and the Traditional Medicine in the Islands (TRAMIL) Programme, which fosters the use of scientifically validated medicinal plants for primary health care.

Table 6.3. Summary of structural indicators

Country	National policy on TCAM	TCAM unit or department within MOH	Regulation of TCAM or herbal products or of both	TCAM practice & integration[a]	Health insurance coverage for treatment and products	TCAM research institute at national or university level	Official education at university level[b]
Argentina	Yes	No	Herbal products	No	No	Yes	No
Bolivia	Yes	Yes	Both	No	No	Yes	No
Brazil	No	Yes	Herbal products	No	No	Yes	No
Canada	Yes	Yes	Herbal products	Yes, in some state hospitals	Partial	Yes	No
Chile	Not explicit	Yes	Both	No	No	Yes	No
Colombia	No	Yes	Herbal products	No	No	Yes	No
Costa Rica	Yes	Yes	Both	No	No	Yes	No
Cuba	Yes	Yes	Both	Yes	Not applicable	Yes	Yes
Dominican Republic	No	No	Herbal products	No	No	Yes	No
Ecuador	No	Yes	Herbal products	No	No	Yes	No
Guatemala	Yes	Yes	Both	Yes, in some hospitals	No	Yes	No
Honduras	No	Yes	Herbal products	No	No	No	No
Jamaica	No	No	Herbal products	No	No	Yes	No
Mexico	No	Yes	Herbal products	Yes, in some hospitals	No	Yes	No
Nicaragua	No	Yes	Herbal products	Yes, in some hospitals	No	Yes	No
Panama	No	Yes	Herbal products	Yes, in some clinics	No	Yes	No
Peru	No	Yes	Herbal products	Yes, in some hospitals	No	Yes	No
Suriname	No	Yes	Herbal products	Yes, in some clinics	No	Yes	No
USA	No	No	Both	Yes, in some state hospitals	Partial	Yes, in some State Universities	Yes
Venezuela	No	No	Herbal products	No	No	Yes	No

[a]TCAM practised at all levels including public hospital; TCAM integrated into national health systems

[b]Official education at university level covering both TRM and CAM for doctors, pharmacists and nurses

Table 6.4. Summary of indicators on structure, budget, and training in TCAM

Country*	A legal framework for TRM	A national management or coordination body	Association(s) of traditional practitioners	National budget allocation for TRM
Argentina	No	No	Yes	No
Bolivia	Yes	Yes	Yes	No
Brazil	No	No	Yes	No
Canada	Yes	No	Yes	No
Chile	No	Yes	Yes	No
Colombia	No	Yes	Yes	No
Costa Rica	No	Yes	Yes	No
Cuba	Yes	Yes	Yes	Yes
Dominican Republic	No	No	No	No
Ecuador	No	No	Yes	No
Guatemala	Yes	Yes	Yes	No
Honduras	Yes	Yes	Yes	No
Jamaica	No	NA	NA	No
Mexico	No	No	Yes	No
Nicaragua	No	No	Yes	No
Panama	No	Yes	Yes	No
Peru	No	No	Yes	No
Suriname	No	Yes	No	No
USA	No	Yes	Yes	No
Venezuela	No	No	Yes	No

*No information is available for the following countries: Antigua and Barbuda, Bahamas, Barbados, Belize, Dominica, El Salvador, Grenada, Guyana, Haiti, Paraguay, Puerto Rico, Saint Kitts and Nevis, Saint Lucia, Saint Vincent and the Grenadines, Trinidad and Tobago and Uruguay.

NA = not available.

AMR has more than 60% of the world's biodiversity, and many countries are trying to develop research and evaluation programmes to identify potential resources. There are ongoing research programmes at national universities, mainly on ethnobotany, chemical and pharmacologic evaluation of medicinal plants, and pharmaceutical technology of herbal products in almost all countries. Gupta (6) has reviewed the status of ethnobotany, bio-prospecting and research into natural products in Latin America.

6.4. TCAM USE

The main form of TCAM therapy in AMR is herbal medicine and the use of medicinal plants for primary health care is widespread in all countries. Even though it is difficult to establish reliable data on the prevalence of other TCAM therapies, homeopathy, naturopathy, acupuncture, chiropractic, massage and bone-setting make up a major proportion of the sector and there are many private clinics in AMR which offer these therapies. It is impossible to know the exact number of TCAM professionals in these countries, as national health ministries do not maintain such statistics. Insurance coverage for TCAM services or products is also unavailable in the majority of AMR countries.

In the United States, a national survey reported by Eisenberg and colleagues (7) indicated that use of at least one of 16 named alternative therapies during the previous year had increased from 34% of the population in 1989 to 42% in 1997. The number of visits to TCAM providers in the United States far exceeds the number of visits to all primary health care physicians and total out-of-pocket expenditure on TCAM, estimated at US$ 27 billion in 1997, was comparable to the projected out-of-pocket expenditure for all physician services for the same year. In Canada, this figure was US$ 2.4 billion (8).

Few other surveys have been carried out in the AMR region although there are some data from Canada (see Chapter 8). In Peru, where a study (9) compared CAM practices to allopathic medicine practices used in the clinics and hospitals in the Peruvian social security system, the results showed that the overall average direct cost of using CAM was less than that incurred using allopathic therapy. In terms of clinical efficacy, user satisfaction and future risk reduction, the efficacy of CAM was higher than that of allopathic treatments. The overall cost–effectiveness of CAM was 53–63% higher than that of allopathic treatments for the selected pathologies.

6.5. Conclusions and Summary

- Of the 20 countries from which information was received, 15 have a department or unit within their health ministries that deals with TCAM. These departments also oversee indigenous health issues. Many countries in AMR also have societies and nongovernmental organizations for TCAM.

- In Argentina, Bolivia, Canada, Costa Rica, Cuba and Guatemala, there are national policies on TCAM. Legal frameworks for TCAM exist in Bolivia, Canada, Cuba, Guatemala, Honduras and Peru. Legislation and regulation of herbal medicine products exist in all countries from which information is available. In Bolivia, Chile, Cuba, Guatemala and the United States, both TCAM practice and products are regulated.

- TCAM is integrated into the Cuban national health system, and provided in some private clinics and hospitals in Canada, Guatemala, Mexico, Nicaragua, Panama, Peru, Suriname and the United States.

- There is partial health insurance coverage for TCAM products and therapies only in Canada and the United States.

- Most countries have ongoing research programmes on medicinal plants and natural products and there are at least two regional research initiatives (CYTED and TRAMIL).

- Only Argentina, Canada, Cuba and the United States have academic programmes for TCAM at universities. In many countries, private institutions and societies offer courses on TCAM, e.g. Society of Traditional Medicine in Bolivia, Homeopathic Medicinal Society in Chile, Juan Corpas School of Herbal Medicine in Colombia, Homeopathic Traditional Medicine National Academy in Mexico.

- Only Argentina, Cuba and the United States (NCCAM) have national budget allocations for TCAM.

- The main form of TCAM in the AMR region is herbal therapy. Other important forms are acupuncture, chiropractic, homeopathy, massage and spiritual therapies.

- PAHO has made a significant effort in gathering information on TCAM and in organizing many workshops and meetings on indigenous people's health, harmonizing legislation on herbal products and in assessing the future needs in this area.

References

1. *La Salud en las Américas [Health in the Americas]*, Vol. I. Washington, D.C., PAHO/WHO, 2002 (in Spanish).

2. *La Salud en las Américas [Health in the Americas]*, Vol. II. Washington, D.C., PAHO/WHO, 2002 (in Spanish).

3. *Sistema de Salud Tradicionales en América Latina y el Caribe: Información de Base.* Serie 13 de Salud de los Pueblos Indígenas (No. 13 of the Health of Indigenous Peoples Series). Washington, D.C., PAHO/ WHO, 1999. Produced in English as: *Traditional health system in Latin America and the Caribbean: baseline information.* No. 13 of the Health of Indigenous Peoples Series. Washington, D.C., PAHO/ WHO, 2000.

4. La Salud en las Américas, Edición de 1998 [Health in the Americas, 1998 edition]. Washington, D.C., PAHO, 1998. (Publicación científica No. 569), (in Spanish).

5. Legal status of traditional medicine and complementary/alternative medicine: a worldwide review. Geneva, World Health Organization, 2001 (WHO/EDM/TRM/2001.2).

6. Gupta MP. Natural products research in Latin America. *Pharmaceutical Biology*, 2001, Supplement, 39:80–91.

7. Eisenberg DM et al. Trends in alternative medicine use in the United States, 1990–1997: results of a follow-up national survey. *Journal of the American Medical Association*, 1998, 280:1569–1575.

8. Perspective on complementary and alternative health care: a collection of papers proposed for Health Canada. Ottawa, Health Canada, 2001.

9. EsSalud/Organizacion Panamericana de Salud. Estudio Costo-Efectividad: Programa Nacional de Medicina Complementaria. Seguro Social de EsSalud [Study of Cost-Effectiveness: National Program in Complementary Medicine. Social Security of EsSalud]. Lima, EsSalud/Organizacion Panamericana de Salud (Pan American Health Organization), 2000.

Bibliography

Iniciativa de Salud de los pueblos Indígenas: Marco estratégico y plan de acción 1999-2002 [Health Initiative of the Indigenous People: Strategic framework and action plan 1999–2002]. Washington, D.C., PAHO, 2000 (in Spanish).

Iniciativa de Salud de los Pueblos Indígenas: Situación de Salud de los Pueblos Indígenas de Perú [Health initiative of the indigenous peoples: health status of the indigenous peoples of Peru]. Washington, D.C., PAHO/WHO, 1998 (in Spanish).

Iniciativa de Salud de los Pueblos Indígenas: Situación de Salud de los Pueblos Indígenas de Referencias [Health initiative of the indigenous peoples: health status of the indigenous people under reference]. Washington, D.C., PAHO/WHO, 1998 (in Spanish).

Iniciativa de Salud de los Pueblos Indígenas: Situación de Salud de los Pueblos Indígenas de Venezuela [Health initiative of the indigenous peoples: health status of the indigenous people of Venezuela]. Washington, D.C., PAHO/WHO, 1998 (in Spanish).

Iniciativa de Salud de los Pueblos Indígenas. Taller Sub-regional para Mesoamérica-Pueblos Indígenas [Health initiative of the indigenous peoples. Subregional workshop for Mesoamerican indigenous peoples]. Washington, D.C., PAHO/WHO, 1998 (in Spanish).

Condiciones de Salud de pueblos aborígenes de Belice, Guyana y Surinam [Health conditions of aboriginal peoples in Belize, Guyana and Suriname]. Washington, D.C., PAHO/PASB/WHO, 1998 (in Spanish).

Fortalecimiento y desarrollo de los sistemas de salud tradicionales: organización y provisión de servicios de salud en poblaciones multiculturales [Strengthening and development of the traditional health systems: organization and provision of health services in multicultural populations]. Serie 6 de Salud de los Pueblos Indígenas (No. 6 of the Health of Indigenous Peoples Series). Washington, D.C., PAHO/ WHO, 1997 (in Spanish).

Hacia el Abordaje integral de la Salud: pautas para la investigación con los Pueblos Indígenas [Towards implementation of integral health: guidelines for research with indigenous peoples]. Serie 2 de Salud de los Pueblos Indígenas (No.2 of the Health of Indigenous Peoples Series). Washington, D.C., PAHO/WHO, 1997. (in Spanish).

Iniciativa de Salud de los Pueblos Indígenas: Reunión de trabajo sobre Políticas de Salud y Pueblos Indígenas: Parlamento Indígena Andino-Parlamento Indígena de América [Health initiative of the indigenous peoples: working group meeting on health polices and indigenous peoples: Indigenous Parliament – Andean Indigenous Parliament of the Americas]. Washington, D.C., PAHO/WHO, 1997 (in Spanish).

Memoria Primer Encuentro Nacional Salud y Pueblos Indígenas: Hacia una Política Intercultural en Salud. [Proceedings of the First Meeting on National Health and Indigenous Peoples: Towards intercultural policy in health]. Serie 7 de Salud de los Pueblos Indígenas [No.7 of the Health of Indigenous Peoples Series]. Washington, D.C., PAHO/WHO, 1998 (in Spanish).

Iniciativa de Salud de los Pueblos Indígenas: Situación de Salud de los Pueblos Indígenas de Ecuador [Initiatives of health of the indigenous peoples: health status of the indigenous peoples of Ecuador]. Washington, D.C., PAHO/WHO, 1998 (in Spanish).

Iniciativa de Salud de los Pueblos Indígenas: Situación de Salud de los Pueblos Indígenas de Guatemala [Health initiative of the indigenous peoples: health status of the indigenous peoples of Guatemala]. Washington, D.C., PAHO/WHO, 1998 (in Spanish).

Iniciativa de Salud de los Pueblos Indígenas: Situación de Salud de los Pueblos Indígenas de México [Health initiatives of the indigenous peoples: health status of the indigenous peoples of Mexico]. Washington, D.C., PAHO/WHO, 1998 (in Spanish).

Promoción de la Medicina y Terapias Indígenas en la Atención Primaria de Salud: El caso de los Maya de Guatemala [Promotion of the indigenous medicine and therapy in primary health care: the case of the Mayas of Guatemala]. Serie 15 de Salud de los Pueblos Indígenas (No.15 of the Health of Indigenous Peoples Series). Washington, D.C., PAHO/WHO, 2001 (in Spanish).

Promoción de la Medicina y Terapias Indígenas en la Atención Primaria de Salud: El caso de los Ngöbe Buglé de Panamá [Promotion of the indigenous medicine and therapy in primary health care: the case of Ngöbe Buglé of Panama]. Serie 14 de Salud de los Pueblos Indígenas (No.14 of the Health of Indigenous Peoples Series). Washington, D.C., PAHO/WHO, 2001 (in Spanish).

Medicinas y Terapias Tradicionales, Complementarias y Alternativas en las Américas: Políticas, Planes y Programas, Informe de un Taller. 19–20 de marzo de 2001. Guatemala. [Traditional, complementary, alternative medicine in the Americas: policies, plans, and programs. Report of a workshop. 19–20 March 2001, Guatemala]. Washington, D.C., PAHO/WHO, 2001 (in Spanish).

Traditional, complementary and alternative medicine and therapies in the Americas: policies, plans and programs. Washington, D.C., PAHO/WHO, 2001.

Traditional health system in Latin America and the Caribbean: baseline information. Washington, D.C., PAHO/WHO, 2000.

Legal status of traditional medicine and complementary/alternative medicine: a worldwide review. Geneva, World Health Organization, 2001 (WHO/EDM/TRM/2001.2).

García M. Cáceres A, ed. Legislación en Iberoamérica sobre fitofármacos y productos naturales, Primera edición [Legislation on phytopharmaceuticals and natural products in Iberoamerica]. San Jose, University of Costa Rica and CYTED, 2000 (in Spanish).

Germosén-Robineau L. Farmacopea Vegetal Caribeña, Primera edición. [Caribbean plants pharmacopeia, First edition]. Ediciones Emile Désormeaux, Martinique, 1997 (in Spanish).

Gupta MP. 270 Plantas medicinales Iberoamericanas [270 Iberoamerican medicinal plants]. Editorial Presencia Ltd., CYTED, Convenio Andres Bello, SantaFé de Bogotá, 1995 (in Spanish).

CHAPTER 7

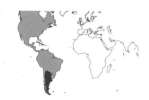

ARGENTINE REPUBLIC

Susana A. Zacchino

Professor of Pharmacognosy, Pharmacy School, National University of Rosario, Suipacha 531-(2000) Rosario, Argentina. E-mail: szaabgil@citynet.net.ar

7.1. INTRODUCTION

The Argentine Republic, the southernmost country in the American continent, with an area of 2.8 million km^2 (*1*) has 37 944 million inhabitants with an average density of 13 people per km^2 (*2*).

The indigenous population comprises only 0.3% of the total population. As a consequence, most of the knowledge about the traditional use of medicinal plants and other practices by Argentina's ethnic groups has been lost. Nevertheless, the use of traditional, complementary and alternative medicine (TCAM) is increasing at a notable rate, especially among low-income populations and among patients whose needs are not met by allopathic health care.

7.2. BACKGROUND INDICATORS

According to the available data, the ten most common causes of morbidity in Argentina are infant diarrhoea, influenza, pneumonia, parotitis, rubella, hepatitis, genital ulcers, tuberculosis, syphilis and HIV (*1*). The ten most common causes of mortality, in descending order of importance are cardiovascular diseases, neoplasm, respiratory infections, cerebrovascular diseases, accidents, infections and parasitic diseases, diabetes mellitus, perinatal conditions, diseases of the urinary system, and others (*1, 3, 4*).

The total number of prescribers in Argentina is about 180 000, distributed as follows: 100 000 physicians; 30 000 dentists; 30 000 nurses; 16 000 pharmacists (*1, 5*). There is no official information available regarding the total number of TCAM providers within or outside the formal health-care system. Nevertheless, unofficial data indicate the following estimates: 800–1500 physicians providing acupuncture (*6*), 600–800 practitioners of homeopathy (*7*) and 400–600 herbal therapists (*8*).

7.3. HEALTH EXPENDITURE

According to data provided by the Ministry of Health (*9*), the Argentinean population of the metropolitan area of Buenos Aires (a crowded zone of middle-income to higher-income people) spends a mean of US$ 12 per month per capita on total health expenditures; in the rest of the country the spending about US$ 8 per month per capita.

There is no information on the expenditure on TCAM systems. TCAM therapies are not covered by any social security programmes, and are not provided in hospitals, with the two exceptions of the Municipal Hospital of Avellaneda, Buenos Aires Province, which provides homeopathy (*7*) and the Nicolas Avellaneda Hospital, Tucumán Province, which provides acupuncture (*6*). However, there are no statistics on TCAM expenditure in these two hospitals. There are no TCAM therapies covered by public health insurance, and no other financing system contributes to the provision of TCAM in the public sector.

7.4. STRUCTURAL INFORMATION

7.4.1. Official National TCAM Policy

The Argentinean Constitution recognizes the ethnic and cultural existence of indigenous populations. It has ratified the Convention on Biological Diversity, and has included regulations for the integration of indigenous peoples into the health programmes of the country since 1985. These regulations state that "in the health plans for indigenous communities, it is necessary to integrate persons who offer empirically based (traditional) health care in the indigenous communities". They also state that:

It is necessary to implement programmes of health prevention and assistance in the indigenous communities, together with the Health Ministry and the different state governments, and to include the knowledge and methodologies of traditional medicine in these programmes (*10*).

There are no general laws applying to all forms of TCAM, but there are specific laws about practitioners of certain forms of TCAM. The National Ministry of Health ruled that acupuncture may be practised only by allopathic physicians (*11*). This resolution was ratified by the Confederation of all Medical Associations of Argentina and is therefore enforced throughout the country. In addition, the Medical Associations of Buenos Aires, Córdoba, La Pampa and Chubut have legalized acupuncture.

Although acupuncture is the only legally-recognized TCAM therapy, in 2001 the Secretary for Health announced that empirical (traditional) health practitioners would be recognized and trained for collaborating in official health-care programmes. Chiropractic, homeopathy and phytotherapy, although not legally recognized, are accepted in some places and forbidden in others.

Herbal products are regulated under the National Administration of Drugs, Foods and Medical Technology and the National Institute of Medicines (INAME) of the Ministry of Health. Homeopathic medicines must be prepared immediately before dispensing, and may be sold only in pharmacies. Pre-manufactured homeopathic products are forbidden.

Table 7.1.   Education and training for TCAM providers outside the formal health-care system

Institution	Course(s)
Argentinean Institute for Natural Therapy (www.verdeynatural.com.ar)	Aromatherapy and Bach flowers (2 months)
Argentinean Society of Anthropologic Medicine (www.sama.org.ar)	Traditional medicine
INCUPO National Institute of Popular Culture (www.incupo.org.ar)	Primary health care
Centre for the Study of Appropriate Technologies of Argentina (CETAAR)	Medicinal plants

7.4.3. Education

A number of different education and training programmes exist, both for TCAM providers outside the formal health-care system (Table 7.1) and health professionals within the formal sector (Table 7.2).

7.4.4. TCAM Control, Information and Education

The main national institution dealing with TCAM control, information and education in Argentina is INAME under the Ministry of Health. It exerts control only on medicinal plants. An expert committee of members from universities, manufacturers and chambers of commerce oversees the acceptance or rejection of plant drugs for clinical use, according to ethnobotanical data, traditional uses and reported toxicities following the WHO guidelines for good manufacturing practices for herbal products (*12*).

Research in the field of TCAM is not considered a priority by Argentinean funding bodies such as the Agency for Promoting Science and Technology (ANPyCT) or the National Council for Scientific and Technical Research (CONICET). Exceptional grants are provided jointly by ANPyCT and some chambers of commerce.

Table 7.2. TCAM education and training for health professionals within the formal health-care system

Institution	Course(s)
Argentinean Medical Association for Homeopathy (www.amha.com.ar)	Homeopathy courses for physicians and veterinarians (2 years), dentists (2 years) and pharmacists (5 months)
Argentinean Scientific Society of Chiropractic (www.quiropraxia.net/scaq.asp)	Courses in chiropractic
Argentinian Society of Acupuncture	Courses in Acupuncture
Argentinian Society of Phytomedicine (www.plantasmedicinales.org)	Phytomedicine
Ayurveda Health Foundation, PREMA (www.medicinaayurveda.org)	Ayurveda practices
Chiropractic Association of Argentina (www.quiropraxia.org.ar)	Courses in chiropractic for kinesiotherapists and physiotherapists
College of Pharmacy, La Plata, Buenos Aires Province	Introduction to herbal medicine
Medical College, District II	Herbal medicine in practice
National Institute of Medicines, Ministry of Health	Courses in quality control of medicines
Private universities in Quilmes	Courses in herbal medicine
School of Pharmacy	Courses in pharmaceutical technology for homeopathic medicines
University of Buenos Aires	Acupuncture; auricular and cranial reflexotherapy; Ayurvedic medicine, including distance learning; therapeutic properties of medicinal plants

7.4.5. Professional Organizations

There are many professional organizations of TCAM practitioners, including:

- Argentinean Association of Phytomedicine (www.plantasmedicinales.org) (www.sinectis.com.ar/u/fitomedicina);

- Argentinean Medical Association of Homeopathy (www.amha.com.ar);

- Ayurveda Health Foundation PREMA (www.medicinaayurveda.org);

- Chiropractic Association of Physiotherapists of Argentina (www.quiropraxia.org.ar);

- Argentinean Scientific Society of Chiropraxis (www.quiropraxia.net/scaq.asp);

- Argentinean Society of Acupuncture (http://welcome.to/acupuntura);

- Argentinean Society of Internal General Medicine (www.samig.org.ar/sociedad.htm);

- Fundacion Puiggros (www.amha.com.ar);

- Argentinean Homeopathic School and Argentinean Homeopathic Association (www.homeopatia.org.ar);

- HOMEOS Foundation (www.elhomeopatico.com.ar);

- Argentinean Society of Anthropologic Medicine (www.plantasmedicinales.org/etno/may2001/3.htm);

- Argentinean Medical Institute of Acupuncture Ramón L. Falcón 2335 - PB A - (1406) - Capital Federal, Argentina. Email: info@imada.com.ar.

Some of these organizations act as voluntary self-regulatory bodies. For example, the Argentinean Societies of Acupuncture and of Homeopathy require that physicians who provide these complementary medicines must have passed a training course in the subject.

7.5. PROCESS INDICATORS

7.5.1. Surveys

There is only one survey of TCAM use by the Argentinean population (*13*), conducted by Franco and Pecci. The target population included all ages and ethnic groups; the method of data collection was face-to-face interviewing; and sampling was done during the patients' first medical consultation at the Clinical Hospital in Buenos Aires. The total number of respondents was 540. The results are illustrated in Figure 7.1.

Fig. 7.1.   Percentage of TCAM consumers using each form of TCAM (24.9% had used two types of therapy; 7.2% had used more than two therapies) (*6–8, 11*).

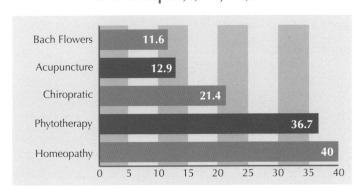

The survey does not show the percentages, but found that all patients using TCAM had chronic pain, which was not relieved by allopathic medicine. Particularly, patients suffering from chronic musculoskeletal pain turn to acupuncture and chiropractic.

Regarding patient satisfaction (*13*), 54% of the consulted patients reported feeling very good after treatment, and 30% said that they felt good. Perceived outcome by phytotherapists and acupuncturists interviewed revealed a very high level of patient satisfaction (over 80%).

Users of TCAM had the following sociodemographic characteristics:

- 65% below the age of 45
- 80% middle class
- 67% have finished secondary school
- 76% lived in Buenos Aires city and surroundings
- 72% women, 28 % men.

The only available estimate for the percentage of the population using any form of TCAM (54.4%) comes from the above survey in Buenos Aires city, and thus it may not be representative of the whole country (*13*). However, no other surveys are available. This survey did not differentiate between visits to a TCAM provider and self-medication.

7.6. DISCUSSION

Argentina has a great percentage of neglected people, including indigenous people, who do not have easy access to the conventional health system. One of the strategies for overcoming this problem would be the development of national health programmes which include TCAM.

It would be necessary to improve the collection of information about the indigenous health care and to make new efforts to incorporate this knowledge into the national primary health care programmes. In turn, it is necessary to take into account the great attempts made by Associations of Alternative Practices to be recognized and incorporated into the National Health System. There is no official position in this matter.

7.7. Conclusion and Summary

It is necessary to have a well-designed plan for the integration of TCAM into the National Health System. Lines of action are urgently needed based on the respect for traditional knowledge and on the recognition of the extensive acceptance by the population of alternative practices.

The integration of both allopathic and traditional health systems will aid in maximizing the gains that can be derived from scarce resources and could lead to the achievement of a more equitable health care system.

References

1. Carlevari IJ, Carlevari RD. The Argentine Republic, Economic and Human Geography. Buenos Aires, Grupo Guía Press, 2003:139–160.

2. Organización Panamericana de la Salud, *La salud de las Américas*, Washington DC. (PAHO: *Health in the Americas*, 2002), Washington DC, Pan American Health Organization, 2002.

3. La salud en las Americas, Organización Panamericana de la Salud, Indicadores básicos de salud. Cuadro 3. [Health in the Americas, PAHO Basic Indicators of Health] (www.econosur.com/docoi/salud0.html, accessed 6 June 2004).

4. Ministry of Health, Argentina (www.deis.gov.ar/Indicadores/Indicadores Básicos 2001/Indicadores de Mortalidad 2001) (www.deis.gov.ar/ Indicators/Basic Indicators 2001/Death indicators 2001, accessed 6 June 2004).

5. Abramzom M. Recursos Humanos en Salud en Argentina OPS (PAHO)/OMS(WHO)-UBA (University of Buenos Aires)-Confederación Odontológica Argentina (Argentine Confederation of Dentists), Buenos Aires, 2001.

6. Information provided by Dr S. Aisemberg, President of the Argentinean Society of Acupuncture (http://www.welcome.to/acupuntura, accessed 22 October 2003).

7. Information provided by Dr A. Zani, Puiggros Foundation (www.fundacionpuiggros.org.ar, accessed 24 October 2003).

8. Information provided by Dr J. Alonso, President of the Argentinean Society of Phytomedicine (www.plantasmedicinales.org, accessed 23 October 2003).

9. www.deis.gov.ar/publicaciones/archivos/serie 10 nro17.pdf, a publication updated March 2004, accessed 8 June 2004.

10. Ministry of Health, Argentine (www.msal.gov.ar/atencion primaria/7.Los encuentros por regiones) (www.msal.gov.ar/primary healthcare/7. Meetings by geographic regions, accessed 6 June 2004).

11. http://welcome.to/acupuntura/Historia Acupuntura Argentina, accessed 8 June 2004.

12. *Good manufacturing practices*: supplementary guidelines for the manufacture of herbal medicinal products. Annex 8 of Guideline of Assessment for the herbal medicines (ISBN 92 4 120863 5), WHO Technical Report Series, No. 863. Geneva, World Health Organization,1996.

13. Survey of Dr J. Franco and C. Pecci, (www.clarin.com). Clarín newspaper, dated 12 July 2003.

CHAPTER 8

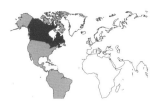

CANADA

Michael J. Smith[1]
and Tracey Spack[2]

[1] Senior Advisor, Natural Health Product Directorate, Health Product and Food Branch, AL 3302D, 2936 Baseline Rd., Qualicum Tower, Tower A, Ottawa, Ontario, K1A 0K9, Canada.
E-mail: michael_j_smith@hc-sc.gc.ca

[2] Policy Analyst, Natural Health Products Directorate, Health Products and Food Branch, AL 3301D, 2936 Baseline Rd., Qualicum Tower A, Ottawa, Ontario K1A 0K9, Canada.
E-mail: tracey_spack@hc-sc.gc.ca

8.1. INTRODUCTION

As in many other countries, people in Canada are increasingly using alternative therapies and taking natural health products such as herbal medicines, nutritional supplements and homeopathic remedies. Over time, the term alternative medicine has evolved into complementary and alternative medicine (CAM), to better reflect the fact that consumers typically use it in tandem with conventional health care. Increased consumer demand is fuelling much activity in this area, with products and practices once considered to be away from the norm now being increasingly acceptable to, or at least tolerated by, the conventional health-care practitioners. While there is still hesitancy on the part of consumers to disclose usage to physicians and pharmacists, there is evidence that this is changing.

A challenge faced when considering CAM is that it is not a single therapeutic approach but rather an umbrella term encompassing many therapies and products. There is much variety between CAM therapies with regard to such things as supporting evidence, regulation, safety, philosophy and acceptance within the political culture. While natural health products such as vitamins and minerals are often included within the definition of CAM, the vast majority of consumers select these without consulting a practitioner.

8.2. BACKGROUND INDICATORS

In Canada, a universal health care system exists, with core medical services, such as hospital admission and family care, being covered by the state. Generally, services such as dental care and prescription drugs are the responsibility of the individual. At present, the ten leading causes of death (all ages) are diseases of the circulatory system, cancer, respiratory diseases, unintentional injuries, diseases of the digestive system, endocrine diseases, diseases of the nervous system, mental disorders, suicide, and genitourinary diseases. (1). Most hospital admissions are due to cardiovascular disease, digestive disorders, respiratory disease, unintentional injuries, genitourinary disorders, psychiatric disease, cancer, musculoskeletal disorders, diseases of the nervous system and endocrine disorders (2).

While physicians and dentists are the primary health-care professionals with authority to prescribe drugs, others such as nurse practitioners, midwives and podiatrists have access to a limited range of formularies in a number of Canadian provinces. In 2000, there were approximately 57 800 physicians in Canada either in clinical or non-clinical practice (3).

Since regulation and title protection of CAM disciplines differs between provinces and territories, obtaining an exact figure for the number of practitioners is challenging. Considering only the regulated CAM practitioners in Canada, there are estimated to be 10 000 registered massage therapists (Canadian Massage Therapy Alliance, personal communication, 2003); 900 naturopathic doctors (Canadian Naturopathic Association, personal communication, 2003); over 6000 chiropractors (4), 2000 acupuncturists and 250 doctors of traditional Chinese medicine (5). These numbers probably make up only a small portion of the CAM providers, with the vast majority of CAM disciplines such as herbalism, homeopathy and Ayurveda being unregulated by any Canadian jurisdiction.

For the fiscal year 2001–2002, the provincial and territorial governments spent a total of C$ 69.1 billion for health, with almost C$ 30 billion provided to hospitals and C$ 14 billion to cover physicians' costs (6). In comparison, in 1997 Canadians spent an estimated C$ 3.8 billion on CAM therapies and products, with approximately C$1.8 billion of this on practitioner visits and the balance on natural health products, books and classes. The largest sectors by far were chiropractic care and massage therapy, with estimated expenditure of C$ 631 million and C$ 419 million respectively. These figures equate to average annual out-of-pocket expenses per person of C$ 60.02 for CAM practitioner visits increasing to C$ 94.69 when natural health products and diet programmes are added (7).

Unlike conventional health care, and with the exception of chiropractic, most forms of CAM are not covered by provincial health-care plans. Consumers must pay for CAM treatments directly and obtain reimbursement from private extended health-care plans. Except for *pro bono* services provided by some community clinics, this means that use of CAM is still largely limited to people in employment and with health-care plans.

8.3. Structural and Process Information

8.3.1. National Policy, Regulation and Research

Practitioners

As with all health-care disciplines in Canada, CAM practitioners are regulated by the provinces and territories. The lack of universal regulation for these practitioners means some are regulated in certain parts of the country and not in others. The vast majority of CAM disciplines are currently unregulated.

Chiropractic is currently the only CAM therapy regulated in all Canadian provinces. Massage therapy is regulated in three provinces (British Columbia, Newfoundland and Labrador, and Ontario) and naturopathy in four (British Columbia, Manitoba, Ontario and Saskatchewan). While acupuncture is licensed in Alberta and Quebec, in British Columbia it is included within a more structured framework that also recognizes doctors of traditional Chinese medicine and Chinese medical herbalists (5, 8). These professions are regulated by bodies set up by the provincial and territorial governments, which are mandated to ensure public safety through development and implementation of such things as standards of practice and effective training for practitioners. For regulation, training institutions must demonstrate that they comply with educational standards determined by the regulatory colleges (8).

Many national associations exist representing the majority of unregulated CAM professions, such as herbalism, homeopathy and aromatherapy. While these associations may demand that members achieve a certain level of education and adopt standards of practice, their authority is not mandated in law. Thus it is important to realize that 'unregulated' does not necessarily mean 'unprofessional' or 'untrained'.

A number of conventional health-care disciplines have adopted a CAM policy for their members, and in some cases have even created specific interest groups. While guidelines vary between disciplines, most allow practitioners to provide CAM if they have received appropriate training in the therapy or therapies; that the therapy falls within their legal scope of practice; and that general guidelines of good practice are maintained.

Natural Health Products

Natural Health Products such as homeopathics, herbal medicines, vitamins and minerals are regulated nationally by the federal government. The Natural Health Products Directorate (NHPD) was established in 2000 to develop a regulatory framework for natural health products to allow Canadians to make objective choices about including them in their health-care options (9). New legislation was passed in June 2003 and implemented on 1 January 2004.

8.3.2. Research

There is no single funding agency dedicated to CAM research. Most CAM research in Canada is supported by agencies responsible for funding health-care research in general. In recent years, a number of research networks have been established to increase research capacity in CAM. In April 2003, the NHPD launched the Natural Health Products Research Programme with the aim to facilitate research in natural health products and promote multidisciplinary research partnerships.

8.3.3. Prevalence and Utilization Patterns

A number of national surveys have been conducted, both amongst the general population and within specific population groups. Depending on the survey and the definition of CAM, national usage ranges from 42% to 73% (7, 10). It appears that only a small proportion of people use CAM to the exclusion of conventional care (6%), while most people consult their doctor before seeking help from a CAM practitioner (49%) (7).

In addition to surveys of the general population, information has been gathered from a number of specific population groups. Amongst breast cancer patients (n=422), 67% of patients used CAM therapies and products (11); among patients with brain tumours (n=167), 24% were users in the previous year (12); among patients suffering from inflammatory bowel disease (n=134), 33% were users in the previous year (13); and among people living with HIV/AIDS (n=657), 39% used CAM in their lifetime (1).

The most common CAM therapies used are chiropractic (36% in lifetime and 13% in last 12 months); relaxation (23% in lifetime and 12% in last 12 months); massage (23% in lifetime and 12% in last 12 months); prayer (21% in lifetime); and herbal therapies (17% in lifetime and 12% in last 12 months). When usage is limited to self-medication, the most popular CAM therapies were folk remedies, prayer, lifestyle changes, diet and consumption of high-dose megavitamins (7).

People also appear to be using CAM proactively for such reasons as boosting the immune system, health promotion, increasing quality of life and gaining control over their illness (15). Typically, people reported using CAM products or therapies 4.4 times a year, primarily to prevent future illness or maintain health (81% of respondents). When used to treat a condition, they were most commonly used by people suffering from back and neck problems (71%), gynaecological problems (70%), anxiety attacks (69%), difficulty in walking (67%), frequent headaches (65%), digestive problems (63%), allergies (60%) and arthritis (60%) (7).

Consumers appear satisfied with the care provided by CAM practitioners and therapies, with the majority responding that they had either 'a lot of confidence' or 'total confidence' in their provider. Most people interviewed who had used CAM thought that their care was helpful (40%) or very helpful (48%) for their condition (7).

CAM utilization varies between Canadian provinces, with British Columbians most likely to use CAM in their lifetime (84%), while those living in the Atlantic provinces (69%) and Quebec (66%) are least likely to use CAM. People living in Ontario appear most likely to have visited a CAM provider in the past year, with an average of 6.6 visits (7).

8.3.4. Sociodemographic Characteristics

When CAM was defined as including both visits to practitioners and self-medication, one survey found that use was most likely by people aged between 18 and 24 years. Consumers in the age group 35–49 years were most likely to see a CAM practitioner (7). There is conflicting information with regard to income; some studies suggested that CAM usage was highest amongst consumers with a higher income (10), while others suggested that this was not the case (7). Usage appeared to be highest among those with at least a post-secondary education (7). Women at any age or income level were found to be more likely than men to consult a CAM practitioner (16).

8.4. DISCUSSION

As use of CAM and natural health products in Canada is increasing, the present political and regulatory framework will need to evolve accordingly. Conventional health-care providers, such as physicians, are becoming more comfortable with these approaches as long as the safety of their patients is not jeopardized, and they recognize the need for more education in the subject. Some CAM therapies are more accepted than others and for those, safety and efficacy will need to be demonstrated.

Given that the regulation of CAM practices differs between provinces and territories in Canada, the development of a national policy will be challenging. Governments at all levels may need to afford increased attention to CAM in order to ensure the safety of the public. Many provinces are reviewing their current laws and regulations, and certain CAM disciplines are increasingly likely to be included under new provincial umbrella laws that apply to all health-care providers. While some CAM disciplines will seek regulation, current evidence suggests that others may fear it, thinking that it will take away the individual nature of their therapy (*17*). A challenge facing many CAM disciplines seeking regulation is the ability to demonstrate effective internal cohesion and establish the professional identity needed to work within the health-care environment. While increasing pressures on the heath-care system make it unlikely that public funds will cover CAM treatments, private health insurers are increasingly exploring this area.

The new Natural Health Product Regulations, implemented in 2004, facilitate informed choice about such products as herbal medicines and vitamins, and are likely to stimulate research and education in the area.

While people in Canada typically use both conventional health care and CAM, it would be premature to consider the two as being truly integrated. This may change over time for certain disciplines such as acupuncture, herbal medicine and chiropractic as new evidence appears. However, it is possible that most CAM therapies will remain as part of the 'other mainstream'.

8.5. CONCLUSIONS

People in Canada tend to use CAM in addition to conventional health care. CAM is a multi-billion dollar industry that is continuing to grow as consumers become more aware and gain greater access to these alternative approaches to address their health-care needs. On 1 January 2004, in response to public pressure for the regulation of, and access to, herbal remedies, the Natural Health Products Regulations came into force. These regulate the manufacture, packaging, labelling and importation for sale of natural health products, including traditional and homeopathic medicines, to ensure that the public has ready access to natural health products that are safe, effective and of high quality, while respecting freedom of choice and cultural and philosophical diversity. CAM practitioners are regulated at the level of the provinces and territories and the use of CAM varies regionally both in patterns of use and in the extent to which its practice is regulated.

References

1. Leading Causes of Death and Hospitalization in Canada (http://www.hc-sc.gc.ca/pphb-dgspsp/publicat/lcd-pcd97/mrt_mf_e.html, accessed 3 June 2004).

2. *Economic Burden of Illness in Canada*, Ottawa, Health Canada, 1998 (http://www.hc-sc.gc.ca/pphb-dgspsp/publicat/ebic-femc98/pdf/ebic1998.pdf, accessed 3 June 2004).

3. *Canada's health care providers*. Ottawa, Canadian Institutes of Health Research, 2001.

4. Canadian Chiropractic Association (http://www.ccachiro.org, accessed 3 June 2004).

5. College of Traditional Chinese Medical Practitioners and Acupuncturists of British Columbia (http://www.ctcma.bc.ca, accessed 3 June 2004).

6. *Preliminary provincial and territorial government health expenditure estimates, 1974–1975 to 2003–2004*. Ottawa, Canadian Institutes of Health Research, 2003.

7. Ramsay C, Walker M, Alexander J. *Alternative medicine in Canada: use and public attitudes. Vancouver*, The Fraser Institute, 1999 (Public Policy Sources No. 21).

8. Boon H. Regulation of complementary/alternative medicine: a Canadian perspective. *Complementary Therapies in Medicine*, 2002, 10:14–19.

9. Health Canada, Natural Health Products Directorate (http://www.hc-sc.gc.ca/hpfb-dgpsa/nhpd-dpsn/index_e.html, accessed 3 June 2004).

10. CTV/Angus Reid Group. *Use of alternative medicines and practices*. Winnipeg, Angus Reid Group, 1997.

11. Boon H et al. The use of complementary/alternative medicine by breast cancer survivors in Ontario: prevalence and perceptions. *Journal of Clinical Oncology*, 2000, 18:2515–2521.

12. Verhoef M et al. Alternative therapy use in neurologic disease; use in brain tumour patients. *Neurology*, 1999, 52:617–622.

13. Hilsden R et al. Complementary medicine use by patients with inflammatory bowel disease. *American Journal of Gastroenterolog*, 1998, 93:697–701.

14. Ostrow M, et al. Determinants of complementary therapy use in HIV-infected individuals receiving anti-retroviral or anti-opportunistic agents. *Journal of Acquired Immune Deficiency Syndrome and Human Retrovirology*, 1997, 15:115–120.

15. Boon H, Verhoef M. Complementary and alternative medicine: a Canadian perspective. In: Ernst E et al, eds. *The desktop guide to complementary and alternative medicine*. London, Mosby, 2001:362–373.

16. Millar W. Use of alternative health care practitioners by Canadians. *Canadian Journal of Public Health*, 1997, 88(3):154-158.

17. Gilmour J, Kelner M, Wellman B. Opening the door to complementary and alternative medicine: self regulation in Ontario. *Law & Policy*, 2002, 24:149–174.

Useful Links

Health Canada, Natural Health Products Directorate
    http://www.hc-sc.gc.ca/hpfb-dgpsa/nhpd-dpsn/index_e.html

CAMline
    http://www.camline.org/index2.html

Canadian Chiropractic Association
    http://www.ccachiro.org/

Canadian Health Network
    http://www.canadian-health-network.ca/

Canadian Massage Therapist Alliance
    http://www.cmta.ca/

Canadian Association of Naturopathic Doctors
    http://www.naturopathicassoc.ca/

Natural Health Products Research Society of Canada
    http://www.nhpresearch.bcit.ca/aboutus.html

IN-CAM
    http://www.incamresearch.ca

CHAPTER 9

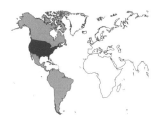

UNITED STATES OF AMERICA

Rowan J.D. Brixey[1],
Joseph Bastien[2],
Karen E. Kun[3]
and Jack Killen[4]

[1] Research Associate, Department of Anthropology, University of Texas at Arlington, Box 19599, Arlington, Texas 76019-0599, United States of America. Email: rjdbrixey@aol.com

[2] Professor of Anthropology, Assistant Chair of Sociology and Anthropology, Director of Anthropology Program, University of Texas at Arlington, Box 19599, Arlington, Texas 76019-0599, United States of America. Email: bastien@uta.edu

[3] Scientific Program Analyst, Contract Staff (Aspen Systems Corp.), National Center for Complementary and Alternative Medicine, National Institutes of Health, 6707 Democracy Boulevard, Suite 401, Bethesda, MD 20892-5475, United States of America. Email: kunk@mail.nih.go

[4] Director, Office of International Health Research, National Center for Complementary and Alternative Medicine, National Institutes of Health, 6707 Democracy Boulevard, Suite 401, Bethesda, MD 20892-5475, United States of America. Email: killenj@mail.nih.gov

9.1. CURRENT STATUS OF CAM IN THE UNITED STATES OF AMERICA

Today, complementary and alternative medicine (CAM) is more widely utilized and readily available in the United States of America than ever before. Particularly over the last decade, there has been a significant increase in usage of CAM by residents of the United States, and physicians, hospitals, and other allopathic health-care organizations have shown a growing interest in the area.

In the United States, CAM practitioners and clients are extremely heterogeneous. CAM is a broad, general term that encompasses a great number of practices and approaches which originated in systems of healing and care of cultures around the world. Furthermore, CAM practitioners vary considerably in their certification, licensing, acceptability, philosophy and approach.

Although usage data are incomplete, recent surveys indicate that most people who use CAM do so in conjunction with allopathic approaches, but often without the knowledge or involvement of their allopathic health-care providers. Very importantly, interest in CAM research continues to grow, and dozens of new studies are being conducted to establish the evidence base required for integration of CAM into routine medical care.

9.2. BACKGROUND INDICATORS

In the United States, the ten most common causes of admission to hospital are pneumonia, congestive heart failure, chronic lung disease, coronary artery disease, urinary tract infection, dehydration, cerebral artery blockage, chest pain, acute pancreatitis, and chronic paranoid schizophrenia. The ten most common causes of mortality are heart disease, cancer, stroke, chronic lower respiratory disease, accidents, diabetes mellitus, pneumonia/influenza, Alzheimer's disease, nephritis, and septicaemia.

Only physicians, dentists, and in some states physician assistants or nurse practitioners under physician supervision, are legally allowed to write prescriptions. The total number of these prescribers is estimated to be 778 400. Exact numbers of CAM providers are not known, since so many sectors are unlicensed and unregulated (see also section *9.3.3*).

Total health care expenditure in 2001 for the allopathic health-care sector was US\$ 1424.5 billion; US\$ 451.2 billion were allocated for hospital care and US\$ 313.6 billion for physician and clinical services. In 1997, the total out-of-pocket expenditure relating to alternative therapies was estimated at US\$ 27 billion (*1*).

9.3. NATIONAL CAM POLICY AND REGULATION

In the United States there is not a separate entity responsible for all aspects of CAM policy, control, education and research. These matters are the responsibility of various governmental and non-governmental entities. A defining feature of the approach to CAM is a substantial commitment to research and integration of proven CAM practices into other mainstream approaches to health care and disease prevention.

9.3.1. Policy and Research

The National Center for Complementary and Alternative Medicine (NCCAM) at the National Institutes of Health, Department of Health and Human Services, is the primary governmental agency addressing scientific aspects of CAM. The United States Congress established the Center in 1998 and its mission is to support rigorous research, to train researchers, and to disseminate information on safety and efficacy of tested CAM modalities. Its long-term goal is to establish the evidence base required for integration of CAM practices into standard medical care (2). NCCAM classifies and supports CAM therapies within five somewhat overlapping domains; alternative medical systems, mind–body interventions, biologically-based therapies, manipulative and body-based methods, and energy therapies (2).

In addition, the Institute of Medicine (IOM) of the National Academies of Sciences has convened a study committee to explore scientific, policy and practice questions arising from the significant and increasing use of CAM by the public in the United States. IOM, which is a non-profit nongovernmental organization, is expected to issue a final report in 2004 (3).

In 2000, a White House Commission on CAM was established and was charged with addressing research, delivery of and access to services, dissemination of reliable information, and appropriate licensing, education and training of practitioners. A final report was issued in March 2002 (4).

9.3.2 Product Regulation

Two regulatory frameworks apply to CAM products in the United States; the Dietary Supplement Health and Education Act (DSHEA; passed by the United States Congress in 1994) and the Food, Drug and Cosmetic Act.

Among other things, DSHEA defines and classifies dietary ingredients, establishes safety frameworks, sets standards for testing, provision of evidence, and labelling, and provides the Food and Drug Administration (FDA), Department of Health and Human Services, with authority to establish good manufacturing practices. DSHEA-defined "dietary ingredients" include vitamins, minerals, herbs, and amino acids, all of which are regulated as foods and not drugs (5, 6).

Under DSHEA, the marketer of a dietary supplement is responsible for determining that the product is safe, and that representations or claims made for it are substantiated by evidence sufficient to show that they are not false or misleading. Thus, except in the case of a new form of dietary supplement where a pre-market review of safety and other information is required, dietary supplements do not need FDA approval before they are marketed.

Other CAM interventions, including drugs and medical devices such as acupuncture needles, are regulated by the FDA through the Federal Food, Drug and Cosmetic Act (7, 8). In these cases, marketers are generally required to provide for FDA review, convincing scientific evidence of both efficacy and safety. Products may be marketed for treatment of specific indications only following FDA review and approval.

The Federal Trade Commission (FTC) regulates dietary supplement advertising. Under the Truth in Advertising Law, advertising must be truthful and not misleading. Before disseminating an advertisement, companies must have adequate objective substantiation of the claims they make for their products (9). The FDA collaborates closely with the FTC in this area, through different laws (6).

9.3.3 Licensing and Practice

Because professional licensure, including that of CAM practitioners, is addressed and regulated at the state level, there is substantial variation from state to state:

- **Acupuncture** is currently licensed in 42 states and the District of Columbia (*10*). More than 14 000 practitioners are licensed (*11, 12*); in addition an estimated 3000 medical doctors have studied formally and incorporated acupuncture into their practice (*11, 13*).

- **Chiropractic** is licensed in every state and the District of Columbia with 70 000 licensed chiropractors currently in practice (*11*).

- **Homeopathy** is licensed in three states (Arizona, Connecticut and Nevada), but then only if practitioners have a medical licence. Arizona and Nevada also license homeopathic assistants who can perform services under the supervision of a homeopathic physician. There are currently 6000 practitioners in the United States (*11, 14*).

- **Massage therapy** is regulated in 33 states (*15*) and there are an estimated 260 000 to 290 000 therapists currently in practice (*16*).

- **Naturopathic physicians** are licensed in 12 states (*17*) and there are an estimated 1500 licensed physicians in practice nationwide (*18*).

Providers for whom no licensure exists in the United States include herbalists, lay homeopaths, unlicensed naturopaths, hypnotherapists, Ayurvedic practitioners, energy healers, mind–body practitioners (biofeedback, hypnotherapy, meditation, visualization, yoga) and Reiki practitioners (*19*). Such practitioners could, in theory, be prosecuted for the unlicensed practice of medicine if they present themselves as physicians (*20*).

9.3.4. National Voluntary Self-regulatory Mechanisms

There are various nongovernmental organizations (mostly professional associations; see Appendix) that exist to facilitate the exchange of information, and in some cases to offer training and/or certification.

9.3.5. Publicly-financed Access to CAM

The Department of Health and Human Services is the federal agency responsible for Medicare, Medicaid, and other publicly financed health-care programmes. In certain cases, coverage is provided for CAM-related services.

Medicare, which serves primarily people over the age of 65, may cover reasonable and necessary alternative treatments proven to be safe and effective, such as spinal manipulation by chiropractors, or massage therapy by physical therapists (*21*). Medicare also provides coverage of biofeedback for muscle re-education of specific muscle groups (*22*) and has begun considering coverage of acupuncture for fibromyalgia and osteoarthritis (*23, 24, 25*).

Medicaid, a health programme that is federally financed and administered by the states and provides medical assistance to low-income families, is giving reimbursement for a growing number of complementary and alternative therapies. A recent survey found that over 75% of state Medicaid programmes provided coverage for at least one alternative therapy; those most commonly covered included chiropractic, biofeedback and acupuncture (*26*).

9.4. CAM Education

9.4.1. CAM Educational Programmes in the United States

CAM-accrediting organizations are national and nongovernmental and include: the Accreditation Commission for Acupuncture and Oriental Medicine; American Board of Medical Acupuncture; Council on Chiropractic Education; Council on Homeopathic Education; Commission on Massage Therapy Accreditation; Associated Bodywork and Massage Professionals; and Council on Naturopathic Medical Education (*11*). Table 9.1 summarizes information on currently-accredited CAM schools and programmes across the United States.

9.4.2. CAM within the Formal Medical Education System

The Liaison Committee on Medical Education, a joint activity of the American Medical Association and the Association of American Medical Colleges (AAMC), is the national accrediting body for allopathic medical schools. This Committee recently reported that 98 of the 126 medical schools in the United States included some CAM instruction in their required curriculum, the purpose of which was to acquaint students with CAM therapies. Additional elective CAM-related courses were offered at 81 schools (*28*). CAM topics taught included, in order of frequency: acupuncture; herbs and botanicals; meditation and relaxation; spirituality/faith/prayer; chiropractic; homeopathy; and nutrition and diet. Surveys have also demonstrated that physicians and medical students want more information about CAM in order to meet the needs of their patients (*29, 30*).

Table 9.1. Accredited CAM Educational Institutions in the United States

CAM system	Accrediting institution	Total no. of programmes
Acupuncture	Accreditation Commission for Acupuncture and Oriental Medicine	41 of more than 70 schools/programmes are accredited and 11 are pending
Chiropractic	Council on Chiropractic Education	16 accredited chiropractic colleges
Massage therapy	Commission on Massage Therapy Accreditation (independent)	63 accredited schools (27)
Naturopathy	Council on Naturopathic Medical Education	3 accredited naturopathic programmes (and one in Canada)

To further support the evolving interest in CAM within allopathic medicine, AAMC has formed an Educational Affairs Special Interest Group in Alternative and Complementary Curriculum Development (*31*). In addition, NCCAM is mandated by law to facilitate the integration of alternative and allopathic medicine and the NCCAM Education project is designed to enhance such integration.

9.5. CAM Usage

9.5.1. Prevalence and Patterns of Use

Within the diverse population of the United States, a wide array of traditional and ethnic CAM practices can be found but many are neither regulated nor licensed, and little research has been conducted to determine their prevalence. Thus at this time, accurate data on the prevalence and utilization of CAM are few.

CAM usage is common and appears to be somewhat more prevalent in more educated and/or upper income groups. Those who seek alternative medicines often cite a desire to avoid the side effects of allopathic treatments; the failure of allopathic treatments to effectively cure or control particular problems; and a desire to be more responsible and in control of one's own health choices. While assimilation of CAM into conventional medical care is clearly occurring, many patients still do not report their CAM usage to their primary care physicians.

According to several studies, CAM is used regularly by up to 43% of the population (*32, 33, 34*). The most recent data on CAM use by adults were obtained in the 2002 National Health Interview Survey (*35*). In a collaborative project by the United States Centers for Disease Control and Prevention and NCCAM, investigators found that 36% of adults use some form of CAM. If the definition of CAM is broadened to include prayer, the number increases to 62%.

For all therapies combined, the estimated number of visits to CAM practitioners in 1997 was 628 825 000; visits to chiropractors (191 886 000) and to massage therapists (113 723 000) accounted for half of all visits (*34*). Other modalities with high rates of usage include various forms of relaxation therapy – primarily meditation (16.3% of the population) – and herbal, mineral or vitamin supplements (12.1% of the population). In 1997, 42% of all alternative therapies used were for treatment of specific medical problems, whereas 58% were used, at least in part, for disease prevention.

Although the greatest numbers of CAM practitioners are found in large cities, the highest ratio of practitioners to population is found in secondary urban areas (e.g. suburbs) (*36*). Rates of CAM usage will obviously be affected by regional availability of practitioners.

9.5.2. Sociodemographic Characteristics

One study (*37*) found that more than 80% of visits to CAM providers were by young and middle-aged adults and that women were more likely than men to use CAM (49% versus 38%). The use of therapies based on self-care is associated with higher educational level. For example, those who seek Reiki and similar energy therapies tend to have a higher level of education than other CAM patients. Surveys indicate that ethnic populations frequently seek out herbal medicine, spiritual healing techniques, and traditional healers, and that they have higher rates of CAM usage than the general population. Use of CAM is also especially high among populations with potentially life-threatening diseases (see below).

9.5.3. Common Uses of CAM and their Effectiveness

Medical conditions for which alternative therapies are most likely to be used include back and neck problems (chiropractic, massage, acupuncture); anxiety (relaxation, spiritual healing); depression (relaxation, spiritual healing, herbal medicine); insomnia (relaxation, herbal medicine); fatigue (relaxation, massage); headache (relaxation, chiropractic); arthritis (relaxation, chiropractic, acupuncture); and digestive problems (relaxation, herbal medicine). According to a recent survey, the most commonly used CAM therapies are: prayer for one's own health, prayer by others for the respondent's health, use of natural products (such as herbs and botanicals), deep breathing exercises, participation in a prayer group for one's own health, meditation, chiropractic care, yoga, massage and diet-based therapies (*35*). Those with the most serious and debilitating medical conditions, such as cancer, chronic pain and HIV/AIDS, tend to be the most frequent users of CAM. Of cancer patients, 63–75% use at least one CAM approach in conjunction with their allopathic treatment. The most frequently used practices include spiritual or relaxation approaches, nutritional therapy, massage, and herbal medicine. Studies of HIV-positive patients show that the most common CAM therapies sought by this group are herbal remedies, massage therapy, acupuncture and nutritional therapy. CAM therapies are chosen more often than allopathic treatments by sufferers of chronic conditions, such as chronic pain (52% of sufferers use CAM versus 34% using allopathic treatments), headache (51% versus 19%), depression (34% versus 25%), anxiety (42% versus 13%), and insomnia (32% versus 16%). Those with recurring psychological problems such as insomnia, depression and anxiety are frequent users of massage, chiropractic, and acupuncture (*38*). CAM is also frequently used by women to treat menopause symptoms; one study found that 22.1% of women surveyed used CAM for this purpose.

Many studies into the perceived effectiveness or helpfulness of CAM treatments have been conducted, and many show high levels (80% or above) of satisfaction with such treatments. In general, however, the studies have been too small and/or inadequately controlled to provide sufficient evidence of efficacy and safety.

9.6. CONCLUSIONS

As the body of knowledge of various CAM practices grows, those proven safe and effective in well-designed scientific studies continue to be assimilated into routine medical care. In this respect, CAM is gaining acceptance in the allopathic medical sector as well as among the public at large. However, there are still numerous challenges to integration, most important among them being the need for more and better research to establish an evidence base for CAM practices, and the need for more researchers who are well-trained in CAM practices. While many in the allopathic medical field view CAM with scepticism, and many CAM practitioners resist research or integration, attitudes on both sides are changing. A better evidence base will facilitate integration by establishing clearly, in the same manner as for conventional therapies, the usefulness and safety of CAM therapies.

References

1. National Center for Health Statistics (http://www.cdc.gov/nchs/fastats/hexpense.htm, accessed 5 July 2004).

2. National Center for Complementary and Alternative Medicine (http://nccam.nih.gov, accessed 5 July 2004).

3. *The Current Projects System: Use of Complementary and Alternative Medicine, Institute of Medicine, January 1*, 2003. Washington, D.C., National Academies, (http://www.nationalacademies.org, accessed 26 August 2003).

4. *Final Report of the White House Commission on Complementary and Alternative Medicine Policy.* Washington, D.C., White House Commission on Complementary and Alternative Medicine Policy, 2002 (http://govinfo.library.unt.edu/whccamp/finalreport.html, accessed 1 April 2004).

5. *Dietary Supplement Health and Education Act of 1994.* College Park, MD, Center for Food Safety and Applied Nutrition, United States Food and Drug Administration, 1995 (http://vm.cfsan.fda.gov/dms/dietsupp.html, accessed 1 April 2004).

6. *Overview of Dietary Supplements.* College Park, MD, Center for Food Safety and Applied Nutrition, United States Food and Drug Administration, 2001 (http://www.cfsan.fda.gov/dms/ds-oview.html, accessed 1 April 2004).

7. *Compliance Policy Guides, Section 400.400, Conditions Under Which Homeopathic Drugs May Be Marketed.* Rockville, MD, Office of Regulatory Affairs, United States Food and Drug Administration, 1995 (www.fda.gov/ora/compliance_ref/cpg/cpgdrg/cpg400-400.html, accessed 1 April 2004).

8. *Product Classification Database.* Rockville, MD, United States Food and Drug Administration, 2004 (http://www.accessdata.fda.gov/scripts/cdrh/cfdocs/cfPCD/classification.cfm, accessed 1 April 2004).

9. *An Advertising Guide for Industry.* Washington, D.C., Bureau of Consumer Protection, Federal Trade Commission, 2001 (www.ftc.gov/bcp/conline/pubs/buspubs/dietsupp.htm, accessed 1 April 2004).

10. *Lists of States with Statutes, Regulations and Bills in Progress.* Gig Harbor, WA. Acupuncture and Oriental Medicine Alliance, 2004 (www.aomalliance.org, accessed 1 April 2004).

11. Eisenberg DM et al. Credentialing complementary and alternative medicine providers. *Annals of Internal Medicine*, 2002, 137:965–973.

12. Mitchell BB. *Acupuncture and oriental medicine laws, 2001 ed.* Gig Harbor, WA, National Acupuncture Foundation, 2001.

13. Diehl DL et al. Use of acupuncture by American physicians. *Journal of Alternative and Complementary Medicine*, 1997, 3:119–126.

14. Ullman D. *The consumer's guide to homeopathy.* New York, GP Putnam, 1995.

15. *Massage therapy laws practice information guide.* Evanston, IL, American Massage Therapy Association, 2003 (http://www.amtamassage.org, accessed 29 August 2003).

16. *Demand for massage therapy.* Evanston, IL, American Massage Therapy Association, 2002 (http://www.amtamassage.org/infocenter/home.html, accessed 1 April 2004).

17. *Licensed states and licensing authorities.* Washington, DC, American Association of Naturopathic Physicians, (http://www.naturopathic.org/licensure/licensing.html, accessed 1 April 2004).

18. *Vision: A healthy world through healthy people.* Washington, DC, American Association of Naturopathic Physician, (www.naturopathic.org/about/aanp.html, accessed 1 April 2004).

19. Cohen MH. *Beyond complementary medicine: legal and ethical perspectives on health care and human evolution.* Ann Arbor, MI, University of Michigan Press, 2000.

20. Cohen MH. *Complementary and alternative medicine: legal boundaries and regulatory perspectives.* Baltimore, MD, Johns Hopkins University Press, 1998.

21. *Testimony of Jeffrey Kang, Director, Office of Clinical Standards and Quality Health Care Financing Administration before the House Government Reform Committee on Integrative Cancer Care.* Baltimore, MD, Centers for Medicare and Medicaid Services, Office of Legislation, 2000 (http://www.cms.hhs.gov/media/press/testimony.asp?Counter=597, accessed 2 April 2004).

22. *Medicare coverage of urinary incontinence therapies. Fact sheet.* Baltimore, MD, Centers for Medicare and Medicaid Services, Office of

Public Affairs, 2000 (http://www.cms.hhs.gov/media/press/release.asp?Counter=386, accessed 2 April 2004).

23. *Medicare Coverage Database*. Baltimore, MD, Centers for Medicare and Medicaid Services, 2003 (http://cms.hhs.gov/coverage/default.asp, accessed 27 August 2003).

24. *Technology Assessment: Acupuncture for Fibromyalgia*. Rockville, MD, United States Department of Health and Human Services, Public Health Service, Agency for Healthcare Research and Quality, 2003 (http://www.cms.hhs.gov/coverage/download/id83.pdf, accessed 2 April 2004).

25. *Technology* Assessment: Acupuncture for Osteoarthritis. Rockville, MD, United States Department of Health and Human Services, Public Health Service, Agency for Healthcare Research and Quality, 2003 (http://www.cms.hhs.gov/coverage/download/id84.pdf, accessed 2 April 2004).

26. Steyer TE, Freed GL, Lantz PM. Medicaid reimbursement for alternative therapies. *Alternative Therapies in Health and Medicine*, 2002, 8:84–88.

27. *Massage education institutions and programs*. Evanston, IL, Commission on Massage Therapy Accreditation (http://www.comta.org/accred.htm, accessed 1 April 2004).

28. *Annual medical school questionnaire, 2002–2003*. Chicago, IL, Liaison Committee on Medical Education, 2003.

29. Corbin WL, Shapiro H. Physicians want education about complementary and alternative medicine to enhance communications with their patients. *Archives of Internal Medicine*, 2002, 162:1176–1181.

30. Kreitzer MJ et al. Attitudes toward CAM among medical, nursing and pharmacy faculty and students: a comparative analysis. *Alternative Therapies in Health and Medicine*, 2002, 8:44–47, 50–53.

31. Gabriel BA. To teach or not to teach: the role of alternative medicine in medical school curricula. *AAMC Reporter*, July 2001, 10(10).

32. Eisenberg DM et al. Alternative medicine in the United States: prevalence, costs and patterns of use. *New England Journal of Medicine*, 1993, 328(4):246–252.

33. Druss BG, Rosenheck RA. Association between use of alternative therapies and allopathic medical services. *Journal of the American Medical Association,* 1999, 282:651–656.

34. Eisenberg DM et al. Trends in alternative medicine use in the United States, 1990–1997: results of a follow-up national survey. *Journal of the American Medical Association*, 1998, 280:1569–1575.

35. Barnes P et al. CDC Advance Data Report No.343. Complementary and alternative medicine use among adults: United States, 2002, May 27 2004.

36. Osborne A. The regional distribution of alternative health care. In: Gordon RJ et al. eds. *Alternative therapies: expanding options in health care*. New York, Springer Publishing Company, 1998:105–116.

37. Palinkas LA, Kabongo ML. The use of complementary and alternative medicine in primary care patients. A SURF*NET study. *Journal of Family Practice*, 2000, 49(12):1121–1130.

38. Krauss HH, et al. Alternative health care: its use by individuals with physical disabilities. *Archives of Physical Medicine and Rehabilitation*, 1998, 79(11):1140–1447.

Useful Links

American Academy of Acupuncture and Oriental Medicine
http://www.aaaom.org/

American Association of Acupuncture and Oriental Medicine
http://www.aaom.org/

American Chiropractic Association
http://www.amerchiro.org/

American Herbalists Guild
http://www.americanherbalistsguild.com/

American Massage Therapy Association
http://www.amtamassage.org/

American Naturopathic Medical Association
http://www.anma.com/

American Osteopathic Association
http://www.aoa-net.org/

Ayurvedic Institute
http://www.ayurveda.com/

The National Center for Complementary and Alternative Medicine
http://nccam.nih.gov/

National Center for Homeopathy
http://www.homeopathic.org/

North American Registry of Midwives
http://www.narm.org/

The White House Commission of Complementary and Alternative Medicine Policy
http://www.whccamp.hhs.gov/

Appendix to Chapter 9: Selected Nongovernmental Self-Regulatory Mechanisms

For information purposes only. This list does not connote recommendation or endorsement.

Acupuncture and oriental medicine
Accreditation Commission for Acupuncture and Oriental Medicine: http://www.acaom.org
Acupuncture and Oriental Medicine Alliance: http://www.aomalliance.org
American Academy of Medical Acupuncture: http:/www.medicalacupuncture.org
American Academy of Acupuncture and Oriental Medicine: http://www.aaaom.org
American Association of Oriental Medicine: http://www.aaom.org
National Certification Commission for Acupuncture and Oriental Medicine:
http://www.nccaom.org

Chiropractic
American Chiropractic Association: http://www.amerchiro.org
Association of Chiropractic Colleges: http://www.chirocolleges.org
International Chiropractors Association: http://www.chiropractic.org
World Chiropractic Alliance: http://www.wcanews.com

Herbalists
American Herbalists Guild: http://www.americanherbalistsguild.com
American Botanical Council: http://www.herbalgram.org
Homeopathic medicine
American Institute of Homeopathy: http://www.homeopathyusa.org
Council for Homeopathic Certification: http://www.homeopathicdirectory.org
National Center for Homeopathy: http://www.homeopathic.org
North American Society of Homeopaths: http://www.homeopathy.org/

Massage therapy
American Massage Therapy Association: http://www.amtamassage.org
American Medical Massage Association: http://www.americanmedicalmassage.com
Associated Bodywork and Massage Professionals: http://www.abmp.com
International Massage Association: http://www.imagroup.com
National Certification Board for Therapeutic Massage and Bodywork:
http://www.ncbtmb.com

Naturopathic medicine
American Association of Naturopathic Physicians: http://naturopathic.org
American Naturopathic Medical Association: http://www.anma.com
American Naturopathic Medical Certification and Accreditation Board: http://www.
anmcab.org

Others
Alexander Technique International: http://www.ati-net.com
American Yoga Association: http://www.americanyogaassociation.org
Feldenkrais Guild of North American: http://www.feldenkrais.com
Reiki Alliance: http://www.reikialliance.com
Reiki Outreach International: http://www.annieo.com/reikioutreach

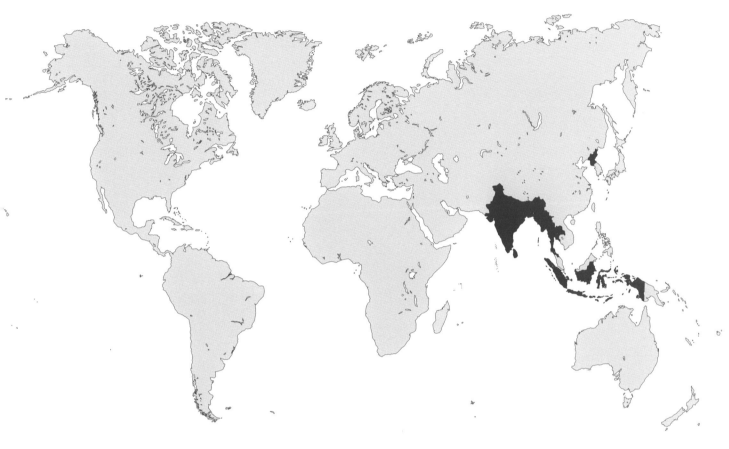

WHO SOUTH-EAST ASIA REGION

REGIONAL OVERVIEW AND
SELECTED COUNTRY CHAPTERS

CHAPTER 10

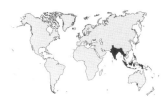

REGIONAL OVERVIEW: SOUTH-EAST ASIA REGION

Bhakaji B. Gaitonde[1]
and Paneerazakathu N.V. Kurup[2]

[1] Former Senior Public Health Administrator (WHO Regional Office for South-East Asia), Banda, Sindhudurg 461 511, Maharashtra, India. Email: bbgaitonde@yahoo.com

[2] Former Vice Chancellor, Gujarat Ayurved University, Chanakya Bhavan, Hospital Road, Jamnagar 361 008, India. Email: ayurveda_uni_jam@hotmail.com

10.1. INTRODUCTION

Allopathic medicine was introduced in South and South-East Asia with colonial rule, starting in the 16th century with Portuguese medicine in Goa, India, followed by Dutch medicine in Java, Indonesia, in the 17th century, and British medicine in India and other British colonies from the 18th century onwards. Prior to these introductions, traditional medicine had been the main source of health care for the general population, as well as for the religious and political elite. Lack of political and cultural support under the colonial rule impeded its use by many leaders, but traditional medicine remained widely used and trusted at the local level.

After the International Conference on Primary Health Care held in Alma-Ata, in the former Soviet Union, in 1978, the countries of WHO South-East Asia Region (SEAR) committed to achieve "Health for All" through approaches which included increased utilization of traditional practitioners and practices. Since then, several countries such as the Democratic People's Republic of Korea, India and Nepal have formulated well-defined national policies on traditional and complementary/alternative medicine (TCAM) and have established departments of traditional medicine. A number of national research councils throughout SEAR promote research in traditional medicine and practices. India and Thailand currently provide resources for drug development, drug standardization and safety and efficacy research on traditional medicines (*1*).

The traditional medical systems of SEAR are recognized nationally and in some cases regionally. Ayurveda, Unani, Siddha, yoga and naturopathy are used and officially recognized in India (*2, 3*). Ayurveda and Unani are recognized in Bangladesh, Nepal, and Sri Lanka. In areas bordering Tibet, China, such as Nepal and Amchi, India, the Tibetan system of traditional medicine, is recognized. In Indonesia, the Jamu medical system is used extensively and partially regulated, and in the Democratic People's Republic of Korea, Koryo medicine is the traditional medical system. Both Myanmar and Thailand formally recognize their traditional medical systems, which are greatly influenced by Ayurveda, traditional Chinese medicine and Buddhist philosophy (*1*).

Despite widespread use of TCAM in different countries of SEAR, there are no consolidated data available on utilization and practices of various modalities of TCAM in the region. Recognizing this need for a comprehensive analysis, the WHO Centre for Health Development in Kobe, Japan, has undertaken activities relating to collection and collation of available information on TCAM.

10.2. BACKGROUND ON THE HEALTH SECTOR

10.2.1. Morbidity and Mortality

With the exception of the Democratic People's Republic of Korea, all countries in SEAR have either tropical or subtropical climate. Thus, the diseases prevalent in this region are those characteristic of tropical regions and include diarrhoea, acute respiratory infections, parasitic infections such as malaria, filariasis and intestinal parasites. These diseases are the major causes of morbidity. Tuberculosis has assumed epidemic proportions in Bangladesh, India and Nepal, and HIV/AIDS is a looming public health crisis in India and Thailand. In the Democratic People's Republic of

Korea, cardiovascular diseases, cancers, and metabolic diseases such as diabetes are the main causes of morbidity (4).

Major causes of mortality, as recorded in country health profiles, are diarrhoea, acute respiratory infections, other infections including tuberculosis, chronic respiratory obstructive diseases, liver disease (acute viral hepatitis and cirrhosis), accidents and poisoning. In the Democratic People's Republic of Korea, cancers, cardiovascular disease and accidents dominate the mortality pattern (4).

10.2.2. Human Resources

Human resource development for health care has been a priority consideration for all countries of the region. All countries except Maldives have established medical, nursing and pharmacy schools offering degree and diploma courses in modern and/or allopathic medicine. The total number of prescribers of allopathic medicine in both the public and private sectors varies from 1.63 to 3.3 per 10 000 population. Maldives, which in 2001 had a population of 299 000, has 171 prescribers who are mostly expatriates, with a few indigenous doctors trained in India, Pakistan, the Russian Federation or Sri Lanka (4).

Compulsory registration of trained and untrained TCAM practitioners was introduced in most countries following the adoption of national traditional medicine (TRM) policies. At the present time, TRM practitioners and traditional healers are required to register with the ministry of health (MOH) in all countries except Indonesia and Maldives. However, there are many unregistered practitioners practising TCAM in Bangladesh, Bhutan, India, Indonesia, Myanmar, Nepal, Sri Lanka and Thailand. The number of TCAM practitioners in each country is shown in Table 10.1 (1). The table includes only those practitioners recorded by surveys or through national registration policies. It is estimated that hundreds of thousands more traditional practitioners remain unregistered and unrecorded throughout SEAR countries.

Table 10.1. Total number of TCAM practitioners recorded in surveys

Country*	Total number of TCAM practitioners	Remarks
Bangladesh	56 000	Includes only those registered
Bhutan	80	Trained at the National Institute of Traditional Medicine
Democratic People's Republic of Korea	NA	Koryo doctors are trained at the Koryo medicine faculties of medical universities
India	490 985	Includes only Ayurveda, Unani and Siddha
Indonesia	281 492	Includes only Jamu
Maldives	1002 (estimate)	Practitioners have almost disappeared
Myanmar	8000	Includes only those registered
Nepal	4000	Registered Ayurveda practitioners
Sri Lanka	1127	Includes only those registered
Thailand	37 157	Registered Thai TRM practitioners

* Data not collected from Timor-Leste; NA = not available

10.3. Health Budgets

In most countries, health care is provided in both public and private sectors. On the basis of the available data for all SEAR countries except Timor-Leste (data not collected), national budget allocations for health do not exceed 7% of gross domestic product (GDP) and health expenditures range from 1.76 to 12.4% of GDP. In smaller countries such as Bhutan or Maldives, health expenditures are 7% and 9% of GDP respectively. India allocates less than 3% of its national budget for health, and its total health expenditure is less than 1% of GDP (4).

Funding for TCAM development in each SEAR country is based within the national health budgets. In Bangladesh, the total amount of spending on TCAM is 550 200 000 Bangladesh takas, which does not exceed 0.02% of the allopathic health care budget. In India, the total government allocation for allopathic health care is 201 155 000 000 Indian rupees – almost ten times that for TCAM. In the Democratic People's Republic of Korea, the majority of primary health care spending is allocated to TRM at the local levels, while at higher levels of health care, the allocation ranges 30–70% of the health budget (4).

The majority of TCAM practitioners charge patients small fees for their services, and patients either buy their medicines directly from the practitioners or from pharmacies. Special treatments such as acupuncture and moxibustion in Chinese medicine, or Panchakarma and Kshar Sutra in Ayurveda are more expensive than common treatments.

10.4. SUMMARY OF INFORMATION ON STRUCTURAL INDICATORS

10.4.1. National TCAM Policy, Legislation and Organization

All the governments in SEAR have declared their commitment to strengthening TCAM policy and practice within their countries. A number of SEAR countries have enacted legislation regarding the registration of practitioners, regulation of traditional medicine production and dissemination, and establishment of facilities for human resource development. These strategies and regulations are monitored in all countries through the MOH. Country-specific policies, legislation and MOH mandates regarding TCAM are given below (1).

Bangladesh: In 1983, MOH established the Board of Unani and Ayurvedic Systems of Medicine to control and regulate education, registration, information and research related to TRM. This board is mandated to register all traditional practitioners, and only those registered are allowed to practise in Bangladesh. In 1990, a separate Directorate of Homeopathy and Traditional Medicine was established under the Ministry of Health and Family Welfare, and in 1998 the National Programme of Unani and Ayurveda was formulated (5).

Bhutan: The Bhutanese National Institute of Traditional Medicine, established under MOH, is mandated to integrate traditional Bhutanese medicine, known as the Himalayan Buddhist system, and allopathic medicine; to conserve and cultivate medicinal plants; improve the production and quality of herbal medicines; oversee research and standardization; and establish training facilities. Bhutanese practitioners in the following categories are officially recognized: (a) persons trained in Tibetan and Bhutanese medical centres; (b) Lamas studying medicine as a part of their religious training; (c) oracle men; and (d) village headman providing treatment in remote areas of the country (6).

Democratic People's Republic of Korea: The Public Health Law of 1980 covers TCAM. The MOH has also established a department for Koryo Medicine, which is mandated to develop Koryo Medicine throughout cities, provinces, districts, counties and factories. All practitioners trained in Koryo Medicine are recognized and registered by the government, and a national expert committee monitors activities for further development of TCAM. Several Koryo Medicine institutes and universities conduct clinical and basic research (1).

India: The Central Council of Medicines Act of 1970 monitors the training and practice of Ayurveda, Siddha, Unani, naturopathy and yoga at national and state levels (3). The Department of Indian Systems of Medicine and Homeopathy was established within MOH in 1995 and was renamed as the Department of Ayurveda, Yoga and Naturopathy, Unani, Siddha and Homeopathy in 2003. It is mandated to regulate education, registration, standardization of TCAM, availability of raw materials, information dissemination, research and integration of Indian systems of medicine in the National Health Programme (2). In October 2002, India's National Policy on Indian Systems of Medicine and Homeopathy received Cabinet approval and is currently going through a parliamentary approval process.

Indonesia: Indonesian health law emphasizes TCAM safety and efficacy. Practitioners of Indonesian traditional medicine (Jamu) are registered under Indonesian law and allowed to use only 54 species of safe and effective plants. The Director General of Food, Drugs and Beverages regulates and registers the manufacturing and sale of Jamu products by factories. The MOH, TCAM Centre provides some primary care services, and the Social Welfare Department provides training in acupuncture (*1*).

Maldives: The Maldivian traditional medical system, Dhivehibeys, has largely disappeared, and there are reportedly only a few surviving practitioners of this medicine. In 1999, MOH established a committee on Maldivian TRM to focus on improving access to local as well as imported herbal medicines, and established a TRM Chair at the Faculty of Health Sciences in the Maldives College of Higher Education (*1*).

Myanmar: The Traditional Medicine Council Law of 2000 and the Department of Traditional Medicine of MOH regulate and control TRM registration, education, research and development. Only registered practitioners of the Myanmar traditional medicine are authorized to practise. MOH also oversees management of the Institute of Traditional Medicine in Mandalay, herbal gardens, hospitals and clinics in the public sector (*7, 8*).

Nepal: The National Ayurveda Health Policy was passed in 1996 to develop and strengthen Ayurveda through human resource development; short-term and college-level training courses; conservation of medicinal plant resources; support for research and development; and expansion of health facilities. The Drug Act of 1978 controls registration and production of Ayurvedic medicines, and only nationally-registered practitioners are allowed to practise TCAM (*9, 10*).

Sri Lanka: The Ministry of Indigenous Medicine and the Department of Ayurveda within the Ministry of Healthcare, Nutrition and Uva Wellassa Development regulate and support local TCAM systems, which include Ayurveda, Siddha, Unani and Desheeya Chikithsa (local Sri Lankan TRM). The Department has the mandate to register practitioners, pharmacists and nurses; regulate and control professional conduct; establish and regulate training facilities; carry out supervision over Ayurveda clinical facilities in the public sector; and promote research. Sri Lanka is the only SEAR country with a separate ministry for promoting and developing the indigenous system of medicine (*1*).

Thailand: Although there is no specific legislation, the Eighth and the Ninth Public Health Development Plans (1997-2001 and 2002-2006, respectively) continue to promote and support Thai TRM. In 1993, the National Institute of Thai Traditional Medicine was established as a division of the Department of Medical Sciences in MOH. Traditional Thai and Ayurvedic practitioners must register with MOH in order to practise Thai massage, reflexology and acupuncture (*1*).

10.4.2. Voluntary Self-regulating Mechanisms

Nongovernmental and self-regulatory organizations are relatively weak in SEAR and do not play a major role in the development and strengthening of TCAM. Exceptions can be found in Bangladesh, India, Nepal and Thailand, where practitioner associations meet periodically to hold seminars, conferences and forums for discussion and review, and to formulate policy recommendations. Private universities and associations throughout India have held various international conferences on research, policy and practice.

10.4.3. Public and Private Funding for TCAM

All governments of countries in SEAR provide some level of financial support for TCAM either through separate MOH budgets, or through provisions to the overall annual health budget. In addition to the national funding, financial support from international organizations such as WHO, UNDP or EC has been allocated to countries including Bangladesh, Bhutan, India, Nepal and Sri Lanka. In some countries, private financing comes from patients, nongovernmental organizations (NGOs) and universities.

10.4.4. Educational Institutions

Having made a policy decision to utilize TCAM practitioners in their health-care programmes, most countries have established facilities for education and training in TCAM with a focus on improving the quality of practice and screening unqualified practitioners.

Table 10.2. TCAM Funding Recipients and Sources

Country*	Recipient of funds	Funding source
Bangladesh	National Board and Research Institute; Unani and Ayurveda Colleges	MOH
Bhutan	All TCAM programmes and institutions; entire population provided treatment free-of-charge	MOH
Democratic People's Republic of Korea	All TCAM programmes and institutions; entire population provided treatment free-of-charge	MOH through national and district allocations
India	Planned and non-planned TCAM activities of the Ninth Plan period	MOH, patients, private and philanthropic institutions, national pharmaceutical industry
Indonesia	None	(see chapter 12)
Maldives	TRM Chair at the Maldives College of Higher Education	MOH
Myanmar	Public sector financing to hospitals through MOH Department of Traditional Medicine	MOH, private donations
Nepal	All TCAM programmes and institutions; entire population provided treatment free-of-charge	MOH
Sri Lanka	The National Institute of Traditional Medicine; Bhandarnayake Ayurvedic Research Institute	MOH, universities, international organizations (WHO, UNDP)
Thailand	Institute of Thai TRM and health centres	MOH, Primary Health Care Directorate, private and religious institutions

* Data not collected from Timor-Leste.

10.5. Summary of information on process indicators

10.5.1. TCAM Surveys and Patterns of Use

There are no systematic surveys on the utilization of TCAM in most countries of SEAR. Utilization data is often collected from hospital outpatient records, which tend to be inaccurate and incomplete. The following summaries of surveys provide some sense of current utilization and practice.

In Bangladesh, a recent sample survey conducted in 1999–2000 in rural areas (5) revealed that 28.7% of the respondents used TCAM for treatment or prevention of disease. Of those visiting practitioners or self-medicating, 26% preferred Unani medicines, while 23% preferred Ayurveda. Of the users of TCAM, 37% preferred practitioner visits, whereas 31% initially self-medicated. Respondents reported using TCAM for five main conditions: fever (1.9% of respondents surveyed), cough and cold (7.1%), high blood pressure (2.5%), stomach pain (3.4%) and dysentery (1.6%).

An Indonesian survey, conducted by the government in 1970, with follow-up in 1995, found a 100% increase in the number of health practitioners over the time period, and 96.2% of these practitioners reported using only Jamu, Indonesian traditional medicine (1).

Table 10.3. Educational Programmes

Country*	Programme	Curriculum
Bangladesh	Nine Unani and Ayurveda institutes under MOH regulation	Four to five-year courses followed by one-year clinical internship.
Bhutan	One programme under the National Institute, MOH	Five and a half -year graduate course, three and a half -year assistant course followed by six months internship. Includes some conventional medicine methods.
Democratic People's Republic of Korea	TRM programme within each medical school (one in each province)	Seven-year course; of the curriculum 30% focuses on conventional medicine.
India	Programmes in 259 undergraduate colleges; 69 postgraduate institutes	Degrees after various lengths of training in Ayurveda, Siddha, Unani, homeopathy, naturopathy and yoga.
Indonesia	One government programme	Training in acupuncture for allopathic physicians and nurses.
Maldives	None	None
Myanmar	One programme in National Institute of TRM in Mandalay; various local programmes	Four-year course followed by one-year internship for diploma; 10-month qualification and two-month refresher course for TRM practitioners.
Nepal	One programme in Tribhuvan University	Bachelor of Ayurvedic Medicine and Surgery.
Sri Lanka	Various indigenous and Ayurveda programmes	Basic medical and PhD degrees.
Thailand	Various public and private, formal and informal programmes	National Institute and national NGO offer three-year courses in pharmacy, Thai TRM, Ayurveda, massage, reflexology; informal primary and secondary school programmes; training provided by wats (religious establishments).

* Data not collected from Timor-Leste

Based on the survey conducted in India by the Central Council for Research in Ayurveda and Siddha (CCRAS), Ayurveda ranks first on the basis of consumer preference; 71.4% of the population studied preferred Ayurveda, 0.01% Siddha, 1.65% homeopathy, 24.67% allopathic medicine and 2.33% others. The most common illnesses for which Ayurveda is used include fever, cold and cough, diarrhoea, neurological diseases, bronchial asthma, menstrual disorders, dyspepsia and skin diseases (3).

In other countries in SEAR it is generally believed that 70–80% of the populations use TCAM, although this may be mainly in the rural and semi-urban areas where allopathic medicine is less available. TCAM is generally preferred for chronic illness, metabolic, skin and mental diseases. In view of unavailability of data on the usage of TCAM, there is an urgent need to undertake well-designed and organized surveys in all countries.

10.5.2. Sociodemographic Characteristics

Sociodemographic characteristics of patients using TCAM have not yet been determined across SEAR by a well-designed survey. It is generally believed that there is greater usage of TCAM by low socioeconomic groups, both in rural and urban areas, because of the low cost of these therapies.

A survey conducted in rural areas of Bangladesh showed that TCAM was used by all age groups, but predominantly in the age group of 21–40 years (56%). TCAM was mainly used by those whose education was limited to secondary school level (66%). Less than 1.4% of graduates and postgraduates seemed to prefer TCAM. People in low-income groups (up to 4000 taka, c.US$ 78.6, per month) constitute 67% of the total users of TCAM in Bangladesh (5). No such data are available from other SEAR countries.

10.6. DISCUSSION

Strong political commitment for, and patronage of, TRM is present throughout SEAR. All countries have enacted legislation on TRM, including strategies for development. Bangladesh, India, Nepal and Sri Lanka recognize Ayurveda, Unani and Siddha and have established institutions to regulate and register TRM practitioners. Nevertheless, there are still a number of unregistered and untrained practitioners. The governments of SEAR countries have taken effective steps to train TRM practitioners through short-term or refresher courses, but efforts must continue if the majority of the traditional healers are to be brought under the registration system (1).

The formalized TRM systems in SEAR possess rich materia medica, treatises and concepts on the pathogenesis of disease and the rationale of therapies which may be of plant, animal or mineral origin. While TCAM is patronized by a large percentage of the SEAR population, thorough efficacy, safety, and cost–benefit analyses of many of these therapies have not been conducted. As TRM is often preferred for chronic illnesses such as arthritis, metabolic diseases like diabetes, neurological diseases and skin infections, possible contraindications to modern medicines must also be systematically assessed.

National policies integrating TRM into the public health infrastructure vary greatly in SEAR. India, Myanmar, Nepal, Thailand and, to some extent, Sri Lanka, have incorporated TRM in their public health infrastructure, while Indonesia, and the Maldives have not yet adopted TRM in their health delivery systems. Bhutan, Democratic People's Republic of Korea and Nepal have outlined strategies to integrate TRM and modern allopathic systems in their national health programmes. Political, religious, social and ethnic groups express divergent views on integration. Some countries have already initiated a process of integration, as in Bhutan, while others, such as India, see difficulties in integration at present and allow the systems to run in parallel. The Democratic People's Republic of Korea provides patients the choice to select either allopathic medicine or TCAM. In India, the official policy is for integration but the lobby of allopathic medicine would oppose such a move. Moreover, Ayurvedic practitioners lobby to preserve the tradition and purity of Ayurveda and not to be associated with allopathic medicine (3).

Despite these activities, no countries except Bangladesh and Indonesia have undertaken surveys on the utilization and practices of TRM; there are no data on the percentage of the population using TRM, nor on the sociodemographic characteristics of TRM users. Since allopathic medicine does not reach more than 20% of the population, especially in rural areas, it is believed that the remaining population seek their health and medical needs through TRM. Furthermore, there are no data on the choice of, or preference for, a modality of TRM.

10.7. CONCLUSIONS

Traditional medicine has been practised in all SEAR countries for many centuries, indeed millennia. It is believed to have survived colonialism in most countries because of its accessibility, affordability and utilization by a large section of the population, particularly in rural areas. The Twenty-Ninth World Health Assembly in 1976 recognized these vast TRM resources, and recommended the collection, collation and exchange of information on TRM. The WHO Inter-Country Project assisted countries to develop and promote TRM, with an emphasis on the provision of TRM for primary health care.

Over the past three decades, most SEAR countries have taken the initiative to develop national policies which include enacting legislation, establishing national institutes, ensuring registration of practitioners, developing training programmes and human resources, and encouraging research.

This overview demonstrates that adequate data exist on the TCAM policy and health infrastructure in SEAR countries (see Chapters 11–14). It remains clear, however, that information about practice, utilization, patient preferences, financial inputs, and socioeconomic or demographic characteristics of users of TCAM is lacking in SEAR countries.

References

1. Chaudhury RR, Rafei UM, eds. *Traditional medicine in Asia.* New Delhi, WHO Regional Office for South-East Asia, 2002 (WHO Regional Publications No. 39).
    Indian systems of medicine & homeopathy. New Delhi, Ministry of Health and Family Welfare, Government of India, 2003 (http://www.indianmedicine.nic.in, accessed 3 February 2004).

2. *Indian systems of medicine and homeopathy in India 1998.* New Delhi, Planning and Evaluation Cell, Department of Indian Systems of Medicine & Homeopathy, Ministry of Health and Family Welfare, Government of India, 1998.

3. *Health situation in the South-East Asia Region 1994–1997.* New Delhi, WHO Regional Office for South-East Asia, 1999.
    Kabir H et al. *Use of traditional medicine in rural Bangladesh – report of a survey.* Dhaka, Directorate of Homeopathy and Traditional Medicine, Ministry of Health and Family Welfare, 2000.

4. Kurup PNV. *Assignment report on medium-term programme for development of traditional medicine in Bhutan.* New Delhi, WHO Regional Office for South-East Asia, 1996 (SEA/TRM/76).

5. Kurup PNV. *Assignment report on development of traditional medicine in Myanmar.* New Delhi, WHO Regional Office for South-East Asia, 1999 (SEA/Trad.Med./79).

6. Mishra SK. *Assignment report on development of teaching curricula for traditional medicine in Myanmar.* New Delhi, WHO Regional Office for South-East Asia, 2000 (SEA/Trad.Med./81).

7. *Annual report 1998–1999.* Kathmandu, Department of Health Services, Ministry of Health, Nepal, 1999.

8. Kurup PNV. *Assignment report on medium-term programme for development of traditional medicine in Nepal.* New Delhi, WHO Regional Office for South-East Asia, 1998 (SEA/TRM/78).

CHAPTER 11

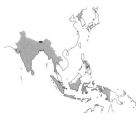

KINGDOM OF BHUTAN

Dorji Wangchuk

Director, Institute of Traditional Medicine Services, Department of Medical Services, Ministry of Health, Kawang Jangsa, Thimphu, Butan. E-mail: dirtms@druknet.bt

11.1. Introduction

The Kingdom of Bhutan is a small landlocked country situated in the eastern Himalayas. According to the 2001 estimates, it has a population of 698 000 and a per capita income of US$ 712 (*1*). It lies between China and India, and is known as Menjong Gyalkhab, meaning 'the land of medicinal plants'.

Above the Indian plain, Bhutan rises gradually from the jungle of the foothills about 100 metres above sea level, to snow-capped peaks at more than 7550 metres (*1*). These differences in altitude, bringing tropical vegetation almost to the base of glaciers, make it possible for plants to grow in extremely diverse environmental and climatic conditions in the same country. Tropical and subtropical forests are found in the south. Temperate and even Mediterranean plants flourish in the valleys, and very rare specimens grow up to 5000 metres above sea level. To date, more than 600 medicinal plants have been identified in Bhutan, and traditional medicine practitioners in the country commonly use about 300 of these plants (*2*).

11.2. Background Indicators

As a result of the effective implementation of successive five-year plans by the Royal Government, Bhutan has achieved significant human development during the last four decades, as highlighted by national health surveys (see Table 11.1).

Table 11.1. Selected health indicators in Bhutan, 1984–2000 (3).

Indicators	1984	1994	2000
Infant mortality rate (per 1000)	102.8	70.7	60.5
Under-five mortality rate (per 1000)	162.4	96.9	84.0
Maternal mortality rate (per 1000)	7.7	3.8	2.5
Life expectancy at birth (years)	48.0	66.0	66.3
Gross fertility rate (%)	169.6	172.7	142.7
Annual population growth rate (%)	2.6	3.1	2.5
Health service coverage (%)	ND	90%	Above 90%
Immunization coverage (%)	80%	90%	Above 90%

ND = Not determined.

Most of the common diseases found in Bhutan are related to poor hygiene and sanitation, and are easily preventable. According to 2002 data, the ten most common causes of morbidity (as % of total morbidity) are: acute respiratory infections (27%); skin infections (9.4%); diarrhoea and dysentery (6.9%); eye diseases (conjunctivitis) (6.5%); peptic ulcer (5.5%); injuries (3.8%); worms and helminthic infestations (3.5%); diseases of the teeth and gums (2.4%); ear diseases (2.3%); pneumonia (1.4%) (*3*).

As of December 2002, there were 29 hospitals, 166 basic health units, 455 outreach clinics and 1023 hospital beds for the provision of primary health care. Regarding human resources for health, there were 122 doctors, 495 nurses, 348 health workers, 252 technicians and 8 dentists, all providing free health-care services in accordance with government policy (3).

Expenditure in the health sector has continued to increase in real terms, with an average annual growth rate of 18%. The strong commitment to the health sector is reflected in an average allocation for health of 10–13% of government expenditure (4).

11.3. BHUTANESE TRADITIONAL MEDICINE

When Shabdrung Ngawang Namgyel came to Bhutan from Tibet in 1616, his Minister of Religion, Tenzing Drukey, who was also an esteemed physician, started to spread the teaching of Sowa Rigpa (Traditional Medicine). Although there had been sporadic instances of Bhutanese being sent by their patrons to study this art in Tibet, it was only after 1616 that traditional medicine was established in Bhutan (2).

Since then, Bhutanese traditional medicine has developed independently of its Tibetan origins; while the basic texts used are the same, certain differences in practice make it a tradition unique to the country. The specific knowledge and experience gained by the Bhutanese over the centuries is still very much alive in this medical tradition that originated in Tibet. The natural environment, with its exceptionally rich flora, also enabled the development of a pharmacopoeia that is without parallel anywhere in the world. The ancient principles and practice of healing were passed on as an oral tradition to younger generations until the system was formalized in 1967 as an integral part of the national health-care delivery system, with the main aim of preserving and promoting this unique system of medical care.

The national policy is to preserve and promote Bhutan's unique system of medicine, through capacity building and the establishment of an effective system within the framework of the national health-care delivery system.

Bhutan 2020: A Vision for Peace, Prosperity and Happiness (5) states the importance of Traditional Medicine as follows:

> We must continue to provide a place for traditional medicine in our system of health care. Traditional medicine embodies knowledge that has been accumulated over centuries and which draws upon the national rich biodiversity and plants with proven medical qualities. As these qualities become substantiated by scientific research, there is a growing need to integrate more effectively traditional medicine with the modern system of health care. The maintenance of traditional medicine not only adds dimensions to the nation's system of health care, but provides an alternative for those who seek one. It should also be regarded as a conscious decision to conserve a part of our rich and varied cultural heritage.
> Therefore, strengthening traditional medicine and integrating it with allopathic health care is regarded as an important policy objective of the health sector.

11.3.1. Development of Traditional Medical Services in Bhutan

From a single Indigenous Dispensary in 1967, the traditional medical service has grown rapidly over the years to cover the entire country. By the end of the Eighth Five-year Plan (1997-2002), traditional medicine units had been established in all 20 districts.

At the national level, the Dispensary was upgraded to a National Indigenous Hospital in 1979 and shifted to its present site in Kawang Jangsa. A small-scale mechanized production unit was started in 1982, with WHO support. The Indigenous Medicine Unit was renamed the National Institute of Traditional Medicine (NITM) in 1988. A new Pharmaceutical and Research Unit was commissioned in 1997 through a project funded by the European Community. In view of its increased functions, the NITM was upgraded to an Institute of Traditional Medicine Services (ITMS) in 1998 (6). There are three units under the ITMS as follows:

- National Traditional Medicine Hospital – responsible for the development and provision of quality medical care;

- National Institute of Traditional Medicine – responsible for development of human resources for traditional medical services;

- Pharmaceutical and Research – responsible for the production of medicines and quality control (QC).

11.3.2. Traditional Medical Services

The Traditional Medical Service functions as an integral part of the national health-care delivery system. It is available in all districts, and is housed under the same roof as the district hospital to enable mutual consultation, treatment and cross-referral of patients. Each District Traditional Medical Unit is staffed by one drungtsho (traditional physician) and one menpa (traditional clinical assistant). Traditional medicine is quite popular especially amongst the older population, and is used daily by about 20–30% of patients visiting the outpatient departments in the district hospitals. The national hospital in Thimphu treats about 200–250 patients per day in summer, and in winter about 150–200 patients per day. Bhutanese traditional medicine is particularly popular for treatment of chronic diseases such as sinusitis, arthritis, asthma, rheumatism, liver problems, digestive problems and diseases related to the nervous system. This is due to its holistic approach.

The main objective of the Traditional Medical Service in future is to improve the quality of health-care provision by conducting operational research and case studies.

11.3.3. Human Resource Development

Since its inception in 1971, the National Institute of Traditional Medicine has trained 36 drungtsho, 34 menpa, 12 pharmacy assistants and 11 research assistants (6). The Institute will continue to train drungtsho and menpa as required by the Department of Medical Services. The Institute has also trained pharmacy assistants and research assistants in collaboration with the Pharmaceutical and Research Unit. The training programmes for degrees, diplomas and certificates are five years for drungtsho, three years for menpa, and two years each for pharmacy assistants and research assistants.

The focus during the next five years will be to improve the quality of training programmes through appropriate faculty development and procurement of the required teaching and learning materials. The Institute will also plan and implement in-service training programmes for qualified drungtsho and menpa to improve the quality of services.

11.4. TRADITIONAL MEDICINE PRODUCTION AND RESEARCH

The Pharmaceutical and Research Unit was established in 1998, for the purpose of manufacturing traditional medicines and conducting scientific research to improve product quality. Unlike allopathic medication, traditional medicines in Bhutan are indigenous products, since most of the raw materials, the processing capabilities and human resource capacity are all available in the country.

The prompt supply of effective traditional drugs in adequate quantities plays a crucial role in the delivery of quality health services. The shortage of traditional medicines has been significantly reduced with the commissioning of the Pharmaceutical and Research Unit. The unit has established links with the environmental sector in Bhutan, including the National Conservation Division, National Parks, the Biodiversity programme and the Renewable Natural Resource Centres of the Ministry of Agriculture. In addition, cooperation and partnerships with farmers and local communities are being strengthened.

11.4.1. Raw Materials

According to Sowa Rigpa, more than 2990 different types of raw materials are used in Bhutanese traditional medicine. Of these, about 260 types are used to produce 103 compounds that constitute an essential list of traditional medicines. About 85% of raw materials are available within the country, and the remaining 15% are imported from India (6). The raw materials are classified (7) into:

- sNgo-sMen – high altitude medicinal plants

- Throg-sMen – low altitude medicinal plants

- Sa-sMen – mineral origin

- Sog-cha-sMen – animal origin

At present, the locally-available raw materials are harvested from the wild, but efforts are being made to promote cultivation of medicinal plants by farmers in order to ensure long-term sustainability.

11.4.2. Manufacturing of Medicines

In the past, all medicines were prepared manually; small-scale mechanized production started only in 1982 with support from WHO. From 1998 onwards, the manufacturing unit was upgraded through European Community funding, and now all products are produced mechanically in accordance with good manufacturing practice (GMP) regulations with a greater emphasis on QC (6). Bhutanese preparations are purely natural, and no synthetic chemicals are used.

The unit currently produces approximately five metric tons (98 products) of traditional medicines, and meets the requirements of 19 District Traditional Medicine Units and the National Traditional Medicine Hospital in Thimphu. In addition, it also produces a small number of herbal products for the local market. To improve patient compliance and administration, dosage forms are standardized. Currently, medicines are manufactured in the form of tablets, capsules, syrups, ointments, medicated oils and powders (6).

11.4.3. Research and QC

The QC section is responsible for assuring quality and assessing the efficacy and safety of the traditional medicines. Research efforts are focused on authentication of species; building quality parameters, both for raw materials and finished products; and standardization of the production processes. Besides routine quality checks, the QC section monitors the stability of traditional medicines on the shelf, coordinates product recalls and assists in the management of adverse drug reactions. It is also responsible for product validation, and oversees the standards for GMP (6).

11.4.4. Marketing

Marketing activities were initiated in 1998. Since then, eight products have been introduced for sale commercially in the local market. Tsheringma Tea and Tsheringma Herbal Incense are two products that are currently popular. There are also several new products in the process of development. However, due to funding constraints, it will take some time to launch these products.

11.5. CONCLUSIONS AND SUMMARY

Due to the dynamic leadership of His Majesty the King and the far-sighted policy of the Royal Government of Bhutan, the traditional medicine system has made considerable progress and is now fully integrated with the allopathic health care delivery system as advocated by WHO. The public can now choose whether they prefer to consult traditional physicians or allopathic doctors, and can receive treatment according to their preference.

As all traditional medicines are manufactured in Bhutan, and human resources are developed within the country, the sustainability of the health sector has improved. There is also a potential for exporting traditional medicine products to other countries, thereby bringing revenue to Bhutan. However, there is a need to improve the quality of the products and their patenting, according to the drug regulatory system. There is also a need to conduct a nationwide survey of different traditional practices, in order to improve the system based on Bhutan's rich culture.

References

1. *Investing in people: Population, development and happiness in Bhutan.* Thimphu, Royal Government of Bhutan and UNFPA, 2003.

2. *An introduction to traditional medicine in Bhutan.* Thimphu, National Institute of Traditional Medicine, Department of Health, 1989.

3. *Annual health bulletin – 2002.* Thimphu, Department of Health Services, Ministry of Health, 2003.

4. *Ninth Five-Year Plan document for the health sector (July 2002–June 2007).* Thimphu, Policy and Planning Division, Ministry of Health, 2002.

5. *Bhutan 2020: A Vision for Peace, Prosperity and Happiness.* Thimphu, Planning Commission, Royal Government of Bhutan, 1999.

6. *Institute at a glance.* Thimphu, Institute of Traditional Medicine Services, 2002.

7. *Traditional medicine: better science, policy and services for health development.* Proceedings of a WHO International Symposium, Japan, 11–13 September 2000. Kobe, WHO Centre for Health Development, 2001.

CHAPTER 12

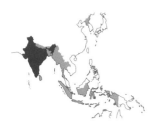

REPUBLIC OF INDIA

Gandhidas S. Lavekar[1]
and Surender K. Sharma[2]

[1] Director, Central Council for Research in Ayurveda and Siddha, Ministry of Health & Family
Welfare, Government of India, 61-65, Institutional Area, D-Block, Janakpuri, New Delhi 110058,
India. Email: ccras@ndf.vsnl.net.in

[2] Adviser (Ayurveda) in the Department of Ayurveda, Yoga & Naturopathy, Unani, Siddha and
Homeopathy, Ministry of Health & Family Welfare, Government of India, Indian Red Cross Society
Building Annex, 1, Red Cross Road, New Delhi 110001, India. Email: adv_ayurveda@yahoo.com

12.1. INTRODUCTION

The Republic of India has a rich, centuries-old heritage of traditional health care systems. Ayurveda
and yoga date back approximately 7000 years. These systems have survived due to their strengths
and the efficacy of their drugs and treatments and have taken care of the health needs of the people. The Indian Government has recognized the codified traditional systems – Ayurveda, Siddha
and Unani – as well as non-drug therapies such as yoga and naturopathy. Ayurveda is a branch of
Atharva Veda, which is the repository of, and treatise, on the knowledge and wisdom of great sages
and seers, acquired, tested and handed down to succeeding generations. Ayurveda is not only a
well-documented system of medicine, but also represents a way of healthy living. It is holistic in
approach and enshrines the complete philosophy of health. Homeopathy, although it originated in
Germany and came to India in the early 18th century, has been completely assimilated, accepted
and enriched like any other Indian system of medicine. These systems and therapies are used to a
large extent to meet the health-care needs of the population. As a result of systematic developments
and improvements, these systems are now being used more widely by the public at national and
international levels. Therefore, India foresees a greater role for these systems and their practitioners
in achieving targets for health care and population stabilization. Traditional health-care systems offer a wide range of safe, cost-effective, natural therapies, which can be used alone or in conjunction
with allopathic health care. They use mainly plant-based drugs, although drugs of mineral, animal
and marine origins are also used to a lesser extent.

After independence in 1947, the Indian Government recognized the merits of each of these traditional systems and made attempts to develop them as viable systems of medicine for the health-
care needs of the people. It was felt that WHO's target of "Health for All" could not be achieved
through the allopathic system alone, and that there was a need to incorporate the Ayurveda, Siddha
and Unani systems and their practitioners into the mainstream in order to reach this goal. The
establishment in 1995, of a separate Department of Indian Systems of Medicine and Homeopathy (ISM&H) under the Ministry of Health & Family Welfare and covering the six recognized
systems of medicine (Ayurveda, Siddha, Unani, yoga, naturopathy and homeopathy), was a major
milestone. This recognition paved the way for the organized development of traditional systems of
health care, each on the basis of its individual philosophy and merits. The broad policy support of
the Government has resulted in a good institutional framework for education, health care, research
and drug manufacture. Some Indian systems of medicine, such as Ayurveda and yoga, are emerging
in the international arena due to global demand and the popularity of holistic approaches.

Public health is a core issue in India. In the last two decades the country has seen an increase in
newly-emerging diseases which have greatly changed the morbidity and mortality scenario. Major
contributors to national mortality and morbidity rates are communicable diseases such as HIV/
AIDS, tuberculosis, malaria, kala-azar and Japanese encephalitis, as well as lifestyle-related and
chronic diseases such as nutritional deficiencies, diabetes, ischaemic heart disease, cancer and certain problems of reproductive and childhood diseases. Despite a relatively good infrastructure for

allopathic primary, secondary and tertiary health care, approximately 70% of the population uses traditional systems of medicine for primary health care needs. In addition, traditional medical systems are widely used for treatment of chronic health problems. There is sufficient awareness and demand for these systems that they are used alongside, or in preference to, allopathic health care. The rural population usually prefers Ayurveda, Siddha and Unani medicines and therapies.

12.2. HEALTH POLICY AND INFRASTRUCTURE

The Indian Government has accorded priority to, and policy support for, the revival and development of Ayurveda, Siddha, Unani, yoga, naturopathy, and homeopathy. Regulatory councils for education and practice have been established under a Statutory Act of Parliament (Indian Medicine Central Council Act of 1970). A central integrated research council later developed into four separate research councils – one for Ayurveda and Siddha, one for Unani, one for yoga and naturopathy, and one for homeopathy. The 1940 Drugs and Cosmetics Act has been broadened, with inclusion of a separate chapter for Ayurveda, Siddha and Unani drugs. The first steps towards mainstreaming traditional health-care systems in the national health system were envisaged in the National Health Policy of 1983, on the basis of the potential role that these systems could play in achieving the goal of "Health for All". This ultimately led to the establishment of an independent department headed by a Secretary in the Government of India, with a mandate to facilitate, encourage, strengthen and promote development efforts and measures for recognition of the traditional medicine sector both within and outside the country.

In 2002, the Indian Government took a major decision to adopt an independent policy for Ayurveda, yoga, naturopathy, Unani, Siddha and homeopathy (AYUSH). The major objectives of this policy are:

- to promote good health and expand the outreach of health care;

- to ensure affordable, safe and efficacious health services and drugs;

- to ensure availability and sustainable use of quality raw materials, particularly those of plant origin, as required under pharmacopoeia standards;

- to facilitate the integration of traditional health systems into national health programmes and health care delivery systems.

In addition, in its endeavour to stabilize population growth, the Government of India adopted a National Population Policy 2000 which includes a full chapter on the mainstreaming and integration of AYUSH and on the utilization of the services of institutionally-qualified practitioners of these systems to fulfil unmet needs and achieve targets in the health sector. The policy also seeks to engage the infrastructure of the traditional medicine sector and enhance its participation in health- and population-related programmes.

The National Population Commission, set up by the Government to address the issue of population stabilization, has further constituted a high-level Expert Advisory Group on mainstreaming of AYUSH into the national health system. This group has been specifically mandated to review the status of the reproductive and child health (RCH) services extended by traditional medical practitioners and infrastructure; to identify areas where these practitioners could be used more effectively by upgrading their knowledge and professional skills; and to identify any legislative or administrative changes required to optimize the utilization of traditional medical systems to augment the existing RCH approach.

Some significant steps that have been taken towards the mainstreaming of Ayurveda, Siddha, Unani and yoga are the:

- introduction of seven Ayurveda drugs and five Unani drugs in the national RCH programme;

- placement of institutionally-qualified traditional medical practitioners in the primary health-care network;

- establishment of general and specialized treatment facilities for traditional medicine in allopathic hospitals;

- provision of health facilities for different medical systems under one roof in the Central Government Health Scheme.

At present, the overall health service infrastructure for Ayurveda, Siddha, Unani, yoga and naturopathy includes 500 000 registered practitioners, with population coverage of 5 doctors per 10 000 people. This incorporates both private and public sectors, at the central as well as the state level. The institutional framework at the central level consists of the Department of Ayurveda, Yoga and Naturopathy, Unani, Siddha and Homeopathy (AYUSH) under the Ministry of Health and Family Welfare; the Drugs and Cosmetics Act; the statutory regulatory council; research councils; national institutes; pharmacopoeia laboratories; and drug manufacturing units. Of the major states of India, 21 have separate departments and infrastructure for AYUSH.

1. **Statutory Regulatory Council:** The Central Council of Indian Medicine (CCIM) of 1970 was set up under an Act of Parliament. Ayurveda, Siddha and Unani systems are within the ambit of the CCIM. It prescribes course curricula, develops and maintains standards of education, and maintains central registers of physicians of Ayurveda, Siddha and Unani. Its main responsibility is to regulate education and practice in these systems of medicine.

2. **Research Councils:** There are three major research councils, namely the Central Council for Research in Ayurveda and Siddha (CCRAS), the Central Council for Research in Unani Medicine (CCRUM) and the Council for Research in Yoga and Naturopathy (CCRYN). These councils conduct research through a number of units, institutes and centres spread throughout the country. They are engaged in clinical research in health care and family welfare, survey and cultivation of medicinal plants, pharmacognosy, phytochemistry, pharmacology, toxicology, drug standardization and research into the ancient classical literature.

3. **Central Pharmacopoeia Laboratory:** The Government has established a Pharmacopoeia Laboratory for Indian Medicine, which is the main laboratory for defining pharmacopoeia standards and testing the quality of drugs used in Ayurveda, Unani and Siddha.

4. **Pharmacopoeias and Formularies:** Pharmacopoeia Committees of Ayurveda, Siddha and Unani, set up by the Government, have an ongoing engagement in developing the standards of drugs. They have published three volumes of Ayurvedic Pharmacopoeia of India containing standards for 326 Ayurvedic drugs, and one volume of Unani Pharmacopoeia containing standards for 45 Unani drugs. The Government of India has also published two volumes of Ayurvedic Formulary of India (636 formulations), one volume of Siddha Formulary (248 formulations) and three volumes of Unani Formulary (746 formulations).

5. **Drugs Regulation:** Ayurveda, Siddha and Unani drugs are licensed and regulated under the Drugs and Cosmetics Act 1940. There is a separate Drugs Technical Advisory Board for Ayurveda, Siddha and Unani drugs. The drugs are manufactured according to formularies and pharmacopoeia standards laid down by the Government. Drug manufacturers are licensed by the State Drugs Authorities. Good Manufacturing Practices (GMP) have been implemented for improving and assuring the quality of manufactured products. Eighteen State Drug Testing Laboratories have already been established and accredited for quality testing of Ayurveda, Siddha and Unani drugs and their raw materials.

6. **Health Budget:** For the Department of AYUSH, an outlay of Rs. 775 crores has been allocated under the Tenth Five-Year Plan (2002–2007). The Plan allocation for 2002–2003 is Rs. 150 crores. There is a separate budget allocation to the states, which is much greater than that of the Department (if summed for all 21 States having infrastructure for AYUSH).

12.3. DEVELOPMENT AREAS

The Government has identified the following areas as priorities for development:

- improvement of educational standards for Ayurveda, Siddha, Unani and homeopathy;

- standardization and quality control of drugs;

- sustained availability of raw materials for Ayurveda, Siddha and Unani medicines, i.e. medicinal plants, metals and minerals, marine and animal products;

- research and development;

- information, public education and communication to raise awareness of the strengths and usage of traditional medicinal products and therapies;

- participation in the National Health and Family Welfare Programmes;

- promotion of Indian systems of medicine, especially Ayurveda and yoga, in other countries;

- establishment and strengthening of health care infrastructure and patient care facilities for Ayurveda, Siddha and Unani;

- mainstreaming AYUSH in the national health-care delivery system.

Some of these are discussed in more detail below.

Table 12.1. Summary of infrastructure available for Ayurveda, Unani, Siddha, yoga and naturopathy in India.

Types of facility	Number of facilities/students in:				
	Ayurveda	*Unani*	*Siddha*	*Yoga*	*Naturopathy*
Hospitals	2 957	312	238	8	23
Beds	43 555	5 023	1 991	150	832
Dispensaries	14 755	961	354	65	56
Registered practitioners	430 263	43 330	17 392	NK	482
Licensed drug manufacturing pharmacies	7 778	450	437	NK	NK
Undergraduate colleges	209	36	6	NK	8
Undergraduate admission capacity	9 250	1 505	320	NK	220
Postgraduate colleges	59	8	2	NK	NK
Postgraduate admission capacity	900	76	90	NK	NK

NK = not known

12.3.1. Education

There are 259 colleges of Ayurveda, Siddha, Unani, yoga and naturopathy in India, of which 69 have postgraduate departments. Undergraduate education, leading to a bachelor's degree (B.A.M.S. – Ayurveda, B.S.M.S. – Siddha, and B.U.M.S. – Unani), has a course curriculum and training schedule of five-and-a-half years, including clinical exposure. It has eight distinct branches of teaching disciplines corresponding to modern systems. Postgraduate courses are of three years' duration. The training in Ayurvedic medicine and surgery is regulated by a statutory body, namely CCIM.

About 30% of the educational institutions are run by State and Central Governments, and the remainder are run by the private sector. The Government has set up national educational institutions in each system as model institutes, to promote excellence in education. The Government is also providing partial financial assistance to private undergraduate colleges for strengthening infrastructure and teacher-training facilities, and for upgrading undergraduate courses and departments for postgraduate specialization. As part of continuing medical education to update skills, a reorientation and training programme for teachers, physicians and paramedics is being implemented.

Diploma and degree courses in Ayurvedic pharmacy are offered by a couple of institutions. There are ongoing efforts to establish regulatory councils for pharmacy and nursing education.

In the field of yoga and naturopathy education, a five-and-a-half-year degree course with a standardized content, and equivalent to that of other traditional medical systems in India, has been introduced. The feasibility of having an independent regulatory body for the education and practice of yoga and naturopathy is under examination. However, a mechanism is being evolved for granting accreditation to institutes conducting diploma and degree courses, pending the establishment of a statutory regulatory body.

12.3.2. Sources of materials for Ayurveda, Siddha and Unani Drugs

The raw materials used in the preparation of Ayurveda, Siddha and Unani drugs are 1000 types of medicinal plants and their parts, 60 types of minerals and metals, and 60 substances of marine and animal origin. About 95% of the drugs are based on medicinal plants. The Department of AYUSH has taken steps to enhance the supply base of medicinal raw materials of plant origin by initiating efforts directed towards the sustainable conservation and cultivation of medicinal plants. The Government has constituted a National Medicinal Plants Board and 29 State Medicinal Plants Boards for organizing this sector. These boards coordinate activities such as conservation and cultivation, demand and supply, marketing and export, quality control and standardization, of plant-based medications.

12.3.3. Research and Development

Research and development related to traditional medicine constitute one of the priority areas, and are implemented under intramural and extramural research programmes. The three central research councils, CCRAS, CCRUM and CCRYN, carry out intramural research activities through their country-wide networks of units, institutes and centres. The CCRAS has patented four drugs and 15 manufacturing processes to date. Its major achievement is the development of an Ayurvedic contraceptive, *Pipplyadi yoga,* and a spermicidal drug based on neem (*Azadirachta indica*) oil. Clinical evaluation of these drugs is underway in the leading modern medical institutes of the country. Automation of therapeutic instruments (Panchakarma) in collaboration with the Indian Institute of Technology, New Delhi, is in progress. CCRUM is engaged in conducting clinical trials on treatments for 18 diseases. Clinical studies on nine new drugs, for diseases such as haemorrhoids, menorrhagia, rheumatoid arthritis and diabetes mellitus, have been completed. During the last two decades, a number of Council of Scientific and Industrial Research institutions, allopathic medical colleges and university departments have also undertaken research projects on Ayurveda, Siddha, Unani drugs and yoga therapy.

The Government has made considerable efforts to popularize Ayurveda and yoga in other countries. There is a scheme for international exchange programmes, seminars and workshops, the objectives of which are to promote and develop Indian systems of medicine and increase the involvement of professionals and researchers in disseminating the results of research and development. Deputation of experts to attend international symposia, seminars and conferences, in order to interact with experts in traditional medicine in other countries, is encouraged. The ISM&H Department (now Department of AYUSH) also hosts delegations from other countries and apprises them of the infrastructure, education and research facilities available in the field of Ayurveda and yoga in India. Delegations from Brazil, Hungary, Malaysia, Myanmar, the Republic of Korea, the Russian Federation and South Africa have visited the ISM&H Department and leading institutions for education, research, health care and drug manufacture. The Government of India has also entered into Memoranda of Understanding with Hungary and the Russian Federation for bilateral cooperation and collaboration in the field of Ayurveda.

12.4. Discussion

India has a rich, centuries-old heritage of traditional medicine systems which have taken care of the health needs of the people and have survived due to their strengths and the efficacy of their treatments. India has the unique distinction of having six recognized systems of traditional medicine: Ayurveda, Siddha, Unani, yoga, naturopathy and homeopathy.

With its wide network of physicians and its infrastructure of medical institutions, hospitals, dispensaries and manufacturing units, Ayurveda is the most widespread Indian traditional medicine system providing health care to the community. The training in Ayurvedic medicines and surgery is regulated by a statutory body, CCIM, which regulates the registration of physicians, and their practice and ethics. Some 209 colleges provide education in Ayurveda, 180 colleges in homeopathy, around eight institutions offer diploma and certificate courses in naturopathy and yoga and six colleges provide education in the Siddha system of medicine.

Drugs are licensed and regulated under the Drugs and Cosmetics Act, 1940, and manufactured according to pharmacopoeia standards laid down by the Government.

The Government of India has set up Research Councils covering each of the Indian Systems of Medicine and homeopathy.

12.5. CONCLUSIONS

In conclusion, it can be said that Ayurveda, Siddha, Unani and yoga are well documented, regulated and utilized in India. The huge infrastructure and human resources available within these systems must be harnessed for achieving the targets set for "Health for All" and bridging the gaps in the health sector.

With official support, the traditional medical systems of India are gradually developing to fulfil their potential. The policy of the Government is to mainstream and integrate them in national health-care programmes and the health-care delivery system. Efforts are also being made to improve the quality and standards of education, drugs and health services. Priority has been given to scientific validation, in accordance with modern scientific parameters, in order to develop traditional medicinal products acceptable to the international market. The full spectrum of traditional medicine in India is thus revitalized and prepared to meet challenges within and outside the country.

Bibliography

National population policy. New Delhi, Ministry of Health & Family Welfare, Government of India, 2000.

National policy on ISM&H. New Delhi, Department of AYUSH, Ministry of Health & Family Welfare, Government of India, 2002.

Annual report 2002–2003. New Delhi, Ministry of Health & Family Welfare, Government of India, 2003.

Essential Ayurvedic drugs for dispensaries and hospitals. New Delhi, Department of AYUSH, Ministry of Health & Family Welfare, Government of India, 2000.

A handbook of domestic medicine and common Ayurvedic remedies. New Delhi, Central Council for Research in Ayurveda & Siddha, 1978.

Ayush-64: a new anti-malarial herbal compound. New Delhi, Central Council for Research in Ayurveda & Siddha, 1987.

Ayush-56: an Ayurvedic anti-epileptic drug. New Delhi, Central Council for Research in Ayurveda & Siddha, 1997.

Report of the task force on conservation and sustainable use of medicinal plants. New Delhi, Planning Commission, Government of India, 2000.

Ayurvedic formulary of India (Part I). New Delhi, Ministry of Health, Government of India, 1978.

Ayurvedic formulary of India (Part II). New Delhi, Ministry of Health, Government of India, 1990.

Ayurvedic pharmacopoeia of India (Part I, Volume I). New Delhi, Ministry of Health, Government of India, 1990.

Ayurvedic pharmacopoeia of India (Part I, Volume II). New Delhi, Ministry of Health & Family Welfare, Government of India, 1999.

Ayurvedic pharmacopoeia of India (Part I, Volume III). New Delhi, Ministry of Health & Family Welfare, Government of India, 2001.

Unani pharmacopoeia of India (Part I). New Delhi, Ministry of Health & Family Welfare, Government of India, 1998.

Siddha formulary of India (Part I). New Delhi, Ministry of Health & Family Welfare, Government of India, 1992.

CHAPTER 13

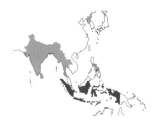

REPUBLIC OF INDONESIA

M. Hayatie Amal[1]
and Hardaningsih[2]

[1] Director, Directorate of Inspections and Certification of Traditional Medicines, Cosmetic and Complementary Product, The National Agency for Drug and Food Control, Republic of Indonesia, Jl. Percetakan Negara No. 23, Jakarta Pusat 10560, Indonesia. E-mail: malti528@indosat.net.id

[2] Head, Traditional Medicine Certification Section, Directorate of Inspections and Certification of Traditional Medicines, Cosmetic and Complementary Product, The National Agency for Drug and Food Control, Republic of Indonesia, Jl. Percetakan Negara No. 23, Jakarta Pusat 10560, Indonesia. E-mail: naningmardjan@yahoo.com

13.1. INTRODUCTION

The Indonesian Archipelago lies between Asia and Australia, covering an area of approximately 1.9 million km^2, with the Pacific Ocean to the north and east and the Indian Ocean to the south and west. As a tropical country straddling the equator, the Republic of Indonesia is very rich in biological diversity. At least 30 000 species of plants grow in the Indonesian islands, of which at least 940 species are recognized as medicinal plants and more than 250 are used by local herbal medicine industries.

Traditional, complementary and alternative medicine (TCAM), including herbal medicine, has been widely used by the Indonesian community since the 15th century, during the era of the Mataram Kingdom. The reliefs on some temples, such as Borobudur, Prambanan and Panataran, show pictures of many medicinal plants in use at that time. Passed on from generation to generation, TCAM is still practised by the people today as part of their daily life, for health maintenance and promotion as well as disease treatment. It serves as an alternative treatment alongside allopathic medicines. The concept of TCAM is based on empirical knowledge, skills and experience implemented beyond their original ethnic settings.

Formally, TCAM has not yet been accepted by allopathic health-care providers. However, Indonesian traditional medicines are being developed and used by the community continuously. Recently, by calling it "back to nature", governments, researchers and local industries have made efforts to develop TCAM so that it can be integrated into existing health systems. In this context, the Government has classified Indonesian indigenous medicines into three groups i.e. Jamu, standardized herbal medicines and phytopharmaca. Herbal medicines will be accepted formally by allopathic medical doctors if their safety and efficacy are scientifically proven.

13.2. SUMMARY OF BACKGROUND INDICATORS

The ten most common causes of morbidity in Indonesia are anaemia (517 per 1000 population), periodontal disease (259 per 1000), upper respiratory infection (234 per 1000), infections (other than respiratory and gastrointestinal) (188 per 1000), refraction (eye problems) (180 per 1000), mental illness (140 per 1000 population), cephalalgia (119 per 1000), gastrointestinal infection (111 per 1000), hypertension (83 per 1000) and deafness (73 per 1000). The ten most common causes of mortality are cerebrovascular and cardiovascular diseases (18.9%), respiratory infections (15.7%), tuberculosis (9.6%), other infections and parasites (7.9%), diarrhoea (7.4%), gastrointestinal infections (6.6%), obstetric complications (5.2%), trauma injuries (5.2%), neoplasm (5.1%) and neuromuscular diseases (2.5%).

In the year 2000, health personnel totalled approximately 171 738 persons, comprising nurses (47.3%), midwives (9.4%), general practitioners (9.0%), specialists (3.5%), dentists (3.2%) and pharmacists (3.5%), etc. However, it is estimated that traditional medicine prescribers number 26 917 persons, including doctors, nurses and pharmacists.

The health survey conducted by the Ministry of Health in 1996 showed that there are approximately 281 492 practitioners of TCAM within and outside the allopathic health-care system. Indonesian TCAM methods are used by 96.2% of these, such as traditional birth attendants (174 263), masseurs (25 077), circumcisers (18 456), tukang jamu (jamu peddler) (18 237), herbalists (14 000), spiritualists (12 498), naturopaths (10 180) and bone-setters (8781). Several other groups of TCAM providers, such as acupuncturists, are also recognized.

The total health expenditure for the allopathic health-care sector is estimated to be around US$ 3 865 664 000. The Government contribution is US$ 1 017 280 000 i.e. around 30%, and the private sectors contribute around 70%. The recent National Survey on Economic and Social Studies (2001) showed an estimated 2.7% of the population using TCAM for outpatient services, with corresponding expenditure around US$ 5.70 per person. The total out-of-pocket spending on TCAM was estimated at around US$ 38 570 853.

13.3. INFORMATION ON STRUCTURAL AND PROCESS INDICATORS

13.3.1. TCAM Policy, Legislation, Organization and Education

There are a number of regulations concerning TCAM provision. Some of these regulate the sector in general, while others focus on specific therapies. All of the regulations have been developed to ensure the safety, efficacy and high quality of TCAM. They include a policy on traditional medicine development; good manufacturing practice, quality, safety and efficacy requirements; regulation of certain traditional medicine providers' registration; industry requirements, product registration, and advertisements. A comprehensive policy framework is still in development, including the National Policy on Indonesian Herbal Medicines Development.

In general, most allopathic health-care professionals are allowed and entitled to provide any TCAM therapy. However, there are certain services, such as acupuncture, that can be provided only by allopathic physicians. At present, all TCAM providers are recognized legally and TCAM is used in parallel with the health-care services. Physicians as acupuncturists who provide acupuncture therapy, and pharmacists who dispense preparations of TCAM (without providing therapy), are professional categories entitled to provide traditional therapies. Other professional categories entitled to provide traditional health-care services are traditional birth attendants; circumcision practitioners; bonesetters; herbalists; religious healers; supernatural healers; Chinese traditional healers; and Arabic traditional healers.

Mechanisms and activities pertaining to TCAM control, education, information and research have been put in place by both the Government and the community to promote and maintain good practices. The Ministry of Health provides guidance and control for TCAM healing services. The control of production and the distribution of traditional medicines is undertaken by a governmental institution, the National Agency for Drug and Food Control (NA-DFC). Education and research are conducted by both governmental institutions (Ministry of Health, NA-DFC, etc.) and the Traditional Medicines Association. Sometimes, research is also supported by the traditional medicines industry.

TCAM associations act as voluntary self-regulatory bodies to ensure the professionalism of practitioners. They organize the provision of specific TCAM therapies. Such associations usually have internal rules covering membership criteria, systems of disciplinary procedures, educational standards, codes of ethics and practice, complaints procedures, organization of traditional medicine practices, and research programme formulation.

There is no financial system that contributes to the provision of TCAM therapies in the public sector. TCAM methods are usually originated locally, hence only certain ethnic groups are familiar with them. The methods vary according to their origin, and it is thus difficult to standardize them. Another constraint is a cultural one; many people believe that TCAM knowledge is a gift and that the provider is prohibited from charging a fixed rate for the services. In the light of the above situation, the development of financial mechanisms will need special effort.

There are educational schools for TCAM in the formal education system, e.g. the School of Acupuncture within the School of Medicine, University of Indonesia, which offers a Masters programme. TCAM services are also integrated into conventional health care, as in the Neurology

Department, where they are offered in conjunction with treatment for patients suffering from cerebrovascular accidents. Gajah Mada University is developing the School of Traditional Medicines Technical Production Programme – a three-year diploma programme. Other forms of education are standardized training for acupuncture, acupressure and traditional birth attendants, and non-standardized training for practitioners such as Jamu sellers and supernatural healers.

Hundreds of TCAM studies are being carried out by separate institutions throughout the country. The studies focus mostly on the confirmation of empirical efficacy using pre-clinical methods. Some studies address ethnobotanical aspects by exploring the utilization of medicinal plants in particular, often remote, areas. The total number of studies undertaken during the last 20 years is estimated to be approximately 100, and there are around 29 studies of traditional medicine users. However, the studies that meet the requirements of Survey Quality Assessment are only around 15 and of these there are four which achieved the highest level of validity (representative sample, instruments pre-tested, training of interviewers) and meet the objectives of the study. Additional effort would be needed to further explore and analyse these studies.

13.3.2. TCAM patterns of use

Despite the huge variety of TCAM practices, the information on these practices is scant. The five most popular individual therapies can be assumed to correspond to the five therapies with the greatest numbers of registered practitioners in 1995; i.e., traditional birth attendants, masseurs, herbalists, providers of traditional medicine based on religious approaches, and traditional medicine based on supernatural or metaphysical powers.

The data on prevalence rates of TCAM use are not available. However, as these data are considered to be important, efforts should be made to include this indicator in the National Economic Survey. The directly-available variables regarding utilization of traditional medicines are herbal medicine use, self-medication use, visits to traditional medicine providers, and visits to allopathic health-care providers.

According to the National Household Health Survey in 1995, the national prevalence of herbal medicine use was estimated to be approximately 50% of the population. The estimated prevalence rates from other studies ranged between 24% and 53%.

In general, the principal reasons for TCAM use can be categorized into: health maintenance and prevention of disease; terminal illnesses; and trivial symptoms or self-limiting diseases. Use is generally by the rural population and by those living in remote areas far from health facilities. There are no studies, even at the local level, designed specifically to obtain information on patient satisfaction or perceived outcomes of TCAM treatment. The most frequent statements of the respondents interviewed were "feeling better", "healed", or "no symptoms any more". It is difficult to quantify the medical determinants of TCAM utilization.

The socio-demographic characteristics of consumers associated with the use of TCAM are available in the annual National Economic Survey. They include age, gender, economic status, education, expenditure, ethnic group, rural/urban population, region and health status. However, nationwide qualitative studies relating to this issue are not available.

The recent Survey on Economic and Social Studies resulted in very rough and underestimated figures for hospital outpatient and inpatient services using TCAM and showed 2.7% of people using TCAM for outpatient services.

13.4. DISCUSSION

In spite of the significant improvements that have been made in the health sector, Indonesia, like many other developing countries, is still characterized by high rates of morbidity and mortality. The number of health personnel is around 84.4 per 100 000 population, and the estimated number of prescribers around 26.9 per 100 000. The number of TCAM practitioners is slightly higher than that of allopathic health personnel. However, along with the trends in population growth, fertility rate and infant mortality rate, the morbidity and mortality rates have been declining over the last two decades and the causes are moving from infectious diseases towards degenerative diseases.

TCAM has been used for centuries by the Indonesian people in rural as well as urban areas, and is part of daily life to overcome their health problems. It has served as an alternative treatment beside allopathic medicine, not only because of its low cost, but also its availability and the existence of traditional as well as empirical evidence for efficacy.

The available data on health expenditure for the TCAM services is scant; however, the rough figures show that out-of-pocket TCAM expenditure was underestimated and far below the expenditure for allopathic health care. The reason for this is the form of payment, which is not always cash. Healers usually consider their practice as a blessing, and do not accept cash payment for this service. In rural areas payment is often in kind for both allopathic and traditional medicine.

The government regulates TCAM to ensure its safety, efficacy and high quality. The Indonesian Health Law considers traditional medicines as an integral part of health care, but they have not yet been integrated into existing formal health-care services. With huge natural resources, and the role of TCAM in providing medication to the community, the Government will support, encourage and facilitate any effort for TCAM development. The Government, together with educational institutions and associations, provides some formal and informal education as well as research to improve practitioners' ability and capacity in public health services and to ensure the safety, quality and efficacy of TCAM.

13.5. Conclusions

TCAM has been practised by Indonesian people for hundreds of years, traditionally and empirically passed on from generation to generation. Some moves have been made to improve and develop traditional medicine practices to ensure quality, safety and efficacy. However, in many cases, no conscious effort has been made to improve traditional health care, as allopathic health-care providers mostly believe in evidence-based medicine. In order for TCAM to be accepted by the allopathic sector for integration into existing health-care services, its safety and efficacy will have to be proven scientifically through clinical trials. To this end, NA-DFC, in collaboration with research institutions, is coordinating clinical trials for nine promising and widely-used Indonesian medicinal plants.

According to the *WHO Traditional Medicines Strategy 2002–2005*, a national policy on TCAM is needed in order to: define its role in the national health-care delivery system; to ensure that the necessary regulatory and legal mechanisms are in place for promoting and maintaining good practice; to provide access to the TCAM practices in an equitable way; and to assure authenticity, safety, quality and efficacy. This policy should cover legislation and regulation of herbal products and practitioners, education, training and licensing of providers, research and development, and the allocation of financial and other resources.

A comprehensive policy framework, namely the National Policy on Indonesian Herbal Medicines Development, Technical Guidance for Good Manufacturing Practices, and Evaluation of Safety and Efficacy of Herbal Medicines, is still in the process of development and finalization. Additional efforts should be made to include indicators that are necessary but not currently available, such as deregulation of TCAM practices and therapies, education and training, intellectual property rights, and promotion and proper use of traditional medicines.

At present, licensing providers of traditional therapies is the local government's responsibility, but as this is not compulsory, the numbers of licensed practitioners are still underreported. The licensing system should be reviewed, and should be followed by standardization of the practices, as well as training and education of practitioners based on standardized qualifications.

Other actions needed to ensure the appropriate and safe use of traditional medicines include information, education and communication for both the consumers and providers, and training guidelines for the various therapies.

Bibliography

Hargono D et al. *Medicinal plants of Indonesia.* Jakarta, Department of Health, Republic of Indonesia, 1986.

Health Law of the Republic of Indonesia, Article 47, No. 23 of 1992. Jakarta, Republic of Indonesia, 1992.

Health survey 1996. Ministry of Health Report. Jakarta, Department of Health, Republic of Indonesia, 1996.

Household survey 1995. Jakarta, National Institute of Health Research and Development, Ministry of Health, Republic of Indonesia, 1995.

Household survey 2000. Jakarta, National Institute of Health Research and Development, Ministry of Health, Republic of Indonesia, 2000.

Indonesian health profile 2000. Jakarta, Ministry of Health, Republic of Indonesia, 2000.

Minister of Health Decree No. 659/Menkes/SK/XI/1991 regarding the Good Manufacturing Practice of Traditional Drug. Jakarta, Ministry of Health, Republic of Indonesia, 1991.

Minister of Health Decree No. 760/Menkes/SK/IX/1992 regarding Phytopharmaca. Jakarta, Ministry of Health, Republic of Indonesia, 1992.

Minister of Health Regulation No. 0371/Birhup/VII/1973 regarding Acupuncturist Registration. Jakarta, Ministry of Health, Republic of Indonesia, 1973.

Minister of Health Regulation No. 038/Birhup/1973 regarding Chinese and Arabic Traditional Healers Registration. Jakarta, Ministry of Health, Republic of Indonesia, 1973.

Minister of Health Regulation No. 246/Menkes/Per/IV/1990 regarding Licenses of Traditional Medicine Industry and Registration. Jakarta, Ministry of Health, Republic of Indonesia, 1990.

Minister of Health Regulation No. 661/Menkes/Per/VII/1994 regarding the Quality Requirement for Traditional Drug. Jakarta, Ministry of Health, Republic of Indonesia, 1994.

Ritiasa K, Handayani L. The role of jamu (Indonesian herbal medicine) for facing the need for drugs. *Folica Medica Indonesiana,* 2002, XXXVIII October–December:282.

Sarjaini I et al. The use of herbal medicines by household members in Java – Bali, based on Household Health Survey 1995. National Institute of Health Research and Development Media. *A journal of National Institute of Health Research and Development,* Vol. VII (March–April), 1998.

Supardi S et al. *The use of TM/CAM at the household at West Java, Central Java and Lampung. Study report.* Pharmaceutical R & D Centre, National Institute of Health Research and Development. Ministry of Health, Republic of Indonesia, 1994.

The national health system of Indonesia 1982. Jakarta, Ministry of Health, Republic of Indonesia, 1982.

WHO Traditional Medicine Strategy 2002–2005. Geneva, World Health Organization, 2002 (WHO/EDM/TRM/2002.1).

CHAPTER 14

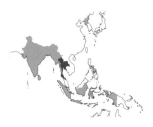

KINGDOM OF THAILAND

Pennapa Subcharoen[1]
and Anchalee Chuthaputti[2]

1 Deputy Director-General, Department for Development of Thai Traditional and Alternative Medicine, Ministry of Public Health, Tiwanont Road, Nonthaburi 11000, Thailand. E-mail: pency@dtam.moph.go.th

2 Senior Pharmacist, Institute of Thai Traditional Medicine, Department for Development of Thai Traditional and Alternative Medicine, Ministry of Public Health, Tiwanont Road, Nonthaburi 11000, Thailand. E-mail: anchalee@dtam.moph.go.th

14.1. INTRODUCTION

The Kingdom of Thailand has her own system of traditional medicine called "Thai traditional medicine" (TTM), which originated during the Sukhothai period (1238–1377) and developed progressively as a means of national health care until the early 20th century when it began to be replaced by modern medicine as the mainstream health-care system. The revival of TTM and the promotion of the use of herbal medicines and medicinal plants for primary health care began again in 1978. The Thai Traditional Medicine and Pharmacy Coordinating Centre was established in 1989 under the Office of the Permanent Secretary of Public Health, as a coordinating organization to develop TTM. The Centre later became the Institute of Thai Traditional Medicine (ITTM) under the Department of Medical Services in 1993 (1).

As a result of Bureaucratic Reform Act 2002, the Department for Development of Thai Traditional and Alternative Medicine (DTAM) was established as a new department under the Ministry of Public Health (MOPH) in October 2002 (2). ITTM was then moved to be an institute under DTAM and the Division of Alternative Medicine was also set up under DTAM (3). The establishment of DTAM showed the commitment of the government to promote TTM and complementary and alternative medicine (CAM) as other means of health care and health promotion for Thai people.

14.2. POLICY

Based on the 9th National Economic and Social Development Plan (2002–2006), the current National Health Development Plan states that MOPH will support the development of the body of knowledge of TTM and CAM and the use of herbal medicines at the general and community hospital levels (4). The Government also pledged in its public health policy to support the promotion and systematic development of the knowledge and standards of TTM and CAM and medicinal plants for their effective and safe use in the health service of the country (5). DTAM and the Medicinal Plant Research Institute under the Department of Medical Sciences are responsible for developing and implementing action plans. As a result of the national policy, a survey by ITTM showed that in the year 2003, 83.3% of regional/general hospitals and 67.8% of community hospitals in Thailand provided at least one type of TTM service.

14.3. REGISTRATION AND CONTROL

Under the Practice of the Art of Healing Act B.E. 2542 (1999), the professional committees, namely the TTM Committee and the Applied TTM Committee are responsible for the registration and licensing of TTM and applied TTM practitioners, respectively. The Division of Medical Registration, Department of Medical Service Support, MOPH, serves as the secretariat of the two committees. In addition, the committees are also responsible for setting standards of professional practice, giving advice to academic institutions on their teaching curricula, and considering professional misconduct of practitioners and appropriate measures of punishment (6).

In 2002, MOPH issued two Ministerial Regulations regarding the types of TTM practices and the personnel who are allowed to practise in the health-care facilities. They include licensed 'Thai traditional medicine practitioners', licensed 'applied Thai traditional medicine practitioners' or persons who have fulfilled the training in the fields of TTM using the curricula of MOPH. Their practice must, however, be under the supervision of a licensed medical doctor.

These personnel are allowed to:

- provide basic health care using herbal medicines listed in the National List of Essential Drugs, household traditional medicines, and herbal medicines from medicinal plants selected for primary health care;

- give massage, herbal steam bath and hot herbal compress services, give advice to the patients on "Ruesi Dud Ton" (Thai-styled series of exercises), and meditation therapy, promote physical and mental health, relieve and rehabilitate certain diseases and symptoms.

14.4. EDUCATION

The systematic teaching of TTM is divided into several different education systems:

1) The system that produces Thai traditional pharmacy practitioners and Thai traditional medicine practitioners. Under this educational system, a student is not required to finish high school. The curriculum is divided into a one-year curriculum in traditional pharmacy, followed by a two-year curriculum in traditional medicine practices in order to become a TTM practitioner. The schools which provide this educational system include:

   - The Society of Schools of Traditional Medicine. Some schools are associated with and located in Thai Buddhist temples.

   - Institute of Thai Traditional Medicine and Thai Traditional Medicine Development Foundation. In addition to teaching TTM and Thai traditional pharmacy, various training courses in Thai traditional massage are also offered.

   - Teacher–student system of teaching and learning. An informal form of education in which a person learns the principles and the practices of Thai traditional pharmacy, medicine, or midwifery from a teacher who is a licensed practitioner.

2) The system that produces applied Thai traditional medicine practitioners commonly called Ayurvedic doctors. In this three-year education system, the students must be high-school graduates. Some basic life science subjects, e.g. anatomy, physiology, biochemistry and botany, are taught together with the courses on Thai traditional pharmacy, medicine and massage. Ayurvedic doctors are allowed to use stethoscopes, thermometers, and sphygmomanometers for physical examination of the patients in order to achieve a better diagnosis and rule out serious illnesses that require modern medical treatment. The schools which offer this system of education include:

   - *Ayurved Vidhayalai (Jevaka Komarapaj) College*, the first school that offered this form of education, founded by Professor Dr Ouy Ketusigh, who contributed significantly to the revival of TTM. The school has recently been moved under the administration of the Faculty of Medicine, Siriraj Hospital, Mahidol University and the curriculum will be adjusted to a bachelor's degree level with more clinical practice training.

   - *Rajamangkala Institute of Technology Pathumthani Campus*. This Institute has offered an applied TTM curriculum since 1999 and the curriculum will be improved to a bachelor's degree level in the future.

3) The system which teaches TTM at a bachelor's degree level. An increased interest in TTM and CAM among the Thai people prompted many universities and academic institutions to offer bachelor's degree education in TTM. In addition to the study of TTM, the curricula also cover basic life sciences and social sciences. The first two universities shown below have already started teaching the course, while the rest will open their bachelor's degree programme soon.

   - *Mahasarakharm University*, Faculty of Pharmacy in Mahasarakharm province in the northeast of Thailand;

- *Rangsit University*, Faculty of Oriental Medicine;

- *Sukhothai Thammathirat Open University*, the first open university that offers the bachelor's degree course in TTM starting from June 2004;

- *Mahidol University*, Faculty of Medicine at Siriraj Hospital;

- *Thammasat University*, Faculty of Medicine;

- *Ramkhamhaeng University*.

In summary, regardless of the system a person chooses to receive an education in TTM, he or she must take examinations given by the Division of Medical Registration in order to become a licensed practitioner. Currently, there are four types of licensed practitioners and, as of the year 2003, the cumulative numbers of these practitioners were as follows (7):

- TTM practitioners — 14 912

- Applied TTM practitioners — 379

- Thai traditional pharmacy practitioners — 18 997

- Thai traditional midwifery practitioners — 2869

14.4.1. Training and education in Thai traditional massage

Thai traditional massage is a branch of TTM which uses manual therapy to treat several diseases and symptoms and for relaxation. It is now becoming popular and well-known worldwide and various institutes offer training courses in Thai traditional massage. Therefore, DTAM together with the Department of Labour have developed three levels of national occupational skill standards of Thai traditional massage, based on the curricula of MOPH, in an attempt to standardize the skill of Thai traditional masseurs and masseuses for consumer protection. Skill tests are then given periodically by the Ministry of Labour in collaboration with DTAM. Moreover, the Division of Medical Registration is now working on a plan to license traditional masseurs and masseuses for consumer protection purposes in the future.

14.5. Financing

DTAM received a fiscal budget of 95 and 120 million bahts (US$ 1 is about 40 bahts) for the fiscal years 2003 and 2004, which was 0.22% and 0.27% of the fiscal budget of MOPH, respectively. In addition, ITTM also receives financial support for some of its activities from the Thai Traditional Medicine Development Foundation, a non-profit organization established in November 1996 to support the development of TTM.

Regarding the national health insurance system, the types of TTM services in public health-care facilities covered by the Universal Coverage Programme are traditional herbal medicine, massage, herbal steam bath and hot herbal compress meant for the treatment and rehabilitation purposes, not for health promotion purposes.

14.6. Research and Information

According to the policies of the National Research Council of Thailand and MOPH, the body of knowledge of TTM and CAM and development of new herbal drugs from medicinal plants are regarded as important areas of health research of the country. Collaborative research projects that pool experienced researchers and resources from various research institutes, and are product-oriented and complete-cycle in nature, are given high priority for funding. Several research and academic institutes in Thailand are actively researching medicinal plants to develop easy-to-use modern dosage forms and to establish the efficacy, safety and quality of the herbal products. In addition, DTAM and universities also conduct research on the bodies of knowledge of TTM and CAM.

Over the years, ITTM has disseminated the information on TTM in various forms, e.g. seminars, books, video cassettes and compact discs, posters, pamphlets, and web pages. The knowledge is distributed to the public at all levels in hospitals and health centres, and through radio, television, newspapers, printed materials, the Internet, exhibitions and road shows.

14.7. Discussion

Regardless of the national policy on the promotion of TTM and CAM in the health-care system, certain laws and regulations still hinder the move. For example, the 2002 Ministerial Regulation and Drug Act B.E. 2510 (1967) will not permit a TTM or applied TTM practitioner to practise in a public health-care facility that has no medical doctor. This has become an obstacle to the provision of TTM services since Thailand does not have enough doctors to work at the health-centre level. Hence, there has been a movement for the amendment of this regulation.

Although several attempts have been made to promote the use of TTM for health care, traditional medicines are still not widely used by the public, as expenditure on locally-produced and imported traditional medicines during the years 1993–1999 was only 1.2–2.5% of that on modern medicines (8). In order to gain greater acceptance by other health professions and the public, more pre-clinical and clinical research must be conducted to obtain evidence-based knowledge to support safe and effective therapeutic practices and to develop quality TTM and CAM products.

14.8. Conclusions

For successful integration of TTM and CAM into the national health-care system in the future, DTAM places great emphasis on research to prove therapeutic efficacy and safety of the products and therapies, development of certified educational systems and training curricula and collaboration with other public and private sectors, both locally and abroad.

References

1. Department of Medical Services Order No. 112/2536. *The Establishment of the Institute of Thai Traditional Medicine and Pharmacy.* 26 March 1993.

2. Bureaucratic Reform Act B.E. 2545. Section 43. *The Organization of the Ministry of Public Health.* 3 October 2002.

3. *Ministerial Regulation of the Ministry of Public Health on the Organization of the Department for Development of Thai Traditional and Alternative Medicine,* B.E. 2545. 9 October 2002.

4. Summary of the National Health Development Plan under the 9th National Economic and Social Development Plan B.E. 2545–2549 (2002–2006). In: *Public Health Calendar 2003.* Bangkok, Saha Pracha Panich, 2003:26.

5. Policy statement of the Cabinet on public health and family addressed to the Parliament on 26 February 2001. In: *Public Health Calendar 2003.* Bangkok, Saha Pracha Panich, 2003:16.

6. *The Practice of the Art of Healing Act B.E. 2542 (1999). Thai Royal Gazette, Vol. 116 Part 39 a.* 18 May 1999.

7. Number of licensed practitioners registered during 2001–2003. In: *Public Health Calendar 2004.* Bangkok, Saha Pracha Panich, 2004:250.

8. Working group on the analytical study of traditional medicines and herbal medicines. In: Wibulpolprasert S, Chokevivat V, Tantiwes S, eds. *Thai Drug System.* Bangkok, Agricultural Cooperative of Thailand Press, 2002: 279.

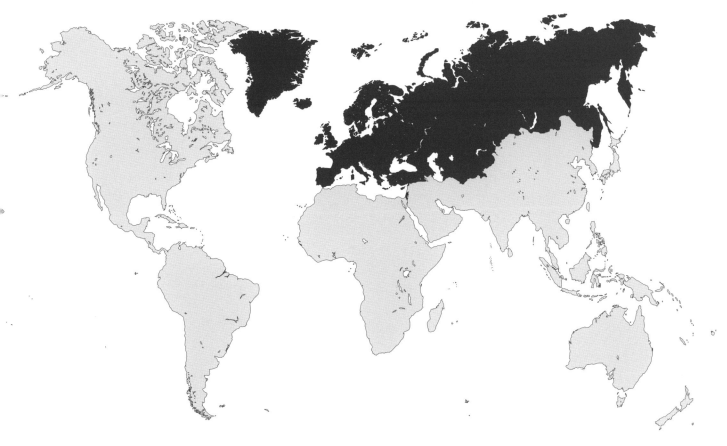

WHO EUROPEAN REGION

REGIONAL OVERVIEW AND
SELECTED COUNTRY CHAPTERS

CHAPTER 15

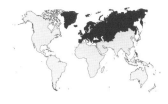

REGIONAL OVERVIEW: EUROPEAN REGION

Chi-Keong Ong[1],
Erling Høg[2],
Gerard Bodeker[3]
and Gemma Burford[4]

[1] Research Fellow in Community and Complementary Medicine, Mansfield College, University of Oxford, Oxford OX1 3TF, United Kingdom. E-mail: paul.ong@ndm.ox.ac.uk

[2] Anthropologist, Department of International Health, Institute of Public Health, University of Copenhagen, Nørre Allé 6, 1st floor, 118, DK-2200 Copenhagen, Denmark. E-mail: e.hoeg@pubhealth.ku.dk

[3] Chair, Global Initiative For Traditional Systems (GIFTS) of Health, and Senior Clinical Lecturer in Public Health, University of Oxford, Green College, 43 Woodstock Road, Oxford OX2 6HG, United Kingdom. E-mail: gerry.bodeker@green.oxford.ac.uk

[4] Research Associate, Global Initiative For Traditional Systems (GIFTS) of Health, University of Oxford, Green College, 43 Woodstock Road, Oxford OX2 6HG, United Kingdom. E-mail: gemmaburford@yahoo.co.uk

15.1. INTRODUCTION

Within the WHO European Region (EUR), there is a wide range of traditional, complementary and alternative medicine (TCAM) currently utilized. However, these systems of health care do not appear to be fully integrated into the formal health services of the respective nations. Within the Region, there are observable and marked differences in the nature and levels of implementation of national policy, legislation, public financing, administration, education and practice.

Changes in the popularity and public perceptions of TCAM in the various countries of EUR have occurred for a variety of different reasons. In western Europe, the advent of the health consumer, with greater disposable income and so-called "green" lifestyle interests, has led to an increased emphasis on the concept of concordance between patient and doctor. Concordance is a process of dialogue between patient and health-care practitioner that leads to the creation of an agreement which respects the beliefs and wishes of the patient. In eastern Europe, there is currently a revival of certain types of TCAM, and growing interest in new therapeutic approaches. There are suggestions that this seems to have followed the easing of social restrictions with the fall of communism. It is also noteworthy that traditional folk medicines still exist and flourish in many countries of EUR.

It is likely that while TCAM is seen as a viable and possibly exotic alternative to allopathic health care in the more industrialized European countries, populations in the newer democracies may resort to traditional systems because they are an accessible and affordable means of health care. It is clear that in many European countries, the use of TCAM is neither a peripheral nor fringe activity. In fact, survey work (1–3) seems to indicate that there is widespread public awareness of recent increases in TCAM utilization and popularity. The concept of concordance will be vital to this era of a modern, pluralistic health-care system.

15.2. BACKGROUND INDICATORS

There is a clear difference in life expectancy between the countries of western Europe (mean 81.4 years for women, 75.1 years for men); those of central and eastern Europe, excluding the former Soviet Union (mean 76.5 years for women, 68.9 years for men); and the emerging economies of the former Soviet Republics (mean 69.3 years for women, 61.0 years for men) (4). The respective differences in life expectancy between western and central/eastern Europe, and between central/eastern Europe and the former Soviet Union, are significant (p<0.05; Student's two-tail t-test) for both men and women. Similar trends can be observed in both infant and maternal mortality.

Data on causes of morbidity are available for only 13 of the 51 countries in EUR. Cardiovascular diseases (disorders of the circulatory system) appear in the top three in all of these countries except Israel, and are the leading cause of morbidity in nine countries. Cancer, respiratory diseases, digestive disorders and accidents also feature highly in a number of countries. It is difficult to determine east–west trends across the Region, because all but three of the countries from which data are available are in western Europe.

Twenty countries have information on causes of mortality, of which 10 are in western Europe, six in central and eastern Europe, and four in the former Soviet Union. Cardiovascular (circulatory) diseases and cancer are ranked first and second, respectively, in all but two of these countries. As in the case of morbidity, no clear east–west trends are evident.

15.3. European Union Initiatives in TCAM

Of the 51 countries in the WHO European Region, 25 belong to the European Union (EU). Prior to 1999, a number of European initiatives had focused their attention on the standardization and harmonization of TCAM at the level of the EU. The 1997 European Parliament Resolution on the status of unconventional medicine in the EU was the result of much work, consultation and compromise between Member States. This reflected the different interests of different nations, as well as the variation between European countries with regard to the nature of governance within the TCAM sector (5–7). The proposed objectives included a clear reference to freedom of health-care choice for patients and practitioners; unified European training and legislation; recognition and professionalization of practitioners; inclusion of TCAM prescriptions into the European pharmacopoeia; and public financing for TCAM. A significant proportion of the proposed objectives were rejected on the grounds of patient safety and the lack of a credible evidence base for TCAM. Research programmes on TCAM were, however, integrated into the European Commission's Fifth Programme Framework for European Research and Development, 1998–2002 (8).

In 1999, the European Parliament made four calls for initiatives to be launched with respect to TCAM. These set out four stages for a comprehensive TCAM programme. First, there was a call for a process of official recognition of various TCAM therapies, with the eventual goal of setting up appropriate commissions for these therapies. Second, with patient and public safety in mind, there was a call to set up a framework to encourage into the safety, efficacy and areas of applicability of different types of TCAM. This remit carried with it the mission to define and categorize the different forms of TCAM. Third, there was a call to initiate a programme to examine and compare different types of national legislation; and finally, there was a call for the development of basic scientific and clinical research programmes into TCAM.

In the same year, the European Commission issued the final report of a five-year project on TCAM carried out under the Cooperation in Science and Technology framework (7). The report emphasized the need for serious consideration of the issue of patient choice, while simultaneously calling upon EU Member States to protect their citizens from under-qualified practitioners in order to ensure patient safety. At its core, it called for safety and efficacy research and a close examination of the system of ethics surrounding TCAM. The report suggested an independent European research office for TCAM, which would encourage the very highest quality research using the tools of evidence-based medicine. The development of research infrastructure for TCAM was also encouraged. The report recommended that TCAM organizations set up boards for licensing and accreditation purposes, and it was hoped that these organizations would oversee guidelines for training, practice and research within their respective fields.

15.4 Structural indicators

15.4.1. Policy and Legislation

The countries of EUR can be divided into three categories, on the basis of their broad legislative approaches to TCAM practice. The first category corresponds to a monopolistic system, which states that only qualified and licensed allopathic physicians may practise TCAM. The monopolistic system prevails in a number of countries throughout Europe, with such legislation being an integral aspect of health-care systems in France, Kyrgyzstan, Latvia, Lithuania, Luxembourg, Poland, Romania, Serbia and Montenegro, Slovenia and Spain. In France, for example, allopathic physicians maintain a strict monopoly over health care, and lay practitioners may be prosecuted, although some continue to practise (9).

The second system would best be described as one which practises tolerance in law, whereby some measure of legislative control, regulation and protection is accorded to non-allopathic TCAM practitioners. Detailed rules for the training and/or registration of non-allopathic providers of named TCAM therapies (other than chiropractic) currently exist in Belgium, Hungary, Kazakhstan, the Netherlands, Tajikistan, Ukraine and the United Kingdom of Great Britain and Northern Ireland.

The final category comprising mixed systems, is a combination of the first two, as exemplified by Sweden, Finland and Denmark. In several cases, chiropractic and acupuncture are regulated separately from other TCAM therapies. Chiropractors have specific licensing requirements and professional or paramedic status in a number of countries, while acupuncture is often restricted to allopathic physicians even when other therapies are unrestricted.

Throughout EUR, there is a general trend towards legalising non-allopathic TCAM practitioners and introducing formal regulation and licensing systems. A number of countries have issued new laws within the past five years, revoking bans on lay practitioners or setting out regulatory frameworks, while others are in the process of developing such legislation. An example is the Czech Republic, where allopathic physicians maintained a monopoly over health care until 2002, when a new Act permitted non-physician homeopaths to practise freely (10). The 2000 Pharmaceuticals Act in the Czech Republic defines medical teas, homeopathic remedies and medicinal plants as pharmaceuticals requiring registration with the State Institute for Drug Control (11). However, the allopathic medical establishment remains generally unsympathetic towards TCAM therapies (L. Bendova, Czech Organization for Traditional Chinese Medicine, personal communication, 2003).

Explicit policies on TCAM exist in five countries of the former Soviet Union — Azerbaijan, Kazakhstan, Kyrgyzstan, Tajikistan and Ukraine. These policies deal primarily with the training and licensing of folk healers, who are permitted to practise without formal medical education in all of the above countries except Kyrgyzstan. In the Russian Federation itself, no official policy exists, although the TCAM sector has been regulated for over ten years. Public health authorities certify potential candidates as having the requisite professional skills in different forms of traditional or folk healing through the issuance of a diploma of healing. This assessment is, however, independent of any formal examination, training or educational requirements. In July 2002, the new Code of Administrative Offences came into force in the Russian Federation, introducing, for the first time, fines for breaching the regulations for practising TCAM. However, since 1993 when the certification system was first introduced, only 3 of 89 regions making up the Russian Federation have enforced the law (A. Goryunov, Institute for Social Development of Natural Abilities, personal communication, 2003).

15.4.2. National Institutions

A variety of national institutions and committees exist in EUR for TCAM control, education and research, although there is no country with a ministry entirely dedicated to TCAM issues. In some countries – Denmark, Georgia, Poland, the Russian Federation, Slovenia, Ukraine and the United Kingdom – there is a TCAM-related department or committee within the Ministry of Health itself. Ireland is in the process of developing a Health and Social Care Professions Council, with a Registration Board for each separate profession. In Kazakhstan, there is a Scientific and Practical Centre of Oriental and Modern Medicine, as well as a Republic Commission for Attestation and Merit Rating of Folk Healers. Belgium, Germany, Latvia, Norway and Ukraine also have TCAM commissions and/or national expert committees, while Sweden, Switzerland and the United Kingdom have national regulatory bodies for chiropractic (and osteopathy in the case of the United Kingdom). Other institutions with TCAM divisions include the National Board of Health in Armenia; the National Institute of Health in Denmark; the National Council for Public Health in the Netherlands; and the Medicines and Healthcare products Regulatory Agency (MHRA) in the United Kingdom.

In countries where there is no dedicated national institution, TCAM issues may be under the remit of other agencies – the Medicines Agency and National Board for Medico-Legal Affairs in Finland;

the National Public Health and Medical Officers' Service in Hungary; and the Ministry of Culture in Turkey. In six countries (Estonia, Israel, Luxembourg, Portugal, the Republic of Moldova and Spain) there is known to be no national institution of any sort whose mandate includes TCAM. There are 22 countries for which information on this indicator is not available.

15.4.3. Professional Organizations and Voluntary Self-regulation

The majority of EUR countries have one or more professional associations of TCAM practitioners. Practitioners of medical acupuncture and/or traditional Chinese medicine are organized into associations in at least 28 countries, and homeopaths in at least 22 countries. In Georgia, there is an association for 'pharmacists, ecologists and producers of medicinal plants' (L. Dateshidze, personal communication, 2003). There are also professional organizations in certain countries for spa/massage therapists, herbalists, reflexologists, chiropractors, osteopaths, nature therapists, folk healers and practitioners of yoga, Reiki, and energy healing, as well as general associations open to all TCAM providers.

There is rarely sufficient information available to determine whether or not these associations function as effective voluntary self-regulatory bodies. Self-regulation implies that membership of the association is restricted to appropriately trained and licensed practitioners; that there is a code of ethics for members; and that individuals who do not maintain appropriate standards of practice will have their membership revoked. Organizations known to fulfil these criteria exist in Denmark, Norway and Sweden (chiropractic); France (osteopathy); Ireland (traditional Chinese medicine); Israel and Latvia (homeopathy); the Russian Federation and the United Kingdom (herbal medicine). There are additional associations working towards voluntary self-regulation in the Netherlands, Norway and the United Kingdom.

15.4.4. Public Financing of TCAM

Virtually all countries in EUR have some form of public financing for TCAM, but the nature, practice and availability varies greatly from country to country. In Germany, the system of reimbursement for TCAM medication changed in 2004 (see Chapter 17). Public health insurance can only reimburse treatments identified within the framework of certain special cases – for example, when allopathic medical treatment has side effects or risks to the patient, or when TCAM would be more cost-effective than allopathic treatment. Public reimbursement is also possible if the aetiology of an illness is known but no allopathic medical treatment is available, or if previous allopathic treatment has failed.

In Italy, part payment of TCAM treatment costs is normal practice, with some variation of proportions by region. The purchase of homeopathic remedies is reimbursable using public funds (*9, 12*).

In certain countries, public finance funds only specific forms of therapy. In Latvia, for example, acupuncture, homeopathy, electro-acupuncture, iridology and bio-resonance therapy are reimbursed by public insurance (*7*). In the Czech Republic (*13*) and Iceland (*14*), allopathic physicians can refer patients for spa treatment – including massage, hydrotherapy, aromatherapy and thalassotherapy – at public expense.

Another relatively common scenario is that national governments reimburse TCAM treatment only when offered by specific types of providers. In Luxembourg, for example, the Government runs acupuncture clinics within public health services, at which treatment is provided free of charge. Costs of acupuncture and other TCAM services obtained privately are not reimbursed. Homeopaths in the Netherlands qualify for reimbursement if they belong to a recognized professional association, whether or not they have a medical degree (*15*). In Finland, public insurance covers treatments provided by registered chiropractors, naprapaths and osteopaths who work in institutions led by physicians or physiotherapists, after referral of patients by a physician (*9*).

In six countries, one or more TCAM therapies can be provided free of charge in standard public hospitals. These are Croatia and Malta (acupuncture), Georgia (herbal medicine), Israel (homeopathy), Romania and the Russian Federation (a variety of treatments including herbal medicine, nutritional therapy, manipulation, light treatment and hydrotherapy). The United Kingdom is the only country in the European Region with dedicated public-sector hospitals for TCAM, in this case homeopathy.

15.4.5. Education and Training in TCAM

There are very wide variations in the way in which education and training in TCAM are implemented within EUR, so that it is difficult to describe general trends within Europe as a whole.

For allopathic physicians within the conventional health-care sector, many countries offer some kind of training in acupuncture and/or traditional Chinese medicine. This varies from optional classes of a few hours' duration within the undergraduate medical curriculum, to full-time or part-time postgraduate diplomas with formal medical speciality status. The Czech Republic has a postgraduate specialization in Balneology and Medical Rehabilitation for physicians (M. Kerpta, Director of Czech Inspectorate of Spas and Mineral Springs, personal communication, 2003). Homeopathy is also a recognized postgraduate medical speciality in several countries, while in others it is incorporated into the undergraduate pharmacy or medicine curriculum.

In Germany, during conventional medical training, the study of naturopathy (including phytotherapy) has become a mandatory subject in medical curricula and examinations since October 2003 (see Chapter 17). Postgraduate medical specializations in TCAM can be obtained in a large number of TCAM practices. State licensing examinations for pharmacists include a compulsory paper on herbal medicines and other "natural healing substances" (*16*, *17*). Likewise, in Georgia, all medical students study the pharmacology and pharmacognosy of certain officially-recognized herbal medicines, licensed by the Ministry of Health's Department for the Activity of Traditional Medicine (L. Dateshidze, NGO Institute of Medicinal Plants, personal communication, 2003).

Hungary has the most highly developed TCAM education programme within EUR. Nationally recognized training is provided in sixteen separate therapies, organized into two categories. Training in so-called higher level therapies such as homeopathy, Ayurveda and traditional Tibetan medicine is restricted to physicians, and taught in medical universities. The Institute for Basic and Continuing Education of Health Workers offers training in nine so-called middle level therapies that do not require a medical degree, including acupressure, massage, reflexology and herbalism. The Public Health Service licenses successful middle level candidates (*7*).

15.4.6. Information and Advisory Services

There are dedicated information centres for alternative and complementary medicine in Denmark (see Chapter 16), Germany (see Chapter 17), the Netherlands and Norway; for homeopathy in the Russian Federation; and for folk medicine in Ukraine. The French Academy of Osteopathy is also in the process of establishing an information centre. The Homeopathic Association of Ireland is a public interest group, aiming to provide unbiased information on homeopathy in Ireland. Bibliographic databases for TCAM are available in the Netherlands and the United Kingdom.

Nine countries – Finland, Georgia, Germany, Hungary, Iceland, Israel, Kazakhstan, Norway and Poland – have national journals or newsletters relating to TCAM, mainly published by professional associations. The British journal, *Homoeopathic Links,* is widely available in Europe, and has been translated into Bulgarian, Croatian, Czech, Portuguese, Russian and Spanish (*18*). A number of professional associations, mostly in western Europe, use websites to provide background information on specific therapies, and have e-mail addresses for enquiries.

15.4.7. TCAM Surveys

Very little data is available for this indicator. For 30 of the 51 EUR countries, no information at all relating to user surveys has been collected. Many of the identified studies in the remaining countries are surveys of sub-populations, e.g. cancer patients or homeopathy users, rather than the general population.

With the exception of Georgia, Israel and Slovenia, the 15 countries in which valid general population surveys have been performed are all in western Europe. Many of these surveys are only just within the 20-year time frame, and only five countries – Denmark (*19*), Georgia (*20*), Germany (*21*), Ukraine (P. Vetrenko, Ukrainian Association of Folk Medicine, personal communication, 2003) and the United Kingdom (*1*, *2*, *22*) – have survey data less than five years old. Another problem is that mainstream literature usually cites findings alone, without describing the methods used, and primary sources have proved difficult to obtain. Population surveys with substantial methodological detail are currently available for only three countries: Denmark (*19*), Israel (*23*) and the United Kingdom (see Chapter 19).

15.5. PROCESS INDICATORS

15.5.1 Most Popular Therapies

Broadly, the most commonly used therapies in Europe are homeopathy, phytotherapy, anthroposophic medicine, naturopathy, traditional Chinese medicine (including acupuncture), osteopathy and chiropractic. However, there is true heterogeneity in terms of which therapies are the most popular in individual countries.

Naturopathy (including phytotherapy) is the most commonly utilized TCAM therapy in Germany, where 52% of surveyed physicians indicated that they used phytotherapy at least occasionally (see Chapter 17). In the United Kingdom, eight therapies were listed as being popular: acupuncture, aromatherapy, chiropractic, homeopathy, hypnotherapy, herbal medicine, osteopathy and reflexology (*1, 22*). The precise definition of what was the most popular therapy was hard to determine in this instance because of methodological flaws in the various surveys conducted in the United Kingdom. These methodological issues highlighted a need to distinguish between practitioner-based therapies, over-the-counter medication and self-practised therapies such as yoga and meditation. Self-medication with over-the-counter products tended to bias the popularity ratings against therapies that were solely dependent on practitioner intervention, such as osteopathy and chiropractic.

There are also particular situations such as pertain in Iceland, where the popularity of different TCAM therapies may be usefully determined only in the years due to major changes in legislation and control structures. Over the past ten years, there have been huge improvements in the availability and official recognition of TCAM services in Iceland. Until the mid-1990s, homeopathy was entirely illegal, and even the import of remedies for personal use was banned. The import of Bach flower remedies was likewise banned, due to their alcohol content. These restrictions have now been removed, and the remedies became available to the general public in pharmacies in early 2002. Iceland is also developing its own herbal industry, based on traditional blended herbal teas and products made from *Cetraria islandica* (Iceland moss), although tinctures are still subject to the strict restrictions on alcohol sales (*14, 24*).

Homeopathy and acupuncture were found to be the most popular therapies in France (*25*), while in the Netherlands, there are now eight formally recognized TCAM professions (presumably reflecting the most popular therapies) – homeopathy, herbal medicine, manual therapies, paranormal healing, acupuncture, diet therapy, natural healing and anthroposophic medicine (*7*).

In Georgia, it would appear that phytotherapy is the most commonly utilized TCAM therapy, probably as a result of its integration into the formal health sector (*20*). Spiritual healing appears to be increasing in popularity. A new private complementary sector is emerging, with qualified doctors taking out licences for herbal creams and ointments, which they use in their own urban clinics (*26*). Within this sector, there is a growing interest in traditional Chinese medicine and particularly acupuncture, provided by practitioners who were educated abroad.

The overall picture is one of great heterogeneity, which suggests that this Global Atlas project is timely in beginning the process of mapping the vast and complex area of TCAM utilization in Europe.

15.5.2. Trends in TCAM Utilization in Europe

Across EUR, there appears to be a trend for TCAM utilization by the general public to increase annually.

In Denmark, the number of persons who have used TCAM at least once in their life has increased from 23% in 1987 to 43.7% in 2000 (*19*). The number who had used TCAM during the twelve-month period preceding the survey increased from 10% in 1987 to 20.6% in 2000. The increase is seen within all gender and age groups, with the exception of women over 67 years of age (see Chapter 16). In the United Kingdom, a survey found that 78% of responders said that they were, or felt that other people were, using TCAM therapies more than they had done five years earlier. Only 6% indicated that they were, or thought other people were, using TCAM therapies less than they had done five years earlier (*1*, *2*). Another study (*22*) estimated that 8.5% of the adult population visited TCAM practitioners in 1993, rising to 10.6% in 1998. Homeopathy was utilized by 16% of the French population in 1982, rising to 29% in 1987 and 32% in 1992 (*3*).

In the Russian Federation, there is evidence of moves to rehabilitate and reintegrate the traditional folk healer after a 70-year ban on healing in any of its forms (A. Goryunov, personal communication, 2003). Recovery of the traditions of ancient folk healing could be linked to a renewed interest in past history, as in Azerbaijan (*27*).

Not all countries within EUR demonstrated a high prevalence of TCAM use. A detailed survey of TCAM utilization in Israel – specifically, visits to TCAM practitioners – was carried out between 1993 and 1994 (*23*) and showed a prevalence rate of only 6%, much lower than other European countries surveyed. The authors suggest that this may be because Israelis are relatively satisfied with the care they receive from the allopathic health system, or because no TCAM practitioners have legal standing and treatment is not covered by public insurance.

15.6. Conclusions

It remains difficult, if not impossible, to give a single clear picture of the status of unconventional, traditional, complementary, and alternative medicines in EUR. The examples presented above give some idea of the complexities that confront any study of TCAM in the Region. Consistency might have been easier to achieve if common research designs (including indicators and terms for surveillance) had been agreed in detail and if more studies, both qualitative and quantitative, had been conducted, at regional and national levels. It is alarming, for example, that so little is known about the numbers of TCAM practitioners on the ground in many countries.

Much TCAM continues to be practised at the grassroots level and criticisms have been levelled at the proposed EU initiatives as being too uniform, broad and unworkable. One need only look to see the multitude of organizational structures that already exist across Europe, each with its own set of professional codes, to realize how complex the task of unifying these organizations will be. The coming years will be a true test of any proposed EU initiative to govern TCAM. Patients, legislators, educators, health professionals, TCAM practitioners, politicians and monolithic national and international organizations will struggle for consensus in their attempt to reform medical legislation within the 25 EU Member States which stretch from the Mediterranean to the Baltic seas. Moreover, within the WHO European Region with its 51 countries, there is even greater diversity of approach to TCAM.

Nonetheless, it is certainly true that TCAM is neither peripheral nor "fringe" in modern Europe. The high levels of consumer investment and interest in TCAM suggest that the evidence base for TCAM needs to be urgently addressed and expanded, in the interest of patient safety within the modern pan-European context. In societies that increasingly value the consumer perspective and the principle of choice in health care, the Global Atlas project provides a basis for discussion of what is meant by a diverse and integrated health service.

References

1. Ong CK, Banks B. *Complementary and alternative medicine: the consumer perspective.* London, The Prince of Wales's Foundation for Integrated Health, 2003 (Occasional Papers No. 2).

2. Ernst E, White A. The BBC survey of complementary medicine use in the UK. *Complementary Therapies in Medicine,* 2000, 8:32–36.

3. Fisher P, Ward A. Medicine in Europe: complementary medicine. *British Medical Journal,* 1994, 309:107–110.

4. *Country statistics.* Copenhagen, World Health Organization Regional Office for Europe, 2001 (http://www.euro.who.int/countryinformation, accessed 15 October 2003).

5. European Parliament. *Resolution on the status of non-conventional medicine.* Brussels, 1997, (http://www.laleva.cc/choice/non_con_medicine.html).

6. Lannoye P. *Report on the status of non-conventional medicine.* Brussels, European Committee on the Environment, Public Health and Consumer Protection, 1997 (Report No. A4-0075/97).

7. Monckton J et al. *COST Action B4: Unconventional medicine in Europe. Final report of the Management Committee, 1993–1998.* Brussels, European Commission Directorate-General for Science, Research and Development, 1999.

8. European Commission. *Fifth programme framework for European research and development, 1998-2002.* Brussels, 1998, (http://www.laleva.cc/choice/non_con_medicine.html).

9. *Legal status of traditional medicine and complementary/alternative medicine.* Geneva, World Health Organization, 2001 (WHO/EDM/TRM/2001.2).

10. Viksveen P, Gordon S. The future of the practice of homeopathy in Europe. *Homeopathic Link,* 2002, 15:77–79.

11. *Pharmaceuticals Act 2000.* Prague, Ministry of Health, Government of the Czech Republic, 2000.

12. Jütte R. *Homöopathie im europäischen trend. [European trends in homeopathy].* Biologische Medizin, 1999, 28:242–247.

13. Thorne S. Spas accepted part of health care in Czech Republic. *Canadian Medical Association Journal,* 1995, 153:94–95.

14. Veal L. Complementary therapies in Iceland. *Complementary Therapies in Nursing and Midwifery,* 1997, 3:12–15.

15. Finne B, Viksveen P. *A survey of ten countries where homeopathy is being practised.* Oslo, Norske Homeopaters Landsforbund *[Norwegian Homeopathic Assocation]*, 1999.

16. Huber R. Symposium: *Übersicht über den Versorgungsschwerpunkt Anthroposophische Medizin in Deutschland [Overview of treatments focusing on anthroposophic medicine in Germany].* München, Forum Universitärer Arbeitsgruppen für Naturheilverfahren und Komplementärmedizin, 2003.

17. Linde K. *Symposium: Übersicht über den Versorgungsschwerpunkt Phytotherapie in Deutschland [State of phytotherapy in Germany]* München, Forum Universitärer Arbeitsgruppen für Naturheilverfahren und Komplementärmedizin, 2003.

18. Anonymous. LINKS going East. *Homoeopathic Links,* 2002, 15:14.

19. Kjøller M, Rasmussen NK, eds. *Sundhed & sygelighed i Danmark 2000 – og udviklingen siden 1987 [Health and morbidity in Denmark 2000 – and the development since 1987].* Copenhagen, National Institute of Public Health, 2002.

20. Dateshidze L. Georgian pharmaceutical market and marketing of pharmaceutical preparations in Georgia. *Caucasus Medical-Biological Journal,* 2000, 1. (http://gps.iatp.org.ge/Stat-Dateshidze3.htm, accessed 13 May 2004).

21. Kahrs M et al. Alternative Medizin – Paradigma für veränderte Patienten–Ansprüche und die Erosion medizinischer Versorgungsstrukturen? *['Alternative medicine' – A paradigm for changed patients requirements and erosion of the medical health care system?]* Arbeit und Sozialpolitik, 2000, 54:20–31.

22. Thomas KJ, Nicholl JP, Coleman P. Use and expenditure on complementary medicine in England: a population based survey. *Complementary Therapies in Medicine,* 2001, 9:2–11.

23. Bernstein JH, Shuval JT. Nonconventional medicine in Israel: consultation patterns of the Israeli population and attitudes of primary care physicians. *Social Science and Medicine,* 1997, 44:1341–1348.

24. Veal L. A comparison of the use of complementary therapies in Australia and Iceland. *Complementary Therapies in Nursing and Midwifery,* 2001, 7:72–77.

25. Ullman D. The French lead: time for Britain to catch up. *Homoeopathy Today,* 1987, 2:7.

26. Waters E. Medicinal plants in Soviet and post-Soviet Georgia. *European Journal of Herbal Medicine,* 2001, 5:5–13.

27. Alakbarov F. Scents that heal: aromatherapy in ancient Azerbaijani medicine. *Azerbaijan International,* 2001, 9:60–63.

CHAPTER 16

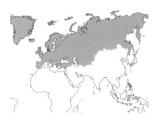

KINGDOM OF DENMARK

Erling Høg

Anthropologist, Department of International Health, Institute of Public Health,
University of Copenhagen, Nørre Allé 6, 1st floor, 117, DK-2200 Copenhagen, Denmark.
E-mail: e.hoeg@pubhealth.ku.dk

16.1. INTRODUCTION

The use of traditional, complementary and alternative medicine (TCAM) (usually referred to as 'alternative therapies') in Denmark has increased significantly since the 1970s. There are no national educational requirements for alternative therapists, but several self-regulating independent associations exist. The most popular therapies are reflexology, massage/manipulation, natural medicinal products, acupuncture, and relaxation therapy. A National Board of Alternative Therapies was founded in 1985, followed by an independent Knowledge and Research Centre in 1998. A law concerning a system of voluntary registration of alternative therapists entered into force on 1 June 2004.

16.2. BACKGROUND INDICATORS

The ten most common causes of morbidity in Denmark are: diseases of the circulatory system; neoplasm; external causes (e.g. injury, poisoning); pregnancy, childbirth and puerperium; diseases of the digestive system; diseases of the respiratory system; 'symptoms' and other ill-defined conditions; diseases of the musculoskeletal system and connective tissue; diseases of the genitourinary system; and diseases of the nervous system and sensory organs. The ten most common causes of mortality are: ischaemic heart disease; cerebrovascular disease; malignant neoplasm (of sites other than larynx, trachea, bronchus and lung); other forms of heart disease; bronchitis, emphysema and asthma; malignant neoplasm of larynx, trachea, bronchus and lung; 'symptoms' and other ill-defined conditions; all accidents (other than motor vehicle accidents); diseases of arteries, arterioles and capillaries; and mental disorders.

In 2001 there were a total of 18 167 physicians and 5319 dentists in Denmark. There are no systematic studies of the number of practitioners of alternative therapies, either within or outside the allopathic health system. In 2003, the Danish Parliament agreed to implement voluntary registration of such practitioners by organizations approved by the health authorities by June 2004. Requirements will focus on membership of professional organizations, education, quality and ethics of practice. It is estimated that 15 000 persons hold some kind of alternative health education, of whom approximately 2000 make a living from their practice.

In 2002, the total health expenditure for the allopathic health care sector was 92.8 billion Danish kroner (c. US$ 14.85 billion).

16.3. STRUCTURAL INDICATORS

16.3.1 Policy and Legislation

Alternative treatments are defined, from a legal point of view, as 'those therapies which are beyond the treatments offered by the state financed health care system and excluded from the supervisory control administered by the Danish National Board of Health'. There is no alternative medicine provision subject to regulation of a general nature in terms of minimum education or standard examinations. However, chiropractors are regulated, and are no longer considered 'alternative' from a legal point of view.

In Denmark the entitlement to provide alternative therapy belongs to everyone, as the quackery chapter in Danish Practise of Medicine Act implies that "anyone may care for the ill", regardless of education, with certain limitations. Persons without medical authorization may not treat venereal diseases, tuberculosis or other infectious diseases; perform surgery or anaesthesia; support delivery; use prescription medicine; perform X-ray examinations or radium treatment; or use electrical apparatus in treatment. Furthermore, there are specific limitations mentioned in other laws concerning authorization of health professionals. Physicians are allowed to use any therapy they deem appropriate to ameliorate illness, based on the wide-ranging legitimacy of their comprehensive medical education and within the limits of their obligation to exercise care and conscientiousness in the performance of their duties. Other professionals, such as nurses and midwives, are permitted to use only the skills included in their legally-recognized education and are obliged to perform their duties within the framework of the regulation concerning their authorization, unless supervised by a medical doctor. In principle, a medical doctor may delegate any task to an assistant, regardless of the education and background of this assistant. Whether a given alternative practice is permissible in a hospital setting varies according to local medical authorities.

16.3.2. Alternative Therapy Control, Education, Information and Research

Currently, all alternative therapies are monitored by quackery laws. In order to remove alternative therapies from these general laws, regulation of TCAM education must begin. This regulation would require a publicly-recognized education system, in which appropriate authorities assess the qualifications needed to practise a health profession. Without such educational requirements, alternative therapies are left uncontrolled until their effects can be scientifically proven.

The Council Concerning Alternative Treatment under the National Board of Health, supplemented by the Knowledge and Research Centre for Alternative Medicine, is engaged with questions on alternative therapies. The Research Centre is an independent institution endorsed and organized under the Ministry of the Interior and Health. The report of a questionnaire-based study carried out in 1995 lists 82 training programmes in alternative therapies (1).

The Danish Medical Research Council decided to take initiatives within the field of alternative treatment in its strategy plan for 1998–2002. A research group has been established, developing its activities in cooperation with alternative practitioners and researchers. Three areas have been prioritized; networking, research methods, and training of researchers.

16.3.3. National Voluntary Self-regulatory Mechanisms

National voluntary self-regulatory mechanisms include the Health Council, the National Organization Council of Nature Health, and the Danish Society for Holistic Health Perception, all in which membership is based on ethical and educational standards. There are several other self-regulatory associations and schools, all of which are permitted in the tolerant Danish system.

16.3.4. Public Sector Financing of Alternative Therapies

All residents in Denmark are entitled to health care, including free hospital care and benefits, under the Health Care Reimbursement Scheme. In general, there is no public financial support for alternative treatment. The exception is acupuncture, which is free if provided by a general practitioner or within the hospital system by an anaesthetist or a rheumatologist. In addition, the Health Care Reimbursement Scheme covers a part of the costs for chiropractic treatment.

16.3.5. Out-of-pocket payments

There are no systematic studies or estimates of out-of-pocket payments or total national expenditure for alternative therapy utilization. A rough estimate suggests that if there are 2000 alternative practitioners making a living from their practice, and their average income is 250 000 Danish kroner per year, then the total out-of-pocket payment for alternative therapies will be 500 million Danish kroner (80 million US dollars).

16.3.6. User surveys

National surveys on the use of alternative and complementary therapies were published in 1987, 1995 and 2000 (2, 3, 4). These surveys were all part of larger studies of health and morbidity in Denmark. The numbers of respondents were 4753, 4668 and 16 690, with response rates being 79.9%, 78.0%, and 74.2% respectively. The methods of data collection were face-to-face interviews and a questionnaire completed by the respondents to elicit their subjectivity (what they feel and experience).

Sampling Methods

Each study describes the size and spread of commonly accepted positive and negative aspects of health. The occurrence of the different study conditions (health risks, resources, morbidity, etc.) is made up for sub-groups in the population, e.g. in different age groups, men and women, etc. Localization variables are: age, gender, occupation and occupational status, and urbanization.

Interviewees were shown a card with 12 different alternative therapies: alternative medicine (e.g. homeopathy); reflexology; relaxation; counselling on diet and/or exercise; needle acupuncture; laying-on of hands; massage/manipulation; use of apparatus (including magnetic therapy and radionic treatment); healing; psychotherapy; hypnosis; other. They were asked: "Have you ever (or within the last year) used practitioners outside the common health system, and for example used some of the treatments shown on this card?". Additionally, interviewees were asked the reason for seeking this kind of treatment and whether they had taken any natural medicine within a two-week period. If they had experienced any of 14 named common symptoms in the past two weeks, they were asked whether they had on that occasion talked to an alternative practitioner or naturopath.

The authors do not explain their choice of alternative therapies, and definitions were not presented to respondents. The questionnaire was submitted to relevant ministries, councils and professionals to test its reliability. The Institute of Social Research performed a pilot test in 1994.

Results

The results of the studies showed that the number of persons who had used alternative therapy at least once in their life increased from 23% in 1987 to 43.7% in 2000, and those who had used it within the 12 months preceding each survey increased from 10% in 1987 to 20.6% in 2000. The increase was seen in both sexes and all age groups, except in women over 67 years of age. The alternative treatments showing the largest increases in use are needle acupuncture, massage/manipulation and reflexology.

The results also showed common trends in alternative therapy use: those most likely to use alternative therapies were younger age groups, women, the working population (with no marked difference between occupations), and sufferers of chronic illnesses. Additionally, the number of persons using alternative treatments increased as self-assessed health status worsened. There were more users among the early retired than among the working population in general, but there was a decrease in use after the age of 67. The lowest rate of alternative treatment use was found among persons with 10 or fewer years of schooling, and the highest rate among business people. There was no significant difference in use between urban and rural areas.

16.4. USE OF ALTERNATIVE AND COMPLEMENTARY THERAPIES

16.4.1. Popular Therapies

The five most popular therapies are reflexology, massage/manipulation, natural medicinal products (e.g. homeopathy), acupuncture, and relaxation therapy. A distinction between use for treatment and for prevention has not been made.   The most common health problems presented to alternative practitioners include illnesses of the motor system and muscle tension, headaches/migraine, asthma, allergy, eczema and stomach–colon problems. Men primarily present with gastrointestinal problems, work-related injuries and sports injuries. Women primarily present with muscle tension, headaches/migraine, asthma, allergy, eczema, psychological problems and inflammatory disorders (5).

16.4.2. Patient Satisfaction

For visits to alternative therapists in general, a 1990 study showed that 23% of the patients reported that they had been totally cured, 45% said that their condition had improved, and 32% said that they found no effect (6). In a later study, 33% were cured; 44% were helped, but not cured; 17% found no effect; and 1% reported that their health problem had worsened (7).

16.5. Discussion

The Danish model characterizes a tolerant system, as it allows unofficial treatment with certain limitations. Historically, this tolerance stems from a revision of the Medical Law in 1934. The Medical Law Commission proposed four options for unauthorized treatment: absolute prohibition, complete freedom, special responsibility legislation for the treatment of disease by non-physicians, and limited authorization to non-physicians (8). The Commission allowed for quackery with certain limitations, since they did not want to hinder "human beings seeking help anywhere they mean to find it". Thus, quacks had certain responsibilities without any form of authorization (8). This remains the current legislation.

In turn, the patient makes choices based on factors such as the practitioner's local reputation, mutual sympathy, treatment costs, accessibility and efficacy. In other words, patients, practitioners, and the general public recognize alternative therapy.

In 2000, the National Board of Health issued a memorandum concerning legal and health problems connected with use in treatment of needle acupuncture by non-physicians. According to the memorandum the resources needed from the National Board of Health, medical officers and the police to examine and unravel the field of non-physicians' use of acupuncture in violation of Section 25 (2) of the Practise of Medicine Act, far outweighed the risks this therapy posed to the population. This assessment was not based on surveillance but on the fact that over several years, no patients have presented to the National Board of Health with damage incurred through treatment by a non-physician.

16.6. Summary and Conclusions

Traditional, complementary and alternative medicine is widely used in Denmark. For every full time alternative practitioner, there are 12 allopathic prescribers (physicians and dentists), while many more engage in informal practice of traditional, complementary and alternative medicine.

The majority of patients present with common illnesses (e.g. muscle tension, headaches, allergies). The estimated out-of-pocket payment for alternative therapies is significant, estimated as 500 million Danish kroner (US$ 80 million) in 2003, yet small compared to the total allopathic health expenditure at 92.8 billion Danish kroner (c. US$ 14.85 billion).

Since 1934, Danish law has considered alternative therapies as quackery. However, the Danish health system tolerates alternative practitioners, as long as no significant harm is done. More research has been conducted over the last decades, while practitioners have become increasingly well organized. Any given alternative treatment is not paid for by the national health security until it has been recognized by law and/or science, like chiropractic and physician acupuncture. This means that all other traditional, complementary and alternative treatments are not paid for by the national health security scheme, which provides free allopathic treatment from general practitioners and hospitals. Ultimately, practitioners of TCAM in Denmark live with the dilemma of their relative freedom and toleration under current medical law and their efforts to regulate and gain independent state recognition, removed from the provisions of quackery law. The National Board of Health points to developments in TCAM in Norway and Sweden, leaving it to the Ministry of the Interior and Health to take decisions on how best to regulate alternative therapies.

Acknowledgement: The review of this chapter by the Ministry of the Interior and Health and the National Board of Health of Denmark with the involvement of Ms Karen Worm of the Ministry is greatly appreciated.

References

1. Hofmeister E. *Alternative Behandleruddannelser i Danmark [Alternative Practitioner Education in Denmark]*. Copenhagen, The Council Concerning Alternative Treatment, 1996.

2. Rasmussen NK et al. *Sundhed og sygelighed i Danmark 1987. En rapport fra DIKEs undersøgelse [Health and morbidity in Denmark 1987. A report from the study by DICE]*. Copenhagen, Danish Institute of Clinical Epidemiology, 1987.

3. Kjøller M et al. *Sundhed og sygelighed i Danmark 1994 – og udviklingen siden 1987 [Health and morbidity in Denmark 1994 – and the development since 1987]*. Copenhagen, Danish Institute of Clinical Epidemiology, 1995.

4. Kjøller M, Rasmussen NK, eds. *Sundhed og sygelighed i Danmark 2000 – og udviklingen siden 1987 [Health and morbidity in Denmark 2000 – and the development since 1987]*. Copenhagen, National Institute of Public Health, 2002.

5. Launsø L. *Brug og Bruger-erfarede Virkninger af Alternativ Behandling – En Sammenfatning [Use and user experienced effects of alternative treatment – a summary]*. Copenhagen, The Council Concerning Alternative Treatment, 1995.

6. Andersen JG. *Overtro eller nytænkning? Befolkningens brug af og holdning til alternative behandlingsformer [Superstition or new thinking? The use of and attitude to alternative forms of treatment in the population]*. Working Paper No. 62. Aarhus, Centre for Cultural Research, University of Aarhus, 1990.

7. Launsø L. *Det alternative behandlingsområde. Brug og udvikling; rationalitet og paradigmer [The field of alternative treatment. Use and development; rationality and paradigms]*. Copenhagen, Akademisk Forlag, 1995.

8. Nehm J, Thorning S, von Magnus M. *Lægeloven. Lov om udførelse af lægegerning med kommentarer [Medical law. Law about the medical practice with commentaries]*. Copenhagen, Jurist- og Økonomforbundets Forlag, 1990.

Bibliography

Akasha ES. *Egen bekendtgørelse – endelig! [Own order – finally!]*. Copenhagen, DAP, 2002 (http://www.dap.dk/pdf/egenbekendt.pdf, accessed 19 March 2004).

Aktive medlemmer i SAB [Active members of SAB]. Danish Association of Alternative Practitioners, 2004 (http://www.alternativ-behandling.dk/SABhjemmeside/allemedl.html, accessed 22 March 2004).

Alternativ behandling: skrappere kontrol og flere tilskudsmuligheder [Alternative treatment: tougher control and more subsidies]. Copenhagen, Gallup Institute, 1993.

Bekendtgørelse om uddannelsen til afspændingspædagog. BEK nr 194 af 2 April 2002 [Departmental order on the educational structure for relaxation pedagogy. Order no. 194 of 2 April 2002]. Copenhagen, Ministry of Education, Denmark, 2002 (http://www.retsinfo.dk, accessed 3 June 2003).

Bekendtgørelse om uddannelser i klinisk biomekanik ved Odense Universitet. BEK nr 870 af 26. november 1997 [Departmental order on education in clinical biomechanics at Odense University. Order no. 870 of 26 November 1997]. Copenhagen, Ministry of Education, Denmark, 1997 (http://www.retsinfo.dk, accessed 4 June 2003).

Health Council. Copenhagen. Health Council, 2004 (http://www.sundheds-raadet.dk/sr/, accessed 22 March 2004).

Health Insurance Denmark. Health Insurance Denmark, 2004 (http://www.sygeforsikring.dk, accessed 22 March 2004).

Johannessen H. *Alternativ behandling i Europa [Alternative Treatment in Europe]*. Aarhus, ViFab, 2001 (http://www.vifab.dk/artikler/alle/alternativ_behandling_i_europa, accessed 22 March 2004).

Johannessen H. *Alternativ behandling i Europa: udbredelse, brug og effekt – et litteraturstudie [Alternative treatment in Europe: dissemination, use and effect]*. Copenhagen, The Council Concerning Alternative Treatment, 1995.

Knowledge and Research Center for Alternative Medicine. *Eksterne Projekter [Research on alternative medicine in Denmark]*. Aarhus, Vifab, 2003.

Knowledge and Research Center for Alternative Medicine. *Forskning [Research]*. Aarhus, Vifab, 2003 (http://www.vifab.dk/forskning, accessed 22 March 2004).

Lov om kiropraktorer m.v. LOV nr 415 af 6 June 1991 [Law on chiropractors, etc., LAW no. 415 of 6 June 1991]. Copenhagen, Ministry of Health, Denmark, 1991 (http://www.retsinfo.dk, accessed 2 June 2003).

Lov om mellemlange videregående uddannelser. LOV nr 481 af 31. maj 2000 [Law on medium length higher education. Law no. 481 of 31 May 2000]. Copenhagen, Ministry of Education, Denmark, 2000 (http://www.retsinfo.dk, accessed 4 June 2003).

Mikkelsen P et al. *Sygesikring. Brugere og fordeling [Health insurance. Users and distribution]*. Copenhagen, Amtskommunernes og Kommunernes Forskningsinstitut, 1988.

National Board of Health. *Vedr.: Lægers benyttelse af medhjælp og lægers samarbejde med lægfolk/ alternative behandlere [Re: Physicians' use of assistants and physicians' co-operation with lay persons/ alternative practitioners]*. Copenhagen, National Board of Health, Fourth Department, 1990.

Percentage who talked to an alternative therapist/healer after suffering pain or complaints within the past two weeks. Copenhagen, National Institute of Public Health, 2003 (http://www.si-folkesundhed. dk/udgivelser/web/SUSY/tabel/649.htm, accessed 22 March 2004).

Retlige og sundhedsfaglige problemstillinger i forbindelse med ikke-lægers brug af nåleakupunktur i behandlingsøjemed. 3. januar 2000 [Legal and health professional problems in connection to the use of acupuncture for treatment purposes by non-physicians. 3 January 2000]. Copenhagen, National Board of Health, 2000.

Ryborg R. *Afspændingsfagets lange vej til anerkendelse [Relaxation therapy: Its long road to recognition]*. Copenhagen, DAP, 2002

(http://www.dap.dk/pdf/langevej.pdf, accessed 22 March 2004).

Skaarup B et al. *Forslag til folketingsbeslutning om en registreringsordning for alternative behandlere. 26 november 2002 [Proposal for Parliament decision on registration of alternative practitioners. 26 November 2002]*. Copenhagen, Danish Parliament, 2002.

Statusrapport om Rådets arbejde 1987–2000. April 2001 [Status report on the Board's work 1987–2000. April 2001]. Copenhagen, The Council Concerning Alternative Treatment, 2001.

Symptoms and complaints. Copenhagen, National Institute of Public Health, 2003 (http://www.si-folkesundhed.dk/udgivelser/web/SUSY/sporg/6.htm, accessed 22 March 2004).

Ugeskrift for Restvæsen. Akupunkturvirksomhed i behandlingsøjemed sidestillet med operativt indgreb i lægelovens forstand. Ikke strafbortfald [Acupuncture activities for treatment purposes compared to surgery as understood in medical law. No exempt from punishment]. *Ugeskrift for Restvæsen*. 1978, 112A:926–932.

Ugeskrift for Retsvæsen. Læge frifundet for straf for samarbejde om akupunkturbehandling [Physician found not guilty in co-operation on acupuncture treatment]. *Ugeskrift for Restvæsen*. 1986, 120A:624–628.

Useful Links

Alternative Info
  http://www.alternativinfo.dk

Association of Alternative Practitioners
  http://www.alternativ-behandling.dk

Chiropractic Education at University of Southern Denmark
  http://www.studieguide.sdu.dk/studier/index.php?uid=15

Danish Chiropractic Association
  http://www.kiropraktor-foreningen.dk

Danish Parliament
  http://www.ft.dk

Danish Relaxation Therapists
  http://www.dap.dk

Danish Society for HOLISTIC Health Perception
  http://www.holistisksundhed.dk

Health Council
  http://www.sundhedsraadet.dk

Health Insurance Denmark
  http://www.sygeforsikring.dk

Knowledge and Research Center for Alternative Medicine
  http://www.vifab.dk

Ministry of Education
  http://www.uvm.dk

Ministry of Interior and Health
  http://www.im.dk

National Board of Health
  http://www.sundhedsstyrelsen.dk

National Institute of Public Health
  http://www.si-folkesundhed.dk

National Organization Council of Nature Health
  http://www.l-n-s.dk

CHAPTER 17

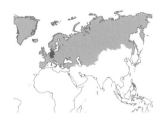

FEDERAL REPUBLIC OF GERMANY

Gudrun Bornhöft[1],
Susanne Moebus[2]
and Peter F. Matthiessen[3]

[1] Chief Coordinator of Centre of Complementary Medicine, University of Witten/Herdecke, Gerhard-Kienle-Weg 4, D-58313 Herdecke, Germany.
E-mail: gudrun.bornhoeft@uni-wh.de

[2] Head, Unit of Complementary Medicine, Institute of Medical Informatics, Biometry and Epidemiology, Medical Faculty, University Duisburg Essen, Hufelandstr. 55, D-45122 Essen, Germany. E-mail: susanne.moebus@uni-essen.de

[3] Chair in Medical Theory and Complementary Medicine, University of Witten/Herdecke, Gerhard-Kienle-Weg 4, D-58313 Herdecke, Germany. E-mail: peter.matthiessen@uni-wh.de

17.1. INTRODUCTION

The Federal Republic of Germany has a long history of practice of traditional, complementary and alternative medicine (TCAM). Since Samuel Hahnemann developed his concept of homeopathy in 1796, and some 50 years later naturopathy was systematized by Sebastian Kneipp, these health care approaches have remained an integral part of the German health-care system. At the beginning of the 20th century, Rudolf Steiner and Ita Wegmann elaborated and extended somatic medicine by incorporating regulative, psychic and spiritual aspects, which gained some importance especially in oncology and paediatrics.

Nowadays, the "traditional" German medicines phytotherapy (as part of naturopathy), homeopathy and anthroposophical medicine, are formally recognized as Besondere Therapierichtungen (special lines of therapy) by a 1978 amendment of the 1976 Medications Law. Physicians can train in homeopathy, naturopathy, manual therapy/chiropractic and balneology as medical specializations. Naturopathy and homeopathy are part of the standard qualifying examinations for medical students, and have become even more integrated in the curriculum by the new form of the German Medical Probationers' Ordinance (Approbationsordnung) which was enforced in October 2003.

Since 1939, in addition to physicians, non-medically qualified healers (Heilpraktiker) have been legally entitled to practise TCAM.

17.2. BACKGROUND INDICATORS

17.2.1. Epidemiology

The population of Germany is more than 80 million. The life expectancy is 80.1 years for women and 73.7 years for men (1), with an infant mortality rate of 3.8 per 1000 live births (2). The main causes of mortality overall are circulatory diseases (47%), cancer (12%), and respiratory diseases (6%). The first two are also the leading causes of morbidity (17% and 12% respectively) followed by injury and poisoning with 10% (2).

17.2.2. Medical Providers

Germany currently has approximately 300 000 physicians, or one physician for every 275 inhabitants (3). Nearly all physicians have undergone further specialist training after the six-year basic training to be a medical doctor. For example, four years of specialist training are needed to train as a general practitioner, and six years for internal medicine or surgery.

There are over 50 000 pharmacists, about 64 000 dentists, 700 000 nurses and midwifes, and about 130 000 physiotherapists, masseurs or medical spa attendants in Germany (3).

Of the 300 000 physicians, over 10% are educated in TCAM, including 13 000 in naturopathy (including balneotherapy), over 12 000 in manual therapy and 4500 in homeopathy (4). About 1000 physicians have been trained in anthroposophical medicine (5). In addition, about 18 000 non-medical TCAM providers (Heilpraktiker) practise in Germany (3).

17.2.3. Health Expenditure

The health expenditure exceeds 3200 (US$ 2654) per capita, or approximately 270 billion (US$ 224 billion) in total (2). This approximates 11% of German gross domestic product (3). There is no detailed information available about the TCAM sector. The expenditure for medications (both allopathic and TCAM) covered by public health insurance increased from 17.1 billion (US$ 14.2 billion) in 1998 to 22.3 billion (US$ 18.5 billion) in 2002. In the same period, the percentage of herbal drugs prescribed decreased from 5% to 3.1% (6). In 2000, the estimated over-the-counter sales of herbal drugs amounted to 1.1 billion (US$ 914 million) (4). In 2002, the market volume of unregulated herbal drugs amounted to US$ 3 billion in Europe, of which Germany accounted for 45% (A. Albrecht, personal communication, 2003)(6, 7).

17.3. STRUCTURAL INDICATORS

17.3.1. TCAM Policy

Until 1999, there was an official TCAM policy. The Federal Ministry of Education and Research funded a number of TCAM research projects between 1981 and 1999 with US$17 million (8). Since then, there has been no further government support.

17.3.2. Regulation of TCAM practice

Professional categories entitled to provide TCAM are physicians, nurses, midwives, physiotherapists, curative eurythmists, painting therapists, music therapists, masseurs and healing practitioners (Heilpraktiker). Qualified physicians are legally entitled to practise homeopathy, naturopathy, acupuncture, and all other forms of TCAM, whether or not they have specific training in the field. Reimbursement, however, is restricted as discussed further in Section 17.3.5. In addition, pharmacists usually give advice with respect to over-the-counter herbal medications.

Non-medical TCAM practitioners (Heilpraktiker) must be licensed. Certain fields and procedures are restricted to physicians, such as anaesthesia, gynaecology, X-rays, autopsy, delivery of death certificates, treatment of venereal diseases and communicable/epidemic diseases, use of prescription-only medications and immunization.

Besides these officially-recognized non-medical practitioners, a number of so-called healers, with no legal recognition, can be found in all parts of the country.

17.3.3. Regulation of TCAM Medications

The German Law distinguishes between foods, dietary supplements (no legal definition), over-the-counter herbal drugs and prescription-only herbal drugs, mainly depending on their potential to harm and the risk of misuse (Arzneimittelgesetz AMG 1976 §48).

The Second Medicines Act (Arzneimittelgesetz AMG, 10th amendment in force since 2000) obliges manufacturers of herbal drugs (as for allopathic drugs) to present pharmacological, toxicological, and clinical data to prove the efficacy as well as the safety of their products. In the case of herbal drugs with well-known constituents only, bibliographic material such as monographs may be accepted in place of primary data. Such monographs are usually provided by the official German Commissions (Commission C for homeopathy, Commission D for anthroposophical medicine, and Commission E for phytotherapy) (7). This is in accordance with the EU Directive (Art. 10.1 (a)(ii) 2001/83/EG) for drugs with "well established medical use" (6, 7).

Alternatively, herbal drugs can be licensed as traditional medicines. They may be indicated only for minor conditions and preventive health care, such as "strengthening", and cannot be prescribed to treat diseases.

Reimbursement by public health insurance (discussed further in Section 17.3.5) is regulated by Social Law (Sozialgesetzbuch V) and special directives.

17.3.4. Regulatory Bodies

Governmental bodies:

  (a) The Federal Ministry of Health and Social Security, which has a legislative function for the entire health service including TCAM, has established three commissions for the CAM specialities: homeopathy (C), anthroposophical medicine (D) and phytotherapy (E) to evaluate the efficacy, safety and suitability of the respective medications. Since their establishment in 1978, they have been situated at the Federal Health Agency (BGA), which became the Federal Institute of Drugs and Medical Devices (BfArM) in 1994. This Institute is charged with reviewing and approving the safety and efficacy of all drugs (*9–11*).

  (b) The Federal Committee of Physicians and Health Insurances issues directives for reimbursement.

  (c) The Federal Ministry of Education and Research can support national research activities. From 1981 to 1999, it focused some of its funding on TCAM research projects.

Nongovernmental bodies:

  (a) The (Federal) Chamber of Physicians regulates postgraduate education of physicians, including TCAM.

  (b) Several voluntary associations of TCAM specialities develop guidelines for training and practice in their respective fields. Some examples are Bund Klassischer Homöopathen (Union of Classical Homeopaths), an umbrella organization for homeopaths; Zentralverein der Ärzte für Naturheilverfahren (Central Society of Physicians for Naturopathy); German Medical Acupuncture Society; German Chiropractors' Association; German Society of Manual Medicine; and German Society of Phytotherapy. The German Society of Phytotherapy works with several pharmaceutical companies to assemble scientific knowledge on medical plants, which is presented to Commission E (see above) for evaluation where required (*12*).

17.3.5. Financing Systems

Until 2003, all herbal drugs were automatically reimbursed unless they were included in a 'negative list' of ineffective or uneconomical medications. From 2004 onwards, however, only prescription drugs will be reimbursed. An over-the-counter list with exceptions (including some herbal, homeopathic, and anthroposophical medications) is generated by the Federal Joint Committee and came into force on 16th March 2004 (*13*).

TCAM treatment by physicians or healing practitioners (Heilpraktiker) must be paid by the patients out-of-pocket, or by private health insurance. Public health insurance can normally reimburse TCAM treatments only in the context of special model projects (§ 63 Social Law) as is currently the case with acupuncture, which is restricted to specialized physicians. Also treated as exceptions are parts of naturopathy such as hydrotherapy which is reimbursed when it is concluded within the scope of a 'regular' rehabilitation treatment. Furthermore, for homeopathy some public insurance systems have made special contracts with (specialized) physicians for reimbursement of time-consuming homeopathic exploration. However, reimbursement may also be made in the following circumstances (*14*) if:

- the aetiology of the illness is unknown, and provided that the treatment has at least a minimum chance of success;

- the aetiology is known but no allopathic treatment is available, or previous allopathic treatment has failed;

- allopathic treatment has side-effects or causes a risk to the patient;

- TCAM is more cost-effective than allopathic treatment.

17.3.6. Education and Research

During the standard allopathic medical training for physicians, naturopathy (including phytotherapy) is an obligatory subject in examinations, and since October 2003 it has been an essential part of the curriculum (*15*). Before that, of the 35 medical faculties in Germany, only 12 provided education in naturopathy (*16*). University departments or chairs exist only in Witten/Herdecke, Berlin, Heidelberg, Freiburg, Rostock, Munich and Duisburg/Essen (the last two include mind/body medicine (*17*). Postgraduate medical specializations in TCAM can be obtained in naturopathy (including phytotherapy), balneotherapy, chiropractic, homeopathy, and from autumn 2004 onwards, also in acupuncture (regulations are still in preparation). Further voluntary training courses in osteopathy, Ayurvedic medicine, and more recently developed areas such as electroacupuncture, bioresonance, Bach flower therapy and others are offered. Anthroposophical medical associations have developed an internationally standardized postgraduate education (*5*).

State licensing examinations for pharmacists include an obligatory paper on herbal medicines and other natural healing substances (*18*). All 22 universities providing pharmaceutical education have established chairs in pharmaceutical biology (*19*).

There is no compulsory TCAM training for nurses or midwives, although voluntary training courses are available.

Most of the healing practitioners (Heilpraktiker) are trained by private Heilpraktiker Schools. There is no mandatory curriculum. The examinations are conducted by local authorities according to federal law, thus standards can vary. The subjects taught include knowledge and diagnosis of specific diseases, and knowledge of legal regulations concerning the profession.

Research is supported by foundations, some health insurances (model projects) and some pharmaceutical companies.

17.3.7. Information

For scientific literature, a centrally organized database (CAMbase) for experts and lay persons has been established (*20*). The Berlin Documentation Centre for Research in Alternative Medicine (*21*) specializes in providing TCAM information. For German-speaking countries, a scientifically evaluated information system will be set up in the near future (*22*). Pharmaceutical companies sometimes provide compilations of information on herbal drugs. Most of the above-mentioned associations (see Section *17.3.6*) have their own journals, which are usually free-of-charge for members and also available to non-members.

17.3.8. Surveys on TCAM Utilization

Some surveys on TCAM utilization have been conducted (*23, 24*), most recently in 2002 (*25*). A health report on the actual situation of TCAM utilization in Germany was published in 2002 (*4*). A general health survey, including considerations of TCAM, was conducted in 1998 (*26*). In 1992 an overview addressed the situation of TCAM research (*27*).

17.4. PROCESS INDICATORS

17.4.1. TCAM Usage

The TCAM therapies used most frequently are: naturopathy (including phytotherapy), acupuncture, and homeopathy, together with nutritional therapies, manipulative therapies and relaxation techniques (*23, 24*). Of approximately 800 physicians interviewed, 52% recommend phytotherapy for their patients at least occasionally (*28*).

The diseases and symptoms most frequently treated with TCAM are cough and/or common colds (24.6%), gastrointestinal disorders (15.3%), cardiovascular disorders (14.3%), anxiety/insomnia (11.8%), pain (7.6 %) and urogenital disorders (7.6%) (*4*).

17.4.2. Sociodemographic Characteristics

In terms of sociodemographic characteristics, 73% of all surveyed people surveyed over 16 years of age had used naturopathic remedies, with a higher percentage of women than men. This represents a considerable increase in use (over 20%) in the last 20 years. In contrast to previous enquiries, the 2002 survey found almost no differences in use of naturopathic remedies between different age groups (in groups over 30 years of age) and education. Even in the youngest age group (16–29 years), 57% of those surveyed claimed to use them at least occasionally. Economic status does not appear to play an important role today: in 2002, more junior employees than executives used naturopathic remedies. Overall, the intensity and frequency of the utilization has increased in the past 20 years, as has the percentage of self-medication. Further increases are expected (*25*). Data show that utilization of TCAM in general varies between 26% and 41% of the population (*4*).

17.4.3. Patient Satisfaction

Of the patients interviewed, 54% stated that herbal drugs or naturopathy improved their conditions. This was particularly true for common colds/cough, cardiovascular diseases, exhaustion and chronic fatigue syndrome and dermatological disorders (*4*). Only 5 % of chronically ill patients who used TCAM stated that they received no benefit (*25*).

17.5. Discussion

TCAM has a long tradition in Germany but despite the constantly-growing demands of patients, TCAM is still under-represented in medical practice, especially in universities. In an enquiry about mind/body medicine, 80% of patients with chronic inflammatory bowel disease expressed a request for "stress resistance therapies", but less than 1% of gastroenterologists knew about these therapeutic options (*17*).

After a governmental TCAM programme supporting research activities (1981–1999), no further special programme has been established to narrow the gap between demand and medical practice. The official policy nowadays seems somewhat inconsistent. On the one hand, naturopathy is increasingly integrated into medical education, while on the other hand, most medications not labelled as 'prescription only' – including many herbal drugs – are no longer refunded by public health insurance.

Despite the fact that many research projects on TCAM have a quality comparable to conventional medical research, acceptance by allopathic physicians is still lacking, especially in universities. One reason seems to be ongoing prejudice and ignorance, so that many studies go unnoticed, including over 1000 randomized controlled trials (RCTs) in phytotherapy, more than 700 in acupuncture and more than 200 in homeopathy (Cochrane CM-Fields database 2002) (*8*). Another reason may be the apparent incompatibility of paradigms; concepts of body energy and spiritual healing are not accepted by the allopathic sector. A third reason is lobbying by pharmaceutical companies, unwilling for their products to be overtaken by cheaper herbal drugs.

The fact that RCTs may be considered as the gold standard may give rise to a number of problems for the TCAM sector. Many TCAM scientists avoid RCTs, not because of ignorance, but because the randomization and blinding procedures interfere with physician–patient interactions and may thus disturb healing processes indirectly. According to this view, the interaction between patient and physician is not considered to bias the outcome assessment, but rather to contribute towards making the benefits of a particular treatment (e.g. herbal drug or acupuncture) manifest. Methods other than RCTs for providing evidence of treatment effects have been discussed in more detail by Kiene (*29*). In addition, it is well known that most patients will refuse randomization when TCAM treatment is available. Furthermore, even when RCTs are considered appropriate, the absence of effective research funding makes their conduct by clinicians and scientific institutions nearly impossible. Even phytopharmaceutical companies, which are mostly small- and medium-seized enterprises, can hardly conduct or support them. For effective utilization of research resources, a Network of German Academic Working Groups for Naturopathy and Complementary Medicine has been established.

Scientific evidence is only one aspect of medicine; economics and everyday life experiences are others. It is the opinion of 60% of the German population that physicians should prescribe drugs and treatment procedures according to their experience; only a minority regards scientific evidence as indispensable (*25*).

The cost–effectiveness of TCAM remains an issue for discussion. On the one hand, TCAM is often used only as an additional treatment for diseases that are already manifest (*25*). On the other hand, with increasing self-medication for disease prevention and minor illnesses, and approaches such as mind/body training for chronic diseases, a significant reduction in medical consultation and expensive medication could be expected (*17*).

There is also a possible ecological aspect to consider, i.e., the increasing water pollution by allopathic drugs such as beta-blockers, currently being investigated at Aachen University of Technology (*30*). Although it appears that there is no acute danger, this phenomenon may occur less if the ratio of herbal to allopathic drugs is increased.

17.6. Conclusions

TCAM is widespread in Germany, especially in the western states. TCAM providers are mainly physicians (about 35 000) and healing practitioners (about 18 000). TCAM is well established in public consciousness, and to a lesser degree in the conventional German health service and medical education. Despite this partial integration, the acceptance of TCAM by the allopathic sector is quite low. The main argument against TCAM is still the conviction of many allopathic physicians that TCAM has no scientific basis. Therefore, one of the major tasks is to establish research methods appropriate to TCAM, which document actual practice and are affordable by physicians and smaller companies. Furthermore, a dialogue between allopathic health care and TCAM—a rational pluralism paying attention to the different lines of thought and the different epistemological vantage points—is necessary. An important step towards a well-balanced relationship between allopathic and complementary medicine in Germany would be the participation of TCAM representatives in official decision-making committees such as federal ministries, research funding societies and other institutions. To overcome their image as a medical fringe group, and to be acknowledged as having equivalent status to allopathic health care, TCAM institutions have to exceed a critical mass. Building up regional and national TCAM centres, and global networking, are essential tasks for the future.

Acknowledgement: An overall review of this chapter by Dr Thomas Hofmann of the Ministry of Health is greatly appreciated.

References

1. *The world health report 2000.* Geneva, World Health Organization, 2000.

2. Favereau F et al. *Healthcare Handbook 4.4, Germany 2003–2004.* Langon, F. Favereau & Associés, 2003.

3. *Health personnel by professions.* Federal Statistical Office, Germany, 2003 (www.destatis.de/basis/e/gesu/gesutab2.htm, accessed 12 March 2004).

4. Marstedt G, Moebus S. *Gesundheitsberichterstattung des Bundes Heft 9: Inanspruchnahme alternativer Methoden in der Medizin [Federal Health Report No. 9: Health care utilization and prevalence of complementary and alternative medicine in Germany].* Berlin, Verlag Robert Koch Institut, 2002 (http://www.rki.de, accessed 10 December 2003), (in German).

5. Huber R. *Übersicht über den Versorgungsschwerpunkt Anthroposophische Medizin in Deutschland [State of anthroposophical health care in Germany].* Forum universitärer Arbeitsgruppen für Naturheilverfahren und Komplementärmedizin, Symposium 07. November. München, 2003 (unpublished document), (in German).

6. Gesetzliche Rahmenbedingungen. *Wissenschaftlicher Informations-Service Dr. Willmar Schwabe Arzneimittel, 2002 [Legal requirements. Scientific information service Dr. Willmar Schwabe Pharmaceuticals, 2002]* (www.schwabe.de/phytothesaurus/content/vortraege/fs_vortraege.html, accessed 12 March 2004), (in German).

7. Steinhoff B. Phytopharmaka in Europa *[Phytopharmaceuticals in Europe]. Deutsche Apotheker Zeitung*, 2003, 44:68–74 (in German).

8. Melchart D. *Viel genutzt, zu wenig erforscht – Zukunft der Naturheilverfahren/Komplementärmedizin an den Universitäten [Often used, insufficient researched – the future of Naturopathic/Complementary Medicine at the universities].* Forum universitärer Arbeitsgruppen für Naturheilverfahren und Komplementärmedizin, Symposium 07. November. München, 2003 (unpublished document), (in German).

9. *German Commission E Monographs (Phytotherapy).* Hamburg, Heilpflanzen-Welt (http://www.heilpflanzenwelt.de/monographien/texts/german_commission_e_monographs_introduction.htm, accessed 31 May 2004), (in German).

10. Steinhoff B. The legal situation of phytomedicines in Germany. *British Journal of Phytotherapy*, 1993/1994b, 3(2):76–80.

11. Steinhoff B. New developments regarding phytomedicines in Germany. *British Journal of Phytotherapy*, 1993/1994a, 3(4):190–193.

12. *Regulatory situation of herbal medicines: a worldwide review.* Geneva, World Health Organization, 1998.

13. Gemeinsamer Bundesausschuss. *[The Federal Joint Committee]*(www.g-ba.de).

14. *Legal status of traditional medicine and complementary/alternative medicine: a worldwide review.* Geneva, World Health Organization, 2001.

15. Bundesgesetzblatt 202 Teil 1 Nr. 44, § 27(1)

16. Stange R. *Komplementärmedizin in Deutschland – Zur Situation in der Lehre [Complementary medicine in Germany – State of the teaching situation].* Forum universitärer Arbeitsgruppen für Naturheilverfahren und Komplementärmedizin, Symposium 07. November. München, 2003 (unpublished document). Parts published as Stange R. *Naturheilverfahren in der Mediziner-Ausbildung – ein Teilerfolg? [Naturopathy in Medical Teaching – a Partial Success?]* In: Kraft K, Resch KL, Stange R, Uehleke B, eds. *Naturheilverfahren und Unkonventionelle Medizinische Richtungen [Naturopathy and Unconventional Medical Therapies]*, Springer Lose Blatt Systeme 2003, 31:1–3 (in German).

17. Dobos G. *Übersicht über den Versorgungsschwerpunkt Ordnungstherapie/Gesundheitstraining in Deutschland [State of mind body therapies/health training in Germany].* Forum universitärer Arbeitsgruppen für Naturheilverfahren und Komplementärmedizin, Symposium 07. November. München, 2003 (unpublished document), (in German).

18. Hartmann J. Naturopathy – definition, importance in the education of physicians and pharmacists. *Öffentliches Gesundheitswesen,* 1991, 53 Suppl. 3:264–267.

19. Linde K. *Übersicht über den Versorgungsschwerpunkt Phytotherapie in Deutschland [State of phytotherapy in Germany].* Forum universitärer Arbeitsgruppen für Naturheilverfahren und Komplementärmedizin, Symposium 07. November. München, 2003 (unpublished document), (in German).

20. *CAMbase – complementary and althernative medicine.* Witten/Herdecke University (www.cambase.de), (in German).

21. *Datadiwan - Bernhard Harrer Knowledge Transfer and Patient Information for Complementary Medicine* (www.datadiwan.de), (in German).

22. *Pan Medion Foundation (knowledge network)* (www.panmedion.org/indexsti.html), (in German).

23. *Naturheilmittel 1997 [Naturopathic remedies 1997].* Allensbach, Institut für Demoskopie Allensbach, 1997 (in German).

24. Kahrs M, et al. *'Alternative Medizin' – Paradigma für veränderte Patienten-Ansprüche und die Erosion medizinischer Versorgungsstrukturen? ['Alternative medicine' – A paradigm for changed patients requirements and erosion of the medical health care system?]* In: *Arbeit und Sozialpolitik 1/2.* 2000, 54:20–31 (in German).

25. Naturheilmittel 2002. *Wichtigste Erkenntnisse aus Allensbacher Trendstudien [Naturopathic remedies 2002. Main outcomes of the Allensbacher trend studies].* Institut für Demoskopie Allensbach, 2002 (http://www.bah-bonn.de/news/Naturheilmittel.pdf, accessed 12 March 2004), (in German).

26. Bellach BM, Knop H, Thefeld W. *Der Bundes-Gesundheitssurvey 1997/98 [The national health survey 1997/98].* Gesundheitswesen. 1998, 60 Suppl 2:59–68 (in German).

27. Matthiessen PF, Rosslenbroich B, Schmidt S. *Unkonventionelle Medizinische Richtungen – Bestandsaufnahme zur Forschungssituation [Unconventional medical trends – State of the research situation].* Materialien zur Gesundheitsforschung. Projektträger Forschung im Dienste der Gesundheit, ed. 21, Bonn, 1992 (in German).

28. Haltenhof H, Hesse B, Buhler KE. Evaluation and utilization of complementary medical procedures – a survey of 793 physicians in general practice and the clinic. *Gesundheitswesen,* 1995, 57:192–195.

29. Kiene H. *Komplementäre Methodenlehre der klinischen Forschung – Cognition-based Medicine [Complementary methodology of clinical research – cognition-based medicine].* Berlin, Springer-Verlag, 2001 (in German).

30. Cleuvers M. Aquatic ecotoxicity of pharmaceuticals including the assessment of combination effects. *Toxicol Lett.,* 2003, 142:185–94.

Useful Links

General Information/Institutes

www.uni-wh.de/komplementaermedizin (*Zentrum für Komplementärmedizin und Lehrstuhl für Medizintheorie und Komplementärmedizin, Univ. Witten/Herdecke [Centre for Complementary Medicine/Chair in Medical Theory and Complementary Medicine University Witten/Herdecke]*), (in German).

http://www.lrz-muenchen.de/~ZentrumfuerNaturheilkunde/ (Centre for Complementary Medicine Research at University Munich/TUM), (in German).

http://www.ukl.uni-freiburg.de/iumwkra/amb_nu/index.htm (University Centre for Complementary Medicine/Section for the Evaluation of Complementary and Alternative Medical Treatment German University Hospital Freiburg) (in German).

http://www.medkur.de/FBK.htm (Forschungsinstitut für Balneologie und Kurortwissenschaft, Bad Elster *[Institute for Research in Balneology and Spa Science Medkur, Bad Elster]*), (in German).

http://www.zdn.de (Zentrum zur Dokumentation für Naturheilverfahren e.V. *[Documentation centre for naturopathy]*), (in German).

www.cambase.de *[CAMbase, University Witten/Herdecke – TCAM scientific literature database]*, (in German).

www.datadiwan.de *[Datadiwan, Patient Information for Complementary Medicine and Bernhard Harrer Knowledge Transfer – database with general information on TCAM]*, (in German).

Phytotherapy

http://www.phytotherapy.org/ *[German Society for Phytotherapy]*

http://www.heilpflanzen-welt.de *[with Commission E monographs in rubric "Heilpflanzen-Infos" – multi MED vision GbR, Hamburg]*, (in German).

http://www.bah-bonn.de/arzneimittel/index.html *[Bundesverband der Arzneimittel-Hersteller e.V. with http://www.bah-bonn.de/news/Naturheilmittel.pdf for Allensbach survey on usage of TCAM 2002]*, (in German).

http://www.bfarm.de *[Bundesinstitut für Arzneimittel und Medizinprodukte: Federal Institute for Drugs and Medical Devices, with http://www.bfarm.de/de/Arzneimittel/bes_therap/index.php for particular therapeutic systems and traditional medicinal products]* (in German). Shortened English version: http://www.bfarm.de/en/drugs/pts/index.php).

http://www.schwabe.de/phytothesaurus *[Dr Willmar Schwabe, Arzneimittel with http://www.schwabe.de/phytothesaurus/content/vortraege/fs_vortraege.html for compilation of indications for medical herbs, legal aspects etc. by Schwabe company]*, (in German).

http://www.madaus.de/cd/frameset_extern/frameset_start.jsp?oid=833 *[Madaus company – database of medical herbs]*.

http://www.g-netz.de/Health_Center/heilpflanzen/ *[Multicom network GmbH]*, (in German).

http://www.heilpflanzen-suchmaschine.de/ *[Biocur company – database of herbal drugs]*, (in German).

Naturopathy including Life Style Management

http://www.zaen.org/ (ZÄN – *Zentralverband der Ärzte für Naturheilverfahren und Regulationsmedizin e.V. [Umbrella organization of physicians for naturopathy, Freudenstadt]*), (in German).

http://www.ugb.de/ (UGB-*Vereine für unabhängige Gesundheitsberatung in Europe [Association for an independent health consulting service]*) (in German).

http://www.dgeim.de/ (*Deutsche Gesellschaft für Energetische und Informationsmedizin [German society for energetic and information medicine, incorporated society]*), (in German).

Homeopathy

http://www.homoepathy.de *Deutscher Zentralverein homöopathischer Ärzte [German umbrella organizations of physicians for homeopathy]*, (in German).

http://www.homoeopathie-aktuell.org/ (*Deutsche Gesellschaft zur Förderung naturgesetzlichen Heilens e.V. [German society for promotion of naturopathic healing, incorporated society, Detmold]*), (in German).

http://www.keimcelle.de *Keimzelle Zukunft – Heilen im Dialog; Niedersächsische Akademie für Homöopathie und Naturheilverfahren – [Lower Saxonian Academy for Homeopathy and Naturopathy, N.A.H.N., Celle]*, (in German).

http://gesundheit.trampelpfad.de/nda/50/Arzneimittel_Hersteller__Lieferanten__Apotheken/ *[Wedekind, Hille – compilation of Companies for homeopathic remedies]*, (in German).

http://www.vkhd.de/ (Verband klassischer Homöopathen Deutschlands e.V.) and http://www.homoeopathie-forum.de/ *Organization klassisch homöopathisch arbeitender Heilpraktijer e.V. – [Professional organization of healing practitioners for classical homeopathy]*, (in German).

http://www.gvs.net *[George Vithoulkas foundation]*, (in German).

http://www.carstens-stiftung.de/ *[Karl and Veronica Carstens foundation]*, (in German).

http://www.homoeopathie-stiftung.de/ *[Foundation of the "Deutscher Zentralverein homöopathischer Ärzte e.V. DZVhÄ" – German umbrella organization of heomeopathic physicians]*, (in German).

http://www.bfarm.de/de/Arzneimittel/bes_therap/am_anthropo/index.php (Bundesinstitut für Arzneimittel und Medizinprodukte – Homöopathika u. Anthroposophika *[Federal Institute for Drugs and Medical Devices]* with Section on "Particular therapeutic systems and traditional medicinal products" (in German). Shortened English version: http://www.bfarm.de/en/drugs/pts/index.php).

Anthroposophic Medicine

http://www.anthroposophische-medizin.org/ (*Medizinische Sektion am Goetheanum mit Informationen zur Anthroposophischen Medizin [Medical Section at the Goetheanum with information about anthroposophic medicine]*).

http://www.bfarm.de/de/Arzneimittel/bes_therap/am_anthropo/index.php (*Bundesinstitut für Arzneimittel und Medizinprodukte - Homöopathika u. Anthroposophika [Federal Institute for Drugs and Medical Devices]* with Section on "Particular therapeutic systems and traditional medicinal products", (in German). Shortened English version: http://www.bfarm.de/en/drugs/pts/index.php).

Acupuncture/Traditional Chinese Medicine

http://www.daegfa.de/ (DÄGfA – *Deutsche Ärztegesellschaft für Akupunktur [German physician's society for acupuncture, incorporated society]*, Munich), (in German).

http://www.atcae.de (*Akupunktur- und TCM-Gesellschaft in China weitergebildeter Ärzte e.V., Wiesbaden [Society of acupuncture and traditional Chinese medicine; WHO accredited incorporated society]*), (in German).

http://www.agtcm.de/ (*Arbeitsgemeinschaft für Klassische Akupunktur und Traditionelle Chinesische Medizin e.V. [Consortium for classical acupuncture and traditional Chinese medicine, incorporated society, Berlin]*), (in German).

http://www.dgtcm.de/ (*Deutsche Gesellschaft für Traditionelle Chinesische Medizin [German society of traditional Chinese medicine], Heidelberg*), (in German).

http://www.dgfan.de/ (*DGfAN Deutsche Gesellschaft für Akupunktur und Neuraltherapie e.V. [German society for acupuncture and neural therapy, incorporated society], Saalburg-Ebersdorf*), (in German).

Osteopathy

http://www.osteopathie-akademie.de/ (*AFO Akademie für Osteopathie e.V. [Academy for osteopathy], Gauting*), (in German).

http://www.osteopathie.de/ (*VOD Verband der Osteopathen Deutschland e.V. [Association of osteopaths, Germany], Wiesbaden*), (in German).

http://www.daao.info (*DAAO Deutsch-Amerikanische Akademie für Osteopathie e.V. [German American academy for osteopathy], Isny-Neutrauchburg*), (in German).

http://www.dgom.info (*DGOM Deutsche Gesellschaft für Osteopathische Medizin [German society for osteopathic medicine], Tenningen*), (in German).

Ayurveda

http://www.ayurveda-gesellschaft.de/ (*Deutsche Gesellschaft für Ayurveda e.V. [German society for Ayurveda], Traben-Trarbach*), (in German).

http://www.mahindra-institut.de (*Mahindra-Institut – The European academy of Ayurveda*), (in German).

http://www.ayurveda-portal.de/ (*Ayurveda-Portal – compilation of useful information and links*), (in German).

CHAPTER 18

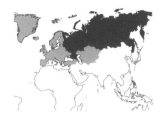

RUSSIAN FEDERATION

Alexey A. Karpeev[1],
Andrey V. Goryunov[2]
and Vladimir V. Tonkov[3]

[1] General Director of the Federal Scientific Clinical-Experimental Center of Traditional Methods of Diagnosis and Treatment, the Ministry of Health and Social Development of the Russian Federation, leading specialist of the Ministry on traditional medicine issues. (Postal address: Russia, 127206, Moscow, Vucheticha str. 12, build.).

[2] Rector of the Institute for Social Development of Natural Abilities (Postal address: Russia, 197198, St-Petersburg, Zverinskaya str., 42 – 22. E-mail: adm@biosens.ru).

[3] Leading specialist of the Institute for Social Development of Natural Abilities on folk medicine issues (Postal address: Russia, 197198, St-Petersburg, Zverinskaya str., 42 – 22. E-mail: tv@biosens.ru).

18.1. INTRODUCTION

Traditional medicine in Russia has a deep-rooted history. Its development is based on traditional methods of healing and recovery to good health predominantly through spiritual healing, the use of medicinal herbs or other natural remedies and bone-setting.

The Russian Federation has a unique basis for the use of traditional medicine in its public health-care system as the country is vast (170 754 000 km²), where live hundreds of nationalities and ethnic groups that have accumulated many cultural traditions in healing and health protection. Thus, there is the Slavic folk medicine, Tibetan medicine that is prevalent in Kalmykia, Buryatia and Tuva, medical practice of Primorie, which is based on traditional Chinese medicine, folk medicine of Yakutia and those ethnic groups that live in north Russia, Povolzhie and northern Caucasus.

There is a significant difference in mechanisms and rules of application between the methods of traditional medicine that are already approved in the public health-care system (i.e. that are scientifically described, studied, examined and officially registered) and applied only by physicians, and the traditional methods of healing, recovery and diagnostics that officially are not allowed in the public health-care system and, therefore, applied only by healers (hereafter referred to as the methods of folk medicine).

18.2. BACKGROUND INDICATORS

In 2002, the population of the Russian Federation was 145.2 million people. Of these, 106.4 million (or 73%) were urban-based and 38.8 million (or 27%) were rural dwellers.

The main causes of mortality in the Russian Federation are circulatory disorders, neoplasm, injuries and poisoning, respiratory diseases, digestive disorders, infectious and parasitic diseases. The leading diseases are respiratory, cardiovascular system diseases, skin and soft tissue diseases, infectious and parasitic diseases, urogenital disorders and digestive conditions. Tuberculosis is again becoming a growing threat for the health of people. Health status varies substantially according to the geographical region, age group and socioeconomic status (1).

At the same time, there is an obvious positive trend in the demographic situation of the country. There has been an increase in marriages and births. The mortality rate has slowed down, the infant mortality rate has noticeably decreased, and overall death rate has declined slightly. In recent years the financial flows to the public health-care system have increased substantially.

The total spending of the state budget for the public health-care system in 2003 was 31.4 billion rubles (c. US$ 1.02 billion); in 2005 more than double this cost is expected. There are no official data about financing of separate sectors of the public health-care system, including the traditional medicine sector. However, it is known that in the traditional medicine sector the government finances only a small part of medical and scientific research on folk medicine methods for the purpose of their application in medical practice.

The total number of medical workers (including physicians, nurses, pharmacists, etc.) is about 2 235 000 people (1). The total number of individuals within and outside the public health-care system, who practice different methods of traditional and folk medicine, is about 40 000 people (2).

18.3 STRUCTURAL AND PROCESS INFORMATION RELATED TO TRADITIONAL MEDICINE

18.3.1. Traditional Medicine in the Russian Federation

Today the Ministry of Health and Social Development (hereafter referred to as the Ministry) recognizes the following traditional medicine classification (3):

1. Types of traditional medicine, recognized by medical science, that are used everywhere in medical practice and classified as medical specialties:

    (a) manual therapy

    (b) medical massage

    (c) reflexotherapy (acupuncture).

2. Types of traditional medicine, recognized by medical science, that are used everywhere in medical practice, but not classified as medical specialties:

    (a) bioresonance therapy

    (b) homeopathy

    (c) naturotherapy (phytotherapy, hirudotherapy, apitherapy)

    (d) osteopathy

    (e) different methods of traditional diagnostics.

The above two groups of traditional medicine relate to medical practice. They are officially approved by the Ministry for application in medical practice and are regularly published in the State Register of new medical technologies (4, 5).

In order to get a license to practice the approved traditional medicine methods, it is necessary to have a high medical education degree, except for massage, for which a secondary medical education degree is sufficient (6).

Types of traditional medicine that are not officially approved for use in medical practice, as they require further study and examination, include separate methods from Tibetan and Chinese medicine, ayurveda, yoga, kinesiology, viscerogenic chiropractic, anthroposophical medicine (Steiner), rebirthing (L. Orr), holotropic breath (S. Grof) and a number of other methods. The Ministry also puts folk medicine into this group (3).

In the opinion of independent research institutions and professional associations of healers, there is a mixing of concepts of folk and traditional medicine and their types. The place of folk medicine in the Ministry classification does not correspond with its actual social status (2) because:

- Folk medicine covers a wider range of healing, recovery and diagnostic methods than the sphere of methods of traditional medicine in the Ministry classification. From olden times it has contained methods that have become the basis for most of the above-mentioned medical methods (groups 1 and 2) and also a variety of unstudied methods of healing and diagnosis, on the basis of which new methods of medical practice can be created (2, 7).

- The place of folk medicine is stipulated by historical and cultural traditions and by its unusual approach to the health of a person that corresponds with the definition of traditional medicine given by the World Health Organization (8). Only the role of folk medicine in the public heath-care system may be numbered and changed, as was done by the Ministry.

- Folk medicine will never become a part of medical activity, which is based on standards, because the effect of its methods depends strongly on the personal abilities of a healer and is directed to the integral regulation of the patient's organism. The methods themselves have a distinct individual nature and at the same time their effectiveness is directly connected with the wishes of a patient (9).

- The title of the Resolution WHA56.31 Item 14.10 in Russian reads as "Folk Medicine", but in English it reads as "Traditional Medicine" (7, 8). Hence, traditional medicine and folk medicine in the Russian Federation must be synonymous. However, in fact in medical practice the term "traditional medicine" is used, but in the society and among healers the term "folk medicine" is used (4, 6, 10).

18.3.2. State Policy in Traditional Medicine

The Ministry, following the WHO recommendations, has taken a number of organizational measures to support, develop and integrate traditional medicine into the country's public health system.

In the infrastructure of the Ministry there is a leading research institution — Federal Scientific Clinical-experimental Centre of Traditional Methods of Diagnosis and Treatment — that works actively on the issues relating to traditional medicine, as well as the Ministry Section of the Academic Council on traditional medicine issues.

A national system of licensing of traditional medicine practices has been established and is currently being implemented. Scientific meetings and practical conferences on topics related to traditional medicine are regularly held under the guidance of the Ministry of Health.

Over 2000 physicians-reflexotherapists and nearly 1000 physicians-manual therapists are currently working in the state system of public health care. There is a steady growth in the number of physicians for whom homeopathy, phytotherapy, hirudotherapy, osteopathy and methods of traditional diagnosis are becoming fundamental medical practice. Over the past five years, the number of licenses granted to the physicians practicing traditional medicine has almost doubled.

The development of traditional medicine requires a considerable increase in the number of trained medical staff. There are 25 postgraduate educational institutions with programmes developed for specialists in traditional medicine and in 2002–2003 over 9000 physicians obtained additional qualifications in specific areas of traditional medicine.

There is no unified professional medical organization (association) in the Russian Federation that would unite and regulate all traditional medicine specialists. There is a number of associations that bring together specialists from different traditional medicine areas, for example: there are three associations of reflexotherapists, three associations of manual therapists, four homeopathic associations, and associations of phytotherapists, hirudotherapists, apitherapists.

18.3.3. Development and Regulation of Medicinal Resources

The creation and use of natural medicines based on the ancient experience of folk treatments is important for further development of traditional medicine. The fact that such treatments are mild, lack side effects, cost comparatively little and have been shown to be effective particularly for chronic illnesses, combined with the fact that people believe in them, means that these medicines are equally attractive to both patients and physicians.

According to the statistics, at least 60% of the Russian population use natural folk remedies, a significant proportion of which are issued without prescription. This raises two issues:

1. First, according to the Federal Law on Medicines No. 86-FZ of 22 June1998, which is currently in force in the Russian Federation, it is compulsory for all medicines to undergo the established registration procedure, which includes pre-clinical and clinical trials, quality control, etc. All medicines without exception, whether they are of animal, plant or mineral extraction, must be submitted to the full registration process. Homeopathic remedies must also be registered in the same way. A registration system has also been established for

biologically-active food ingredients, the majority of which also contain medicinal plant extracts;

2.   Second, is the availability of vast resources of natural remedies. It is well known that biologically active substances extracted from medicinal plants are found in over 65% of all medicines. However, according to the statistics issued by specialists, nowadays only 10-15% of existing medicinal plants are being used for that purpose (for example, over 2500 different medicinal plants were used in Russian folk medicine, but the state pharmacopoeia contains only 250 of them).

The study, development and use of natural substances applied in traditional medicine are opening up opportunities for developing economically beneficial, accessible, safe and effective natural medicines for local production.

18.3.4. Scientific Research in Traditional Medicine

According to the results of a wide range of scientific studies in the area of traditional medicine, the majority of methods have proved themselves effective in the treatment of certain illnesses. There is no doubt of the analgesic effects of acupuncture and manual therapy that are used successfully in neurology, orthopaedic and traumatology. Phytotherapy, homeopathy, certain methods of osteopathy and bioresonance therapy have significant effects in the treatment of chronic diseases. There is a real potential for expanding the opportunities for treatment and diagnosis available to practicing physicians, through widening the application of these methods.

18.4. Structural and Process Information related to Folk Medicine

18.4.1. Social Development of Folk Medicine

Today most aspects of folk medicine — its history, methods, effectiveness, achievements, problems and legal status are not well known in the Russian society. The influence of religion on the application of folk medicine is sufficient. The Russian Orthodox Church is the main traditional religious body in society; it accepts the application of Christian healing — with prayers and herbs, but only in accordance with its canons. Moreover, unlike other religions (Islam, Buddhism, Hinduism, Judaism and others) it forces its position to high society.

Basically, the media does not form a positive perception of folk medicine. Yet the majority of people in their day-to-day life use the simple and effective methods and recipes of folk medicine for stress relief and for the treatment of minor illnesses, such as flu and colds, stomach disorders and minor injuries. Between 60% and 70% of people, when they fall sick, prefer self-treatment with the application of the remedies of both official medicine and folk methods (11).

In the 20th century the gap between folk and official scientific medicine has expanded substantially. Folk medicine was officially recognized only in 1993 in the Law No. 5487-1 (10). The problems of development and regulation of folk medicine in the Russian Federation are still not completely solved. Furthermore, there are no officially adopted norms regulating the consumer market and services provided by folk medicine experts, which create the grounds for speculative practice.

18.4.2. Regulation of Folk Medicine

Folk medicine encompasses the methods of health promotion, prevention, diagnosis and treatment based on the experience of many generations, firmly established in folk traditions and not formally registered according to the procedures set out by the legislation of the Russian Federation (10).

Those practitioners who have received a Diploma in Healing, issued by regulatory bodies of public health care of the federal regions of Russia, are entitled to practice folk medicine. The decision to issue the Diploma in Healing is made on the basis of application by the practitioner and recommendation of a professional medical association (10). To receive the Diploma in Healing it is not obligatory to have a professional medical education degree; it is sufficient for folk medicine practitioner to have relevant experience and the innate abilities (12). By the term "healing" is meant the practice of folk medicine itself — rendering of medical services, i.e. treatment and diagnostics with the help of its remedies and methods (12, 13).

In practice, the transfer of the direct regulation of folk medicine to the regions, taking into account the independence of regional public health-care authorities from the federal Ministry, has adversely affected the development of folk medicine in the Russian Federation. Due to this, it was necessary to create a clear federal policy in the sphere of professional, scientific, educational and methodological issues in the folk medicine area.

Unfortunately, the legislative base as well as the professional, qualifying, social, labour and educational criteria for folk medicine practice are not developed, which seriously complicates its practice. At the same time in the Russian Federation, by the most conservative estimate, about 5000 healers practice folk medicine and this figure is constantly growing (*2*); citizens who practice folk medicine are partly legalized and represented in the society by at least seven professional public associations. Also, in the sphere of folk medicine there are a lot of ideologically- and methodologically-separate small public associations and organizations cut off from the common development and modern ideas of folk medicine (*2*).

18.4.3. Folk Medicine Classification

The uniqueness of Russian folk medicine, linked to the country's vast territory and many ethnic groups, is that it combines a large number of different systems. The methods of folk medicine include:

- Contact-less methods of treatment, disease prevention and diagnostics: spiritual healing that uses prayer, laying-on of hands, affectionate attitude to the patient, bioenergetic effect (contact-less massage, correction of psychic and physical state of a person, correction of energy-exchange processes). There are grounds to consider the processes of energy-informative interactions as the basis for all the above-mentioned methods. They may be referred to as different directions of shamanism, Reiki and cosmoenergetics.

- Folk recipe medicine based on the use of medicinal herbs (herbal medicine) and other substances of natural origin.

- Bone-setting and other physical contact folk methods (massage, Russian baths, etc).

- Use of traditionally well-known qualities of the place (nature), favouring the treatment and recovery (lakes, caves, mountains, forests).

- Systems of self-healing, such as Slavic water hardening (diving into ice-holes, snow rubbing etc.), Detka (the system of well-known Russian healer P. Ivanov), yoga, Chi Gong (*2, 12*).

18.4.4. Scientific Research in Folk Medicine

Academic science does not welcome the activity of folk healers. Mainly, this can be explained by the absence of sufficient cumulative objective information about folk medicine methods. This is due to a number of issues:

- The lack of scientific studies of the effectiveness and safety of folk medicine methods, which is connected with the low level of financing.

- The absence of a system of gathering of obligatory statistical information about the results of healing practice. Consequently, most healers do not keep any documentation of their patients, since there are no required legal documents and forms; the regulatory system for supervision and control of healing practices is not implemented.

- The insufficient number of clinical trials of folk medicine methods due to the absence of legal regulation of interaction between physicians and healers, as well as the existing reciprocal professional scepticism and traditionally different approaches to the health of people.

- An insufficient level of information distribution between scientists about folk medicine methods and the low level of information distribution between healers about the possibilities of scientific research.

It is established that by means of personal abilities, innate or acquired, a person can influence other people without any physical contact. In many cases the healing effect of these people is beyond any doubt. The nature and the mechanisms of their actions are very difficult (if not impossible) to explain with modern methods. Except for patients' references, there is no other officially-implemented criteria that allow differentiation between those who are genuinely able to heal people and those who are simply dishonest; a situation which happens quite often. There are no official statistics of the results of healing. There is no established registration procedure for folk medicine methods and systematic scientific research is not conducted. This is the reason why the system of license issuance, the same as for physician's activity, cannot be established for healers, because the public health-care authorities may not guarantee to society the effectiveness and safety of methods applied by healers.

18.5. Discussion

It should be noted that Russian traditional medicine has always been used alongside official medical practices, particularly in rural areas. However, with time, due to the development of free public health-care services and the broadening of public access to modern medicine, as well as the change of peoples' worldview, traditional methods and healing practices have ceased to be the main form of medical help. In spite of that, cultural traditions and the biological predispositions have allowed the preservation of the good memories of folk medicine, its experience, knowledge and skills.

When a considerable proportion of the population began to express distrust in the approaches of official medicine and concern grew over side-effects of chemical substances in pharmacological medications, the interest of the Russian society in traditional folk practices of healing and recovery revived. In addition, the undoubted influence of religious and other beliefs and persuasions of the population today determine public support of the development of traditional folk methods of healing in the Russian Federation.

It is likely that the economic development of the Russian Federation, viz. lack of budgetary funds and modern social processes, will not allow a solution to the problems of expansion and application of traditional folk methods of healing, diagnosis and treatment within the next few years.

In the opinion of independent research institutions and professional associations of healers, there is a growing problem of exclusion from folk medicine practice those methods that are officially approved for application in medical practice in the public health-care system (see section 25.3.1). This has arisen because, to apply these methods, the healer must meet a great number of official requirements on education, certification, equipment, etc. These often create an insurmountable barrier for the healer's further work and actually its prohibition (4, 6). For example, manual therapy and osteopathy forces out bone-setting, phytotherapy forces out folk herbal practice, reflexotherapy replaces traditional acupuncture, psychotherapy forces out the methods of spiritual healing, etc., (3, 11).

It is necessary to create the legal and social conditions that would guarantee the knowledge, terminology and application of traditional folk methods of healing, recovery and diagnostics, as well as the conditions regulating the parallel and complementary existence of folk medicine practice and medical practice of public health care system (2).

18.6. Summary and Conclusions

Thus, the application of approved traditional medicine methods in the Russian Federation is developing dynamically with the support of the state system of public health care. Active scientific research is being conducted on the problems of application of traditional medicine methods. A system of preparation of specialists in the traditional medicine sphere has been created. The Ministry considers it necessary to conduct deep and fundamental scientific research of healing.

There is insufficient legal regulation of almost all aspects of folk medicine practice, which creates obstacles for expansion and application of traditional methods of healing in Russian society. However, taking into account that there is a sufficient number of physicians in the society, the Ministry considers the integration of healing into the system of public health care to be untimely, while there is no convincing data that prove the safety and effectiveness of traditional folk methods of healing.

Professional associations of healers have a different vision of folk medicine perspectives in the Russian Federation; they see folk medicine as an independent direction in the sphere of health protection of the population. The process of implementation of folk medicine methods in medical practice is necessary, but it does not have to be an obstacle to the process of development of folk medicine, nor to the growth of opportunities for professional healing practices and the broadening of access to the services of healers (2).

References

1. *[Annual reports 2001–2003]*. Moscow, Russian State Committee on Statistics, 2003.

2. *[Overview report of folk medicine]*, (in Russian), St. Petersburg, Institute for Social Development of Natural Abilities; Professional association of folk medicine, Russia, 2004.

3. *[Terminological aspects of medical and pharmaceutical activity in the sphere of traditional medicine and homeopathy]*, Volume 1. Moscow, Ministry of Health of the Russian Federation. Scientific practical centre of traditional medicine and homeopathy, Russia, 2000.

4. Order of Russian Ministry of Health No. 238 of 26.07.2002: *[Organization of licensing of medical activity, 2002]*.

5. *[State Register of new medical technologies (edition 3)]*, Ministry of Health of the Russian Federation, 2002.

6. Regulation of Russian Government No. 499 of 04.07.2002: *[Adoption of regulation on licensing of medical activity]*. Moscow, Government of the Russian Federation, 2002.

7. *WHO Traditional Medicine Strategy 2002–2005*. Geneva, World Health Organization, 2002 (WHO/ EDM/TRM/2002.1).

8. Resolution WHA56.31. Traditional medicine. In: *Fifty-sixth World Health Assembly, Geneva, 19–28 May 2003*. Geneva, World Health Organization, 2003.

9. *COST Action B4: Unconventional medicine in Europe. Supplement to Final report of the Management Committee, 1993–1998*. Brussels, European Commission Directorate-General for Science, Research and Development, 1999.

10. Federal Law of the Russian Federation No. 5487 of 22.07.1993: *[The fundamentals of Russian legislation on the protection of health of citizens]*. Moscow, Government of the Russian Federation, 1993.

11. Social research. *[Estimation of the market of paid services of traditional medicine in St. Petersburg]*. St. Petersburg, Institute for Social Development of Natural Abilities, 2004.

12. *[Classification of occupations of the Russian Federation 010-93, Article 324]*. Moscow, Government of the Russian Federation. 1993.

13. Industry standard. *[Terms and definitions of standardization system in the public health care]*. Moscow, Ministry of Health, Government of the Russian Federation Order No.12 of 22.01.2001.

Useful Links

Institute for Social Development of Natural Abilities
http://www.isres.ru
http://www.biosens.ru

Professional association of folk medicine
http://www.panm.ru
http://www.biosens.ru

NarMed
http://www.narmed.ru (in Russian)

Biomind Portal
http://www.biomind.ru (in Russian)

Centre of Folk Medicine ENIOM
http://www.eniom.ru

LightPlanet Reiki Portal
http://www.lightplanet.org

CHAPTER 19

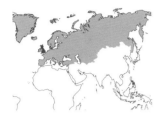

UNITED KINGDOM
OF GREAT BRITAIN
AND NORTHERN IRELAND

Chi-Keong Ong[1],
Gerard Bodeker[2]
and Gemma Burford[3]

[1] Research Fellow in Community and Complementary Medicine, Mansfield College,
University of Oxford, Oxford OX1 3TF, United Kingdom.
E-mail: paul.ong@ndm.ox.ac.uk

[2] Chair, Global Initiative For Traditional Systems (GIFTS) of Health, and Senior Clinical Lecturer in
Public Health, University of Oxford, Green College, 43 Woodstock Road, Oxford OX2 6HG,
United Kingdom.
E-mail: gerry.bodeker@green.oxford.ac.uk

[3] Research Associate, Global Initiative For Traditional Systems (GIFTS) of Health,
University of Oxford, Green College, 43 Woodstock Road, Oxford OX2 6HG, United Kingdom.
E-mail: gemmaburford@yahoo.co.uk

19.1. INTRODUCTION

An editorial in the *British Medical Journal* of 15 February 2003 (*1*) discussed the concept of concordance – "the creation of an agreement that respects the beliefs and wishes of the patient" – and also stated that "when the medicines that doctors prescribe fail to produce benefit they expect, they often respond by selecting an alternative medicine". The United Kingdom of Great Britain and Northern Ireland represents the face of modern health care in an industrialized European country. Pluralism is becoming a norm, with consumers voting, with both feet and wallets, for the types of health care that they want and expect.

One report and three surveys (*2–5*) identify the most common trends and patterns of complementary and alternative medicine (CAM) use in the United Kingdom. These studies provided the basis for the material utilized in completing structural and process indicators for the United Kingdom for purposes of the WHO Global Atlas on Traditional, Complementary and Alternative Medicine.

In the United Kingdom, eight types of CAM were indicated as the most commonly utilized; acupuncture, aromatherapy, chiropractic, homeopathy, hypnotherapy, herbal medicine, osteopathy and reflexology. The survey of most commonly utilized therapies also highlighted a need to distinguish between practitioner-based therapies, over-the-counter medication and self-practised therapies such as yoga and meditation.

Osteopathy and chiropractic are statutorily regulated professions in the United Kingdom. The registered practitioners of these therapies are recognized as official health-care providers who can work in the National Health Service (NHS). However, most practitioners prefer to work as independent contractors and have NHS patients referred to them. Some non-statutorily regulated CAM practitioners (e.g. traditional acupuncturists) also take NHS referrals.

19.2. IMPORTANT BACKGROUND INDICATORS

In the United Kingdom there are 60 300 national health service (NHS) hospital and dental staff, and an additional 31 000 general practitioners. The total health expenditure of the NHS is approximately £39 billion (US$ 70.78 billion) per year.

The CAM sector is about 3.8% of the total size of the formal conventional health economy in the United Kingdom (*2, 5*).

19.3. Structural Indicators

19.3.1. Regulation of CAM

In the United Kingdom, CAM practitioners are encouraged to be covered by insurance and adhere to a Code of General Ethics (6, 7). Under United Kingdom common law, any individual is entitled to carry out medical acts not specifically forbidden by Parliament. Parliament recognizes homeopathy, osteopathy and chiropractic. However, practitioners of these types of CAM may not advertise treatment of cancer, tuberculosis, glaucoma, diabetes, venereal diseases or epilepsy, and may not make claims with respect to these conditions. In addition, they may not prescribe controlled drugs.

The Prince of Wales's Foundation for Integrated Health (PWFIH) collaborated in the publication of two reports (8, 9) in September 2003 with the Herbal Medicine Regulatory Working Group (HMRWG) and the Acupuncture Regulatory Working Group (ARWG), which looked at the nature, scale and recommendations for the regulation of these two CAM professions. HMRWG was commissioned by the Department of Health, PWFIH and the European Herbal Practitioners Association. ARWG was commissioned by the Department of Health, PWFIH, the Acupuncture Association of Chartered Physiotherapists, the British Academy of Western Acupuncture, the British Acupuncture Council and the British Medical Acupuncture Society. These reports have been sent to the Ministers and based upon these reports, the proposal for statutory regulation has been formulated for wider consultation by the Government and subsequently for the legislation (10). Alongside this, the Medicines and Healthcare products Regulatory Agency (MHRA) has consulted on proposals for updating the regulation of unlicensed herbal medicines made up for use following a one-to-one consultation.

There are currently two regulatory routes for herbal medicines to reach the British market. Licensed medicines require safety, quality and efficacy criteria to be met. Herbal remedies exempt from licensing requirements are required to meet the conditions set out in Section 12 of the Medicines Act 1968. Medicinal claims are not permitted. Most herbal remedies on the British market are unlicensed.

In the United Kingdom, homeopathic products are regulated by Directive 2001/83EEC. This Directive incorporates 92/73EEC (11, 12). The European Directive on Traditional and Herbal Medicine Products, 2004/24/EC which amends 2001/83/EC will introduce a simplified registration scheme for over-the-counter traditional herbal remedies by October 2004. Under the new scheme, traditional herbal medicines will have to meet the same specific standards of safety and quality as licensed products. The normal requirement for medicines to demonstrate efficacy will be replaced by evidence of traditional use. Minor claims will be permitted. Products already on the market on 30 April 2003 will be able to benefit from a seven-year transitional period which will end on 30 April 2011. A "Partial Regulatory Impact Assessment (Third Draft) on the Proposed Directive on Traditional Herbal Medicine Products" has been developed by the MHRA (13).

Within the MHRA there is a Herbal Policy Unit responsible for the Herbal Medicinal Products Directive and reform of the regulation of unlicensed herbal remedies made up to meet the needs of individual patients.

19.3.2. Education and Training in CAM

Within the conventional health-care education system, short courses on CAM are offered as part of the undergraduate curriculum in many medical schools including CAM familiarization training for medical students (14). The Faculty of Homeopathy also has accredited training centres for registered health-care professionals (16). The United Kingdom Government House of Lords has recommended clearer guidelines for CAM training of doctors and nurses (cited in 7).

Outside the allopathic health-care system, there are a wide variety of initiatives that address concerns about education and training in CAM in the United Kingdom. The European Herbal Practitioners' Association has developed a core curriculum for herbal medicine, together with specific curricula for the Western, Chinese and Ayurvedic herbal traditions, and has established an accreditation board to assess training standards (15). The Society of Homeopaths also has an education policy and is working towards accreditation of courses (16). The PWFIH is actively developing a network for people involved in TCAM education and accreditation and this has resulted in the formulation of the two reports, previously mentioned, on the regulation of acupuncture and herbal medicine as professions (*8, 9*).

19.3.3. National Voluntary Self-regulatory Bodies and Professional Organizations

The European Herbal Practitioners' Association is an umbrella body working with the Department of Health towards statutory regulation. This is, however, complicated by the fact that a large number of professional bodies and associations already exist. The September 2003 report (*9, 15*) recommended that the herbal medicine community consider a rationalization of the associations and professional bodies.

The British Acupuncture Council's Executive Committee was mandated in 2001 to pursue a suitable route to statutory regulation (*8, 10*). An independent working group consisting of lay members, members from the Council, and organizations representing doctors, nurses and physiotherapists who practise acupuncture, produced a report on the statutory regulation of acupuncture that was published in September 2003 (*10*). The House of Lords Select Subcommittee stated in 1999 that "in time, such statutory regulation may become appropriate for homeopathy".

19.3.4. Nature of Information and Advisory Services Relating to CAM

Several British institutions have high-quality databases on TCAM. The British Research Council on Complementary Medicine, a nongovernmental organization, has a specialised research database known as CISCOM. The British Library in London also has a high-quality database on TCAM, known as the Allied and Complementary Medicine Database (AMED), which is widely distributed to many libraries in the United Kingdom, including university and medical-school libraries. In addition, the various Royal Colleges governing different specialities within the medical profession have working groups to look at CAM within their specialities or sub-specialities.

19.3.5. Public Financing of CAM

The United Kingdom is the only country in the European Union with public-sector hospitals for CAM. There are NHS homeopathic hospitals, in London, Glasgow, Liverpool, Bristol and Tunbridge Wells. Decisions on funding of CAM are now made at the local level and are, therefore, not a matter of national policy.

Currently 79% of CAM is paid for directly by the patient with a mean expenditure calculated at approximately £13.62 (US$ 24.72) per month as out-of-pocket spending per person. The NHS accounts for around 10% of consultations, at an estimated cost of £50–55 million (US$ 90.74–99.82) in 2001. Total expenditure for consultations with CAM practitioners was estimated at £580 million (US$ 1052.63 million) by one survey (*4*). However, other estimates suggested that with the inclusion of over-the-counter products, expenditure on CAM in the United Kingdom could be as high as £1.47 billion (US$ 2.67 billion) per annum (*2, 5*).

19.4. CAM Surveys and Patterns of Use

There are four studies that include large-scale population data (*3–5*). Eleven other patient-specific and/or therapy-centred surveys, which were excluded for the purposes of the Global Atlas study, have also been identified (*17–27*). The majority of these have not been published in conventional peer-reviewed literature, but are available directly from the centres concerned. A recent project undertaken by the Medical Care Research Unit at the Sheffield University and funded by the Department of Health (*28*), examined the impact of the reorganization of primary care services in 1999 on policy development and the provision of NHS CAM therapy services.

19.4.1. Medical Determinants and Reasons for CAM Use

The major presenting conditions for CAM use were found to be musculo-skeletal problems, especially of the neck and back; injuries; bowel problems; indigestion; mental health problems (specifically, stress, anxiety and depression); migraine and asthma. The maintenance of well-being (lifestyle use) was also found to be a significant reason for CAM use. Reasons for choosing CAM included poor outcomes from conventional allopathic medical treatment, experiences of adverse effects from pharmaceuticals, negative experiences of the patient–doctor relationship, and health beliefs which were not in keeping with the allopathic medical models. According to survey results (3–5), there is evidence of a belief in the right to a personal approach and a positive relationship with the health-care practitioner.

Patient expectations can be expressed as four major factors, which impact on all health care interventions, whether allopathic or CAM:

- a comprehensive examination

- a satisfactory diagnosis

- effective treatment interventions

- freedom from unwanted side-effects.

These studies offer health care providers the first comprehensive picture of patients' expectations of their health-care provision and a clear understanding of why consumers are turning to CAM.

19.4.2. Sociodemographic Characteristics of Consumers of CAM

Women were found to be greater users of CAM than men, both in terms of practitioner interventions and over-the-counter purchases of homeopathic and herbal remedies. This pattern was found to be broadly similar to that of women's use of general practitioner and outpatient services. CAM users were also most likely to fall within the 35–44 age group. In terms of social class, those from groups AB (professional and white collar workers) and C1 (clerical, junior managerial and administrative workers) are more likely to be users of CAM, while those from groups C2 (skilled working class) and DE (unskilled and manual workers) were more likely to be non-users. This profile applies in a setting where the majority of CAM treatments are paid for out-of-pocket, and are therefore more likely to be utilized by people with sufficient disposable income.

Stringent estimates of use suggested that between 6.6% and 20% of the population has utilized CAM in the previous 12 months. The average number of visits to a practitioner ranged from 2.8 to 5.3 per year, leading to an extrapolation that around 5.3 million people aged over 18 made 31.7 million visits to practitioners of the eight most popular CAM therapies in the previous 12 months. There were also indications that the use of CAM had risen between 1993 and 1998. Excluding over-the-counter use of CAM products, lifetime use of any of the eight most popular CAM therapies was estimated to be 32.1%. This estimate rose to a figure of 46.6% if over-the-counter products were included in the equation.

19.4.3. Patient Satisfaction and Outcomes

In the United Kingdom, patients generally appear to have their expectations met by CAM. Their health outcomes appear to be positive and there are also reports of economic outcomes, notably, evidence of a decrease in medication and use of general practitioner time.

Positive health outcomes for palliative care, including in cancer patients have been reported, in terms of both primary and secondary symptoms. Other reported benefits include improved coping mechanisms, greater acceptance of end-stage illness and increased self-esteem.

Negative outcomes were also reported, notably some dissatisfaction with CAM methods and health outcomes. For example, some patients assumed that the speed of recovery using CAM would be similar to that expected of allopathic health care. However, the biggest cause of dissatisfaction was that there were not enough CAM sessions, or that CAM sessions did not last long enough. These are important factors when considering integrating CAM into the NHS, in which the amount of contact time between the practitioner and the patient is typically reduced to a minimum.

19.4.4. Conclusions drawn from CAM Studies

There are some strong developments indicated by these studies which would merit close examination in future health and economic outcome research and patient satisfaction surveys. The findings provide some explanations for the increasing use of CAM, and the tendency for some treatments to be increasingly mainstreamed, which therefore warrants their legislation and regulation as professions in their own right. They also point to dissatisfaction with elements of the delivery of allopathic health care, notably the quality of the doctor–patient relationship and the time available for thorough examination and diagnosis.

These studies highlight implications for integrating CAM practice into the NHS, and act as a warning against the reduction of two of the most valued aspects of the CAM experience: the practitioner–patient relationship, and time. Legislated CAM professions would do well to avoid the trap of compromising the practitioner–patient relationship through inappropriate controls and regulation, whilst pursuing greater professionalism and efficacy.

19.5. Discussion

In a society that increasingly values the consumer perspective and the principle of choice in health care, these findings provide a basis for discussion of what we mean by a diverse and integrated health service.

Clearly, the use of CAM is neither peripheral nor "fringe" within the United Kingdom today. The high levels of consumer investment and interest in CAM suggest that the evidence base for CAM needs to be urgently addressed and expanded in the interest of patient safety. Therefore, more investment in CAM clinical and basic scientific research is to be encouraged. Several outstanding projects have been demonstrated by the Department of Health including the national investment of CAM infrastructure for research activity promotion (*29*), research projects on the use of CAM for cancer (*30*) and the studies of therapies including acupuncture, aromatherapy, chiropractic, herbal medicine, homeopathy, hypnotherapy, and massage (*31*).

The UK Research Council for Complementary Medicine is being funded by the Department of Health to reshape its comprehensive database of CAM research studies to categorise the evidence according to the individual health conditions that are a priority for the NHS.

The University of Westminster has been funded by the Department of Health and the Kings Fund to produce some initial guidelines on the clinical governance of CAM in the NHS. These will include suggestions for assembling evidence of clinical and cost-effectiveness, and will be supported by an electronic network of CAM and NHS organizations that are interested in sharing information and experiences.

A modern but diverse and integrated health service will have implications for the way in which responsible consumers of health care interact with their general practitioners to appraise therapeutic options and alternatives. Putting concordance into practice does indeed appear to be of central importance for the future of a modern pluralistic system of health care.

Acknowledgement: The review of this chapter by Ms Judith Thompson, Herbal Policy Unit, Medicines and Healthcare Products Regulatory Agency, is greatly appreciated.

References

1. Bodeker G. Lessons on integration from the developing world's experience. *British Medical Journal*, 2001, 322:164–167.

2. Ong CK, Banks B. *Complementary and alternative medicine: the consumer perspective*. London, The Prince of Wales's Foundation for Integrated Health, 2003 (Occasional Papers No. 2).

3. Ong CK et al. Health status of people using complementary and alternative medical practitioner services in four English counties. *American Journal of Public Health*, 2002, 92:1653–1656.

4. Thomas KJ, Nicholl JP, Coleman P. Use and expenditure on complementary medicine in England: a population based survey. *Complementary Therapies in Medicine*, 2001, 9:2–11.

5. Ernst E, White A. The BBC survey of complementary medicine use in the UK. *Complementary Therapies in Medicine*. 2000, 8:32–36.

6. *Legal status of traditional medicine and complementary/alternative medicine*. Geneva, World Health Organization, 2001 (WHO/EDM/TRM/2001.2).

7. Walker LA, Budd S. UK: the current state of regulation of complementary and alternative medicine. *Complementary Therapies in Medicine*, 2002, 10:8–13.

8. *The Statutory Regulation of the Acupuncture Profession.* London, The Acupuncture Regulatory Working Group, September 2003 (http://www.advisorybodies.doh.gov.uk/acupuncturerwg/, accessed 9 July 2004).

9. *Recommendations on the Regulation of Herbal Practitioners in the UK, A Report from the Herbal Medicine Regulatory Working Group.* London, September, 2003 (http://www.advisorybodies.doh.gov.uk/herbalmedicinerwg/, accessed 8 July 2004).

10. *Regulation of herbal medicine and acupuncture, Proposal for statutory regulation. London,* Department of Health, UK, March 2004. (http://www.dh.gov.uk/Consultations/LiveConsultations/fs/en, accessed 28 June 2004).

11. McDermott A. The EHPA and the EU. *European Journal of Herbal Medicine, 1999, 4:15–18.*

12. *Council Directive 92/73/EEC of 22 September 1992 widening the scope of Directives 65/65/EEC and 75/319/EEC on the approximation of provisions laid down by law, regulation or administrative action relating to medicinal products and laying down additional provisions on homeopathic medicinal products.* Brussels, Council of the European Communities, 1992.

13. *Partial Regulatory Impact Assessment (Third Draft): Proposed Directive on Traditional Herbal Medicinal Products.* London, Medicines and Healthcare products Regulatory Agency, Department of Health, September 2003.

14. Barberis L et al. Unconventional medicine teaching at the universities of the European Union. *Journal of Alternative and Complementary Medicine, 2001, 7:337–343.*

15. Lampert N. *Briefing document on statutory self-regulation for herbal medicine in the UK.* London, European Herbal Practitioners' Association, 2001.

16. Finne B, Viksveen P. *A survey of ten countries where homeopathy is being practised.* Oslo, Norske Homeopaters Landsforbund *[Norwegian Homeopathic Assocation]*, 1999.

17. Richardson J. *Complementary therapy in the NHS: A service evaluation of the first year of an outpatient service in a local district hospital.* Lewisham, The Lewisham Hospital NHS Trust Health Services Research and Evaluation Unit, 1995.

18. *Complementary therapies in general practice.* Glastonbury, Somerset Trust for Integrated Healthcare, 1998.

19. Stedman C. *Assessing herbal treatment within a primary care setting by means of a patient satisfaction survey.* London, Edmonton NHS Health Centre, 1999.

20. *Survey of patient satisfaction with inpatient care at the Glasgow Homeopathic Hospital (UK), utilisation of conventional medication and self-assessment of overall well-being three months after discharge.* Glasgow, International Data Collection Centre for Integrative Medicine, 1998.

21. Alexander L. *Why patients don't come back* (dissertation). London, The British School of Osteopathy, 2000.

22. *1997 client survey results.* Oxford, McTimoney Chiropractic Association, 1997.

23. Masson A. *New Park Medical Practice – audit of acupuncture service.* Dunfermline, New Park Medical Practice, 1999.

24. Sharples F, Van Haselen R. *Patients' perspective on using a complementary medicine approach to their health: A survey at the Royal London Homeopathic Hospital NHS Trust.* London, The Royal London Homeopathic Hospital NHS Trust, 1997.

25. *Audit of patient satisfaction (osteopathy).* Ipswich, Gilmour Piper & Associates, 1999.

26. Pirie Z. *Magic or medicine? Delivering shiatsu in general practice* (thesis). University of Sheffield: Institute of General Practice and Primary Care, 2001.

27. Burns E et al. *The use of aromatherapy in intrapartum midwifery practice: An evaluative study.* Oxford, Oxford Brookes University: Oxford Centre for Health Care Research and Development, 2000.

28. K. Thomas et al. *Complementary Therapies under Primary Care Groups, Final Report to Department of Health.* University of Sheffield, UK, 2003. (http://www.shef.ac.uk/scharr/mcru/reports.htm, accessed 2 July 2004).

29. *National Personal Award Schemes.* London, Department of Health, UK (www.dh.gov.uk/PolicyAndGuidance/ResearchAndDevelopment/ResearchCapacity/fs/en, accessed 2 July 2004).

30. *NHS R&D Programme - Research on the Role of Complementary and Alternative Medicine (CAM) in the Care of Patients with Cancer.*

London, Department of Health, UK, (http://www.dh.gov.uk/PolicyAndGuidance/ResearchAndDevelopment/ResearchAndDevelopmentAZ/NationalNHSRDFunding/NationalNHSRDFundingArticle/fs/en?CONTENT_ID=4032132&chk=WEtKt0, accessed 2 July 2004).

31. The National Research Register, London, Department of Health, (Information available at http://www.update-software.com/National/default.htm, accessed 2 July 2004).

Useful Information

A copy of the consulation document – MLX299: Proposals for the reform of the regulation of unlicensed herbal remedies made up to meet the needs of individual patients can be found on http://www.medicines.mhra.gov.uk/ourwork/licensedmeds/herbalmeds

Further information on the Traditional and Herbal Medicines Registration Scheme can be found on http://www.medicines.mrha.gov.uk/ourwork/licensingmeds/types/thmpd

A copy of the Partial Regulatory Impact Assessment can be found on http://www.medicines.mhra.gov.uk/ourwork/licensingmeds/herbalmeds

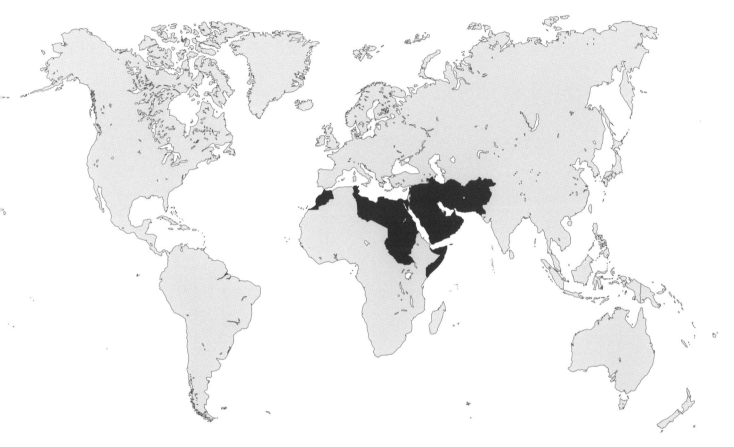

WHO EASTERN MEDITERRANEAN REGION

REGIONAL OVERVIEW AND
SELECTED COUNTRY CHAPTERS

CHAPTER 20

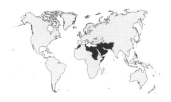

REGIONAL OVERVIEW: EASTERN MEDITERRANEAN REGION

Ahmed Regai El-Gendy

Secretary General Assistant, Islamic Organization for Medical Sciences, P.O. Box 31280, Sulaibekhat 90803, Kuwait. E-mail: ioms@islamset.com

20.1. INTRODUCTION

Traditional, Complementary and Alternative Medicine (TCAM) is culturally accepted and widely used throughout the WHO Eastern Mediterranean Region (EMR) for treating a variety of disorders. In some of the more isolated rural areas, the only available practitioners are traditional healers. Even where allopathic health services are available, some patients prefer TCAM for psychological or religious reasons (1), including a reluctance to seek treatment from strangers (2). Hence, TCAM provides an important mechanism for increasing access to health services. However, few countries in the Region have specific policies or infrastructure for TCAM, or systematic programmes for its integration into formal health services.

While reliable data on TCAM practices and utilization in EMR are not available, an overview of the literature suggests that there are four broad categories of TCAM service provision within the Region. These are (a) popular or folk medicine; (b) the 'traditional-oral' sector, or non-codified traditional medicine; (c) the 'traditional-written' sector, or codified traditional systems of medicine; and (d) complementary and alternative medicine (CAM).

The popular sector, sometimes called the folk sector, is based on self-medication at home. Older family members often have stores of simple herbal remedies for common illnesses and preventative hygiene (3), and may also offer dietary treatments, such as elimination of a certain food group or addition of specific foods (2). Popular or folk medicine is generally unregulated.

The traditional-oral sector includes practitioners of herbalism, bone-setting, cauterization, cupping, bloodletting, massage, leech therapy, circumcision and traditional midwifery. This sector also encompasses religious and supernatural healers who cure through recitation of the Quran and magic formulae, learned by heart (1). Knowledge is transmitted orally, usually from one generation to the next, as many practitioners are illiterate or have only elementary schooling (1, 4). Healing is not always their sole occupation. In Afghanistan, for example, bone-setting may be practised by farmers or craftsmen, and cauterization by barbers or blacksmiths. Health-care providers in this category are not usually recognized or regulated by their respective governments, although there are occasional exceptions.

The foundations of traditional-written medicine (Unani and Ayurveda) are systems of health care from ancient Greece, India and China. There are also Persian and Arabic influences, through Islam (1). Practitioners of these forms of medicine are well-educated members of the community who enjoy high prestige. Healing is usually their main occupation. In Pakistan, where these systems of medicine are most prominent, the Government has passed legislation on training and registration.

In a number of countries in EMR, including Egypt, Jordan, Kuwait, Saudi Arabia and the United Arab Emirates, herbal medicine is being taken out of its traditional contexts (both oral and written) and incorporated, alongside allopathic medicine, into national health services. The herbal product registration policy developed in Kuwait has been reviewed and endorsed by the WHO Regional Office for the Eastern Mediterranean, together with the Islamic Organization for Medical Sciences. On this basis, regional standards for the registration of herbal medicines have been established (5).

WHO/EMR Guidelines for the minimum requirements for the registration of Herbal Medicinal Products based on a series of WHO Technical Guidelines for Safety, Efficacy and Quality Control of Herbal Medicines were developed, as a result of adoption of resolution EM/RC49/R.9, through two Regional Workshops in 2002 and 2003 in Tehran (the Islamic Republic of Iran) and Abu Dhabi (United Arab Emirates), respectively.

There has been a growing interest in complementary and alternative therapies within the Region over the past decade. Homeopathy is popular in Pakistan, where it is regulated alongside Unani and Ayurveda (see Chapter 22). In the United Arab Emirates, traditional Chinese medicine, homeopathy, chiropractic, osteopathy and naturopathy are all formally recognized (see Chapter 24). Other widely-used TCAM practices include spiritual therapy, reflexology, aromatherapy and commercial weight-loss programmes.

20.2. Background Indicators

WHO/EMR consists of 22 Member States: Afghanistan, Bahrain, Djibouti, Egypt, Iran, Iraq, Jordan, Kuwait, Lebanon, the Libyan Arab Jamahiriya, Morocco, Oman, Pakistan, Palestine, Qatar, Saudi Arabia, Somalia, the Sudan, the Syrian Arab Republic, Tunisia, United Arab Emirates and Yemen.

There is a wide range in population among the countries of the Region, from 595 000 in Qatar to 148 600 000 in Pakistan. The total population of the region is over 487 million. Some countries – namely Bahrain, Kuwait, the Libyan Arab Jamahiriya, Oman, Qatar, Saudi Arabia and the United Arab Emirates – have a very large expatriate population.

Both extremes of gross domestic product (GDP) per capita are present in the Region, from 555 international dollars in Somalia to 26 304 international dollars in Qatar. The countries with the lowest per capita GDP (Afghanistan, Djibouti, Somalia and Sudan) are also those with the lowest life expectancy, the highest infant and maternal mortality rates, and the lowest numbers of physicians per 10 000 population (6). Exact figures are not available for the total number of TCAM practitioners.

Diseases of the respiratory system are a major cause of morbidity throughout EMR, together with conditions related to pregnancy and childbirth, but there is wide variation in causes of mortality between countries.

20.3. Structural Indicators

20.3.1. Policy and Legislation

In Kuwait, herbal medicines have been integrated into the official health sector since 1978 (5). The Kuwaiti legislation on herbal products has acted as a model for the development of standards in EMR. Under this legislation, no herbal remedy may be sold in the country unless registered with the competent authority. Medicinal plants are categorized into three groups, ranging from those used on a daily basis to those requiring further study, and each group has specific registration requirements. A licence is required for the importation, manufacture, distribution, sale and export of herbal remedies, which must be fully labelled. No exaggerated claims are permitted in advertising, and all sales promotion must be based on data evaluated by the competent authority (Ministry of Health of Kuwait, personal communication, 2003).

In Egypt, all herbal products must meet the same standards as manufactured chemical preparations. They must be manufactured in a licensed pharmaceutical plant according to local and international good manufacturing practices; registered with the Central Administration of Pharmaceutical Affairs; and priced according to the law. They may be distributed only to pharmacies (5). Legislation on the registration of herbal products is also in place in Jordan, Saudi Arabia and the United Arab Emirates (see Chapters 23 and 24).

In Pakistan, the Unani, Ayurvedic and Homeopathic Practitioners Act, passed in 1965, regulates qualifications and provides for the registration of practitioners (5). The Act established the Board of Unani and Ayurvedic Systems of Medicine to maintain adequate standards, and fixed the duration of approved training at four years. Practitioners with not less than seven years of practice were automatically entitled to registration without further examinations, while those with between five and seven years of practice were required to satisfy the Board of their knowledge and skill (National Institute of Health, Pakistan, personal communication, 2003).

Several countries of the Region have specific policies and legislation relating to integration of TCAM into primary health care. In Djibouti, traditional birth attendants, trained by staff of the Ministry of Health, work in primary health care and receive supplies from UNICEF (7). Likewise, in Jordan, certain TCAM doctors and professionals have been granted approval to practise in primary health care (5). In the Libyan Arab Jamahiriya, one of the Government's health objectives is to strengthen existing traditional primary health care, provided that it has proven efficacy (8). The Syrian Arab Republic has a draft law concerning the use of herbal medicine in primary health care (5).

Complementary and alternative therapies are regulated in a minority of Member States within the Region. The Ministry of Health of Saudi Arabia regulates chiropractic, and has approved new guidelines restricting acupuncture licences to persons who have at least 200 hours of training; are anaesthetists, rheumatologists or orthopaedists; and comply with hygienic standards (see Chapter 23). The United Arab Emirates restricts TCAM practice to individuals who pass a qualifying examination set by the Ministry of Health in one of eight named specialities (see Chapter 24).

20.3.2. Research and Development

During the last few decades, many institutes have been established to undertake research into plants used in traditional medicine in EMR (5). In Sudan, for example, the Medicinal and Aromatic Herbs Research Institute was created 25 years ago, and has trained a considerable number of specialists in different fields of medicinal plant research. It has compiled an Atlas of Medicinal Plants, recording the scientific names of more than 2000 herbs (Federal Ministry of Health of Sudan, personal communication, 2003).

The Government of Kuwait has opened a Centre for Research on Herbal Treatment, incorporating departments of microbiology, pharmaceutics, pharmacognosy, biochemistry, phytochemistry, pharmacology, toxicology and quality control. The Centre has a clinical division, where patients are treated with herbal formulations, and a Drug Manufacturing Unit. Promoting TCAM research is also one of the aims of the Islamic Organization for Medical Sciences, founded by a Decree of the Amir of Kuwait (Ministry of Health of Kuwait, personal communication, 2003).

The Ministry of Health of Somalia has also established a centre to promote and research medicinal plants, now under the control of the National Agency for Importation and Manufacturing of Drugs. Traditional herbalists and conventionally-trained allopathic physicians work together in this centre to prepare herbal therapies. Both the Somali National University and the National Academy of Sciences and Arts have research programmes to promote the integration of the use of herbs into modern medicine (9). Other countries with active TCAM research programmes include Egypt, Islamic Republic of Iran, Morocco, Pakistan and the United Arab Emirates.

20.3.3. Education and Training

In the 'traditional-oral' sector, medical knowledge is usually obtained from ancestors (4) or through apprenticeships under the guidance of a master (1). This knowledge is fiercely protected, and many practitioners are reluctant to share information. In the 'traditional-written' sector and CAM, and increasingly also in the field of herbal medicine, a number of formal education and training programmes are offered in the Region.

Pakistan has the most highly developed system of TCAM education, with 30 colleges and two universities offering diploma courses in Unani and Ayurvedic medical systems, while 119 colleges and two universities offer a Diploma in Homeopathic Medical Sciences (see Chapter 22). There are, as yet, no facilities for acupuncture training, but a minority of doctors with a private income or scholarships travel to China to study the subject. The Registered Association for Promotion of Acupuncture in Pakistan has recommended the establishment of training institutes with a standardized syllabus and qualifications (10).

In 1991, a National Academy of Traditional Medicine was established in the Islamic Republic of Iran (5). It is mandated to recommend an education plan to the Ministry of Health and Medical

Education, including the incorporation of TCAM training and research into allopathic medical programmes. In 2001, the Academy recommended that the Ministry of Health and Medical Education officially begin training allopathic medical students in Iranian traditional medicine.

In Somalia, TCAM has been included as a core subject in the medical curriculum. Future physicians from the Faculty of Medicine travel to rural areas to meet TCAM practitioners (9). Likewise, first-year medical students in the United Arab Emirates attend a twelve-hour programme on TCAM, visit a herbal centre and have discussions with qualified practitioners (11). The official pharmacy curriculum in the Syrian Arab Republic includes a syllabus on herbal medicines.

20.4. PROCESS INDICATORS

Surveys relevant to TCAM utilization have been carried out in five countries of the Region: the Islamic Republic of Iran, Morocco, Pakistan, Sudan and the United Arab Emirates. None of these surveys offer quantitative data on the use of individual therapies, or full sociodemographic profiles of users, but they all provide some insight into public perceptions and utilization of TCAM in the respective Member States.

A 2001 study of treatments provided by 15 traditional healers in the Qazvin region of the Islamic Republic of Iran (12) showed that herbal remedies, bone-setting, massage therapy, cupping and leech therapy are all used. Despite an adequate number of physicians practising in the region, traditional healers continue to be consulted. Another survey carried out in the same year (4) showed that medicinal plants remain the only accessible form of health care for many rural people in the West Azerbaijan region of the Islamic Republic of Iran.

In Morocco, the prevailing situation is one of health care pluralism. A study on knowledge and practices relating to childbirth in Morocco revealed that women often alternate between home and hospital births, depending on the circumstances of pregnancy and labour. Women who exclusively go to hospital tend to be educated, urban and have easy access to health centres (13). In 1989, an estimated 80% of the Moroccan population used traditional medicine concurrently with allopathic medicine, and factors influencing the decision to visit a herbalist included cost, convenience, beliefs, personal prestige of the practitioners, and the patient's own self-esteem (14).

In Pakistan, a study found that urban households preferred to visit qualified medical practitioners, specialists and private hospitals, who were seen to provide a proper diagnosis and rapid relief (15). A similar study (16) showed that educated people with a high socioeconomic status found allopathic doctors to be the most accessible and effective. In this survey, TCAM methods ranked for accessibility and effectiveness showed homeopathic practitioners to be highest, then hakims (herbalists), and spiritual healers lowest.

A further study (17) was undertaken of patients with histologically-proven cancer who visited an oncology service in Pakistan. Just over half of the surveyed patients concomitantly used TCAM, most of them influenced by family members to do so. Herbal therapies and homeopathy were the most popular methods, and spiritual healing and nutritional supplements were also widely used. Most patients used TCAM therapies for three months or less, but a substantial number used them for longer than a year. TCAM was generally thought to be beneficial, although many people had discontinued use because of an apparent lack of effect.

Villagers in the Shendi area of Sudan generally use and trust allopathic medicines for childcare, according to a 1998 study on childhood diseases. Traditional medicine is rarely the first choice of therapy, but is often taken concurrently with conventional methods or utilized after allopathic treatment has failed (18). In central Sudan, a 1999 survey (19) found that most of the visitors to traditional healers were aged 21–40 (61%) and were women (62%). Visitors were less educated than the general population in the area. The main reasons given for attending traditional healers were treatment (60%) and blessing (26%).

In the United Arab Emirates, a study (11) of physicians' and medical students' attitudes towards TCAM and its incorporation into the national health system found that there was widespread use, but many were unsure of the effectiveness and possible side-effects of TCAM. The existence of TCAM was generally acknowledged and supported by physicians, although therapies differed in their levels of acceptance, and spiritual therapy was least likely to be accepted. The majority of physicians had attended educational sessions on herbal medicine, and many said that they would refer patients to TCAM providers, particularly for chronic ailments and non-specific disorders such as headaches.

20.5. Discussion

The countries of the Eastern Mediterranean Region exhibit considerable diversity in the types of TCAM used, the circumstances of utilization, and the extent of official acceptance and recognition. Given the importance of TCAM in health care delivery throughout the region, it is a matter of some concern that very few countries have a national TCAM policy. National policies are required to create the necessary regulatory mechanisms for maintaining good practice; promote equitable access; and ensure the authenticity, safety and efficacy of therapies. It is encouraging, however, that steps are being taken at a regional level to establish guidelines for the registration of herbal products, based on Kuwaiti legislation. The examples of Pakistan, Saudi Arabia and the United Arab Emirates (see Chapters 22, 23 and 24) also provide regulatory models that could potentially be adopted by other Member States.

As in most other WHO Regions, there are enormous folk and 'traditional-oral' sectors that remain largely unregulated. These sectors constitute the principal sources of health care for a majority of the rural population, in areas with little or no access to allopathic health services. In the drive towards greater professionalization and state regulation of TCAM, it will be important to ensure that the affordability and accessibility of these providers are not compromised.

20.6. Conclusions and Summary

In general, a concerted effort is required to define the role of TCAM in national health delivery systems and promote high-quality services. The WHO Regional Office for the Eastern Mediterranean aims to collaborate with Member States in the following priority areas:

- formulating national policies directed towards the proper recognition, promotion and propagation of TCAM;

- developing model legislation to promote the safety, efficacy and quality of TCAM, including good manufacturing practices;

- encouraging dialogue between practitioners of various systems;

- promoting integrated research on TCAM;

- designing culturally appropriate allopathic medical curricula that incorporate information about TCAM;

- developing educational institutions to impart teaching/training in TCAM therapies, leading to the award of diplomas and degrees in specialized areas;

- building TCAM human resources, including researchers;

- providing coverage of TCAM therapies by state health insurance.

References

1. Penkala-Gawecka D. Two types of traditional medicine in Afghanistan. *Ethnologia Polona,* 1987, 13:91–127.

2. Helander B. Getting the most out of it: nomadic health care seeking and the State in southern Somalia. *Newsletter of the Commission on Nomadic Peoples,* 1990, 25:122–132.

3. *An act and notes for guidance aiming at ensuring the safety and quality of herbal remedies (The Herbal Remedies* Act). Kuwait, Islamic Organization for Medical Sciences and World Health Organization Regional Office for the Eastern Mediterranean, 1986.

4. Miraldi E, Ferri S, Mostaghimi V. Botanical drugs and preparations in the traditional medicine of West Azerbaijan (Iran). *Journal of Ethnopharmacology,* 2001, 75:77–87.

5. *Legal status of traditional medicine and complementary/alternative medicine: a worldwide review.* Geneva, World Health Organization, 2001 (WHO/EDM/TRM/2001.2).

6.   *Country statistics* (http://www.who.int via individual country links). Cairo, World Health Organization Regional Office for the Eastern Mediterranean, 2001.

7.   Hatem MM. Health development in Djibouti. *World Health Forum*, 1996, 17:390–391.

8.   Salem SF. The health care delivery system in Libya with special emphasis on public health care services in Benghazi. Libyan Studies, 1996, 27:99–123.

9.   Elmi AS. Present state of knowledge and research on the plants used in traditional medicine in Somalia. *Journal of Ethnopharmacology*, 1980, 2:23–47.

10. Ul-Hassan Z. Acupuncture and developing countries. *American Journal of Chinese Medicine*, 1984, 12:56–59.

11. Hasan MY, Das M, Behjat S. Alternative medicine and the medical profession: views of medical students and general practitioners. *Eastern Mediterranean Health Journal*, 2000, 6:25–33.

12. Asefzadeh S, Sameefar F. Traditional healers in the Qazvin region of the Islamic Republic of Iran: a qualitative study. *Eastern Mediterranean Health Journal*, 2001, 7:544–550.

13. Obermeyer CM. Pluralism and pragmatism: knowledge and practice of birth in Morocco. *Medical Anthropology Quarterly*, 2000, 14:180–201.

14. Bellakhdar J. A new look at traditional medicine in Morocco. *World Health Forum*, 1989, 10:193–199.

15. Parvez A, et al. Medication attitudes – household survey of Faisalabad Tehsil. *Journal of the Pakistan Medical Association*, 1989, 39:290–291.

16. Qidwai W. Accessibility and effectiveness of healthcare providers. *Journal – College of Physicians and Surgeons of Pakistan*, 2003, 13:174–175.

17. Malik IA, Khan NA, Khan W. Use of unconventional methods of therapy by cancer patients in Pakistan. *European Journal of Epidemiology*, 1999, 16:155–160.

18. Ali BH, El Mahi I, Roese PM. Children's diseases and curing methods in a population of the Shendi Area (Sudan). *Annals of the Náprstek Museum*, 1998, 19:1–11.

19. Ahmed IM, Bremer JJ, Nouri AMH. Characteristics of visitors to traditional healers in central Sudan. *Eastern Mediterranean Health Journal*, 1999, 5: 79–85.

CHAPTER 21

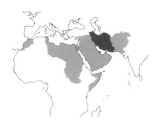

ISLAMIC REPUBLIC
OF IRAN

Mahmoud Mosaddegh[1]
and Farzaneh Naghibi[2]

[1]Dean,Traditional Medicine and Materia Medica Research Centre, Shaheed Beheshti University of Medical Science, Tehran, Islamic Republic of Iran. Email: mmosaddegh@itmrc.org

[2] Associate Professor and Deputy of Research, Traditional Medicine & Materia Medica Research Centre Shaheed Beheshti University of Medical Sciences , P.O. Box 14155-6354, Tehran, Islamic Republic of Iran. Email: fnaghibi@itmrc.org

21.1. INTRODUCTION

Knowledge of medicine in the Islamic Republic of Iran dates back more than 6000 years (*1*). The Gondi Shapoor University was established in 241–272 AD, based on such knowledge and after Iran became an Islamic nation, this university served as an important centre for medical sciences in the region. The teachings of Islam, which promote the acquisition of knowledge, prompted Iranian Muslim scientists such as Avicenna and Razes to theorize medical knowledge in Iran. Their works were translated into different languages, and some of them, such as Avicenna's *Canon of Medicine*, were used in European scientific centres for more than 600 years (*2*).

Although Iranian traditional medicine has been influenced by the introduction of allopathic health care, it is an integral part of the culture of the Iranian people, and thus has continued to prevail despite great pressure from the allopathic sector. Scientists working in universities as well as state officials have been paying greater attention to Iranian traditional medicine in the past two decades and there are ongoing efforts to establish a place for it within the formal health-care system.

21.2. BACKGROUND INDICATORS

21.2.1. Demography of the Islamic Republic of Iran

The Islamic Republic of Iran, with an area of some 1.6 million km^2, has 28 provinces. There is significant natural and geographical diversity with habitats including mountains, forests and deserts. According to the most recent census in 1996, the Islamic Republic of Iran had a population of over 60 million. Of these people, 32.1% were below 15 years and 13.4% over 50 years of age, and the literacy rate was 81.4% (*3*). The current population, based on the latest estimate of the Iranian Census Centre, amounts to 64 500 000. The life expectancy for the Iranian population as a whole was 69.0 years in 2000 (68.0 years for men and 70.0 years for women) (*4*). The estimate for healthy life expectancy for the Iranian population at birth was 57.6 in 2002 (*5*). The per capita gross domestic product of the Islamic Republic of Iran was US$ 1648 in 2000, or US$ 5884 taking into account purchasing power parities (Tehran, Management and Planning Organization, Islamic Republic of Iran, unpublished data, 2003). The total expenditure on health was 5.6% of gross domestic product in 2003 (Ministry of Health and Medical Education, Islamic Republic of Iran, unpublished data, 2003).

21.2.2. Health Care in the Islamic Republic of Iran

The health-care system of the Islamic Republic of Iran is unique in the world. After the foundation of the Ministry of Health and Medical Education in 1985, and a number of subsequent modifications in its management, health and medical services were combined with medical education. Subsequently, universities of medical sciences were established, and were entrusted with the responsibility to offer health and medical services and to train medical students. In this way, the students practice health monitoring and health care outside hospitals in the society, while receiving the necessary instruction.

Under this new system, the national policy has shifted from "treatment only" to a more inclusive policy of "care for healthy people and treatment of patients". Physicians have a responsibility for monitoring the health of different sections of society, in addition to their duty to treat patients. In the primary health-care network, the health houses in small villages and the health centres in larger villages and towns offer the first level of service. Rural and urban health centres represent the second level of service; specialized hospitals and polyclinics represent the third level; and the fourth level consists of sub-specialization in hospitals. Over time, the first and second levels have proven to be the most successful.

The Iranian system of health has many achievements (6), which include:

- easy access to primary health facilities in the villages;

- reduction of the infant mortality rate from 51 per 1000 live births in 1987 to 28.6 per 1000 in 2000;

- reduction of the mortality rate of children under five years of age from 70 per 1000 live births in 1985 to 30 per 1000 in 2000;

- reduction of the maternal mortality rate from 140 per 100 000 in 1985 to 37.4 per 100 000 in 1996;

- reduction of the population growth rate from 3.2% in 1985 to 1.2% in 2000;

- increase in the average immunization coverage against infectious diseases from 28.8% of the population in 1985 to 97% in 2002; and

- increased life expectancy from 59 years in 1985 to 69.0 years in 2000.

21.2.3. Data on Mortality and Numbers of Health-care Providers

The mortality rates due to the ten most common causes of death in Iran in 2002, are given in Table 21.1 (2). Data on the ten most common causes of morbidity have not yet been reported by the authorities. The total number of human resources in health sector is given in Table 21.2 (6).

Table 21.1. The ten leading causes of mortality in the Islamic Republic of Iran in 2002 (2)

Cause of mortality	Deaths per 100 000 population
Cardiovascular diseases	181.44
Unintentional injuries	58.95
Cancers	55.81
Pulmonary diseases	22.77
Neonatal conditions	16.01
Gastric diseases	11.68
Urinary diseases	8.28
Congenital and chromosome disorders	7.78
Nutritional, metabolic and endocrine disorders	7.17
Intentional injuries	6.37

21.3. HISTORY OF IRANIAN TRADITIONAL MEDICINE

Medicine has always played a significant role in Iranian (previously Persian) culture and civilization. Archaeological finds at the site of the "Torched City" in Sistan–Baluchestan Province attribute to a surgical operation on the skull of a 13-year-old girl suffering from hydrocephalus some 4850 years ago. Physicians and hospitals were of great significance in Iran during the Median, Achaemenian,

Parthian and Sassanid dynasties. In the Achaemenian dynasty, the most important medical reference was Avesta, a collection of sacred Zoroastrian writings. Other sacred books also dealt with medicine. Zoroastrians believed that Thrita was the first physician in Iran, and that Mazdaism led by Zoroaster would teach people about the practical and scientific treatment of diseases (1).

In later centuries, with the dawn of Islam, Gondi Shapoor University proved instrumental in promoting Islamic Science, which rapidly swept the world. This opened a new chapter in the medicine practiced in Iran and other Islamic countries. Iranian sciences absorbed Islamic concepts when Islam found its way into Iran (2).

Table 21.2. Human resources in health sector in 2003 (6)

Type of practitioners	Number
Physicians	82 393 (of whom 62 150 are general practitioners)
Dentists	15 236
Pharmacists	11 331
Nurses	87 353 (of whom 17 164 are midwives)

21.3.1. The Basis of Iranian Traditional Medicine

Iranian traditional medicine originated from a combination of the following:

- The medicine practised in Ancient Iran.
- The medicine of the Iran Plateau, which was mainly based on the Zoroastrian teachings and Avesta.
- Oriental medicine – likely to have originated from Indochinese philosophies and faiths – which made its way to Iran via the Indian subcontinent and central Asia.
- Mesopotamian medicine, which found its way to the west and south-west of Iran over a long period of time.
- Egyptian medicine.
- Greek medicine, which was first encountered after Alexander's invasion, and which continued to be incorporated into Islamic civilization during its westward expansion.
- Folk medicine, based on the experience of the Iranian people over centuries.
- Islamic medicine.

21.3.2. Endurance of Iranian Traditional Medicine

The traditional medicine of Iran gradually began to decline at the beginning of the 18th century. The main causes were the development of allopathic health care in Iran together with the establishment of medical and pharmacy schools based on the biomedical paradigm, and the absence of official support for traditional medicine. Swift treatment, new drugs and advanced diagnostic and therapeutic devices encouraged the people, particularly the educated elite, to seek treatment for their ailments in the allopathic sector.

Despite the pressure from the allopathic system, traditional medicine never completely disappeared from the lives of ordinary people. The reasons for its endurance include:

- the popular belief in traditional medicine and efforts undertaken by a small number of traditional practitioners;
- the continued existence of attaris (medicinal herb shops), which meet the public demand for herbs;

- the inability of the allopathic health-care system to cure certain diseases, particularly chronic ailments;

- the advent of the Islamic Revolution, which aroused people's interest in turning to their own national capabilities and knowledge;

- the inclusion of courses on medicinal herbs in the syllabus and as selected dissertation topics in pharmacy schools in Iran;

- global interest in the therapeutic value of medicinal plants, which has encouraged physicians, researchers and the Ministry of Health and Medical Education to pay attention to Iranian traditional medicine.

21.4. Structural and Process Indicators

21.4.1. Legislation and Regulation

Iranian traditional medicine has not been legally recognized, although there is no law against its practice. According to the law, only physicians who are graduates of universities of medical sciences which have been officially approved by the Ministry of Health and Medical Education are authorized to practice medicine. Nevertheless, there are individuals, particularly in small towns and villages, who treat people using traditional medicine. Many of these have been taught by their fathers or other instructors, although some have no training, and practise only to earn money. There are no accurate statistics on the number of people practising traditional medicine. Medicinal herbs are sold to the public in traditional herbal shops known as attaris.

The manufacture of herbal products is controlled by a law, with which the producers are obliged to comply. Recently, an advisor to the Minister has been appointed by the Minister of Health and Medical Education to oversee traditional medicine issues, remove impediments and regulate the traditional health-care sector.

In the Islamic Republic of Iran, the National Drug Policy has been promulgated as an essential part of the National Health Policy. Within the framework of the National Drug Policy, reforms have been carried out in many areas, particularly in the production and rational use of herbal medicine and herbal products. To achieve the rational use of herbal medicine, the Herbal Medicine Bureau was established in 1981 and the National Expert Committee for herbal medicine was established in 1996. The responsibilities of the Committee include drawing up national strategies, legislating and regulating, standardizing and cataloguing herbal medicine. After an application to the Herbal Medicine Bureau, herbal medicines are analysed by the Food and Drug Central Laboratory of the Ministry of Health and Medical Education. If a herbal product is approved, it will be licensed and monitored.

21.4.2. Education

There is no faculty or school offering traditional medicine education. However, due to the increased public attraction to traditional medicine over the last decade, physicians and medical students have become interested in learning about it. Therefore, the Education Department of the Ministry of Health and Medical Education is developing a strategic plan for teaching traditional medicine. The plan, which is expected to be implemented soon, intends to establish faculties of traditional medicine, or at least introduce a number of credits on traditional medicine into the curriculum of universities of medical sciences.

In addition, the Islamic and Traditional Medicine Group, which is part of the Islamic Republic of Iran Academy of Medical Sciences, is one of the strongest groups in the Academy. This group, established in 1989, has taken significant steps to revive and promote Iranian traditional medicine by publishing old Iranian books on traditional medicine, compiling different books on phytotherapy, and by making strategic plans and proposing them to the Ministry of Health and Medical Education.

21.4.3. Research

The Islamic Republic of Iran's special climate and the diversity of its ecosystems supports the growth of over 8000 plant species; indeed botanists call Iran's flora "green gold". Over the last two decades, the amount of research on Iranian traditional medicine, especially on medicinal herbs, has grown considerably. In addition to carrying out research on medicinal herbs at the Iranian faculties of pharmacy, a large number of research institutes have also been established. These include the Traditional Medicine & Materia Medica Research Centre, affiliated to Shaheed Beheshti University of Medical Sciences. Such centres are intended not only to undertake research on medicinal herbs, but also to revive and promote Iranian traditional medicine (7).

It should also be noted that a herbal-medicine network has been established recently, by the Ministry of Health and Medical Education, undersecretary for research and technology, to conduct and harmonize herbal medicine research activities.

21.4.4. Iranian Traditional Medicine Providers

No information is available on the total numbers of Iranian traditional medicine providers, either within or outside the allopathic health-care system. However, there are many attaris which offer their own treatment to the public. Furthermore, it has been noted that a few allopathic physicians are trying to increase their knowledge of traditional medicine, and even to treat their patients by using Iranian traditional medicine principles and products.

Recently, the Health Department at the Ministry of Health and Medical Education formally authorized and licensed 26 practitioners having valid degrees in chiropractic (6).

21.5. CONCLUSIONS

People in the Islamic Republic of Iran have a great deal of trust in Iranian traditional medicine, which has thousands of years of history, and hundreds of books. In spite of its relatively long absence from the Iranian health-care system, very serious attempts have been made recently to revive and promote traditional medicine. Care is being taken to avoid possible abuses of the system, and there is a commitment to introduce traditional medicine into the official health-care system through planning in the educational and research fields.

Among the measures taken to revive and promote traditional medicine are:

- establishing the necessary laws and regulations for medicinal herbs and manufacture of herbal products;

- establishing related industries;

- establishing farms for cultivation of medicinal herbs, to preserve wild stocks;

- planning systematic education in Iranian traditional medicine.

The above measures promote the scientific and rational integration of Iranian traditional medicine into primary health care and the formal health system. Research conducted in institutions such as the Islamic and Traditional Medicine Group within the Iranian Academy of Medical Sciences continues to provide an evidence base to support this policy. However, numerous challenges remain to be confronted.

Acknowledgement: The review of this chapter by Dr Majid Cheraghali, Advisor to the Deputy for Food and Drug Affairs, Ministry of Health, Iran, is greatly appreciated.

References

1. Sarmadi MT. Medicine and treatment in ancient Iran. In: *Research on the history of medicine and treatment up to present era, volume 1.* Tehran, Sarmadi publisher, 1999:131–156 (in Persian).

2. Velayati A. Sciences in Islamic civilization. In: *Culture and civilization of Islam and Iran, volume.1.* Tehran, Ministry of Foreign Affairs, Islamic Republic of Iran, 2003:125–243 (in Persian).

3. *Population and health in the Islamic Republic of Iran.* Tehran, Ministry of Health and Medical Education and United Nations Children's Fund, 2000.

4. *The Work of WHO in the Eastern Mediterranean Region; Annual Report of the Regional Director.* WHO Regional Office for the Eastern Mediterranean 2001:170.

5. *The World Health Report 2003: Shaping the Future.* Geneva, World Health Organization, 2003.

6. *Statistical Calendar*. Tehran, Ministry of Health and Medical Education, Islamic Republic of Iran, 2003.

7. Mosaddegh M, Naghibi F. Iran's traditional medicine, past and present. In: Mosaddegh M, Naghibi F, eds. *Traditional medicine and materia medica, volume 1*. Tehran, Traditional Medicine & Materia Medica Research Center, 2002:1–20.

Useful Link

Traditional Medicine & Materia Medica Research Center, Shaheed Beheshti University of Medical Sciences (http://www.itmrc.org, accessed 28 October 2004).

CHAPTER 22

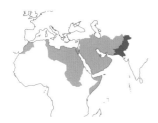

ISLAMIC REPUBLIC OF PAKISTAN

Farnaz Malik[1],
Shahzad Hussain[2],
Athar S. Dil[3],
Abdul Hannan[4]
and Anwarul H. Gilani[5]

[1] Chief/ National Program Manager, Drugs Control and Traditional Medicine Division, National Institute of Health, Islamabad, Pakistan. Email: farnazmalik@yahoo.com

[2] Officer-in-Charge, Chemical Research and Therapeutic Drug Monitoring Section, Drugs Control and Traditional Medicine Division, National Institute of Health, Islamabad, Pakistan.

[3] Executive Director/ National Coordinator, National Institute of Health, Islamabad, Pakistan. [4]Dean, Faculty of Eastern Medicine, Hamdard University, Karachi-74600, Pakistan. Email: Huvc@cyber.net.pk

[5] HEC Distinguished National Professor and Director, Natural Products Pharmacology Programme Department of Biological and Biomedical Sciences, The Aga Khan University Medical College, Karachi-74800, Pakistan. Email: anwar.gilani@aku.edu

22.1. INTRODUCTION

Traditional medicine has been a conspicuous component of the cultural heritage of the Islamic Republic of Pakistan and has played a significant role in providing health care to a large portion of the population. Traditional medicines and practices in Pakistan primarily belong to two categories i.e. Tibb-e-Unani and Homeopathy. Ayurveda is not very common in Pakistan though included in the Act. Acupuncture and Reiki, are also emerging on the scene. Spiritual and mind-body therapies are also prevalent in Pakistan.

22.1.1. Tibb-e-Unani

According to the basic principles of Tibb-e-Unani (Greco-Arab) the body is made up of four basic elements; earth, air, water, and fire, with different temperaments i.e. cold, hot, wet and dry. The body organs get their nourishment through four humors; blood, phlegm, yellow bile, and black bile. The concept of health in Tibb-e-Unani is a state of body in which there is equilibrium in the humors, and the functions of the body are normal in accordance with its own temperament and the environment. When the equilibrium of the humors is disturbed and the functions of body are abnormal, that state is called disease. Tibb-e-Unani takes a holistic approach towards prevention of disease, cure, and promotion of health. Tibb-e-Unani relies on drugs made from medicinal plants, herbs, minerals, or of metallic or animal origin, for the treatment of diseases.

22.1.2. Homeopathy

The homeopathic system of medicine is gaining popularity in Pakistan. It was introduced to this part of the subcontinent a little over a century ago and has blended well with the traditional concepts. Homeopathy simply means treating diseases with remedies, prescribed in minute doses, which are capable of producing symptoms similar to the disease when taken by healthy people. It is based on the natural law of healing—Similia Similibus Curantur—which means 'likes are cured by likes'. Dr Samuel Hahnemann (1755–1843) gave it a scientific basis in the early 19th century.

22.2. DEMOGRAPHY OF PAKISTAN

Pakistan has an area of 796 095 km², which is 0.6% of the total area of the world. It has four provinces; federally-administered areas. Pakistan shares borders with Afghanistan, China, India and the

Islamic Republic of Iran. It is the sixth largest country after China, India, United States of America, Indonesia and Brazil, having surpassed Japan, Bangladesh, Nigeria and the Russian Federation, and has population of 148.6 million, which is 2.36% of the world's population. Of this population 43.2% are less than 15 years old, 53.4% from 15-64 years and 3.4% are 65 years of age or more. The per capita income is US$ 492. Of the population, 33% lives in urban areas and 67.0% lives in rural areas. The population growth rate is 2.06% (*1*).

22.3. HEALTH CARE IN PAKISTAN

Health is the priority area of the Government activities. The high correlation between the expenditure on health and productivity in developing countries like Pakistan is evidence of the importance of increasing health services as an aid to growth. Hence in the health sector, poverty and ill health needed to be brought into sharp focus.

According to a recent survey, childhood and infectious diseases were responsible for two-thirds of the burden of disease in Pakistan (*2*). The specific causes of morbidity include hypertension, injuries, eye diseases, malnutrition, maladies relating to parturition, congenital malformations, dental disease, ischaemic heart disease, anaemia (in adult women) and mental retardation.

Many of the deaths in Pakistan are due to diarrhoea, lower respiratory infections (pneumonia) in childhood, and tuberculosis (*2*). Other causes of mortality featuring among the most common are perinatal conditions, injuries, hypertension, congenital malformations, chronic liver disease, ischaemic heart disease and rheumatic heart disease.

The relatively low life expectancy (63 years), high child mortality rate under 5 years (110 per 1000), high infant mortality rate (83.3 per 1000), and high population growth rate (2.06%) provide the basis for national health priorities (*3*).

The concept of health care includes not only freedom from communicable and other diseases, but also the availability of facilities for maternity-care and child-care. The infrastructure of the health sector therefore covers the establishment of hospitals, dispensaries, basic health units and maternal and child health-care centres, together with their staffing with adequate numbers of doctors, pharmacists, nurses, health visitors and midwives (Table 22.1).

Table 22.1. Facilities in the health sector

Health Facilities	Number
Hospitals	906
Dispensaries	4525
Rural health centres	550
Basic health units	5308
Total number of beds	98264

The details of the registered medical and paramedical personnel are shown in Table 22.2 and the expenditure on health for the last five years (*4*) in Table 22.3.

Table 22.2. Registered medical and paramedical personnel* and expenditure on health (calendar year basis)

Registered personnel	1998	1999	2000	2001	2002
Doctors	82682	87105	91823	96248	101635
Dentists	3444	3867	4175	4622	5068
Nurses	32938	35979	37623	40019	44520
Midwives	22103	22401	22525	22711	23084
Lady Health Visitors	4959	5299	5443	5669	6397
No. of people per Doctor	1590	1578	1529	1516	1466
No. of people per Dentist	38185	35557	33629	31579	29405
No. of people per Nurse	3992	3822	3732	3639	3347

* Registered with Pakistan Medical, Dental and Nursing Councils

The Pakistan system of health has a number of achievements (5), which include:

- enactment of "Anti-smoking Ordinance";

- enactment of "Protection of Breast-feeding and Child Nutrition Ordinance";

- Blood Transfusion Ordinance;

- easy access to primary health facilities in the villages;

- increase in the average immunization coverage against infectious diseases and addition of Hepatitis-B vaccine in the routine immunization coverage;

- increase in the life expectancy to 63 years in 2003;

- final efforts towards the eradication of polio from our country.

Table 22.3. Expenditure on health

Expenditure (million PKR)*	1998	1999	2000	2001	2002
Development	5491.81	5887.00	5944.00	6688.00	6609.00
Non-development	15315.86	16190.00	18337.00	18717.00	22205.00

* US$ 1 = PKR c.57.27

22.4. Current Situation of Traditional Medicine in Pakistan

The following is a list of principal activities of the National Institute of Health and Ministry of Health in the traditional medicine sector in Pakistan.

- The National Advisory Committee on traditional medicine has been established to look into the affairs of this important sector.

- The recommendations for national traditional medicine policy and regulation have been prepared, with consensus amongst the stakeholders of the traditional medicine sector of all the provinces, and submitted to Ministry of Health for formal approval.

- The Bill to regulate the manufacture, storage, import and export of Tibb-e-Unani, Ayurvedic, homeopathic, herbal and non-allopathic medicines has been prepared in consultation with the stakeholders of the traditional medicine sector.

- Monographs of individual Unani medicinal plants have been published.

- The list of essential traditional medicines has been published.

- Work on the development of standards and a specification of individual medicinal plants is in progress and will form the basis for a Pharmacopoeia.

In Pakistan, about 457 Tibbi dispensaries and clinics provide medication to the public. About 95 dispensaries have been established under provincial departments of Local Bodies and Rural Development.

The National Council for Tibb is responsible for developing the curriculum, education and examination of Tibb-e-Unani and for registration of practitioners (Tabibs). Out of 22 council members, 14 are elected through a procedure of postal ballot, and the Federal and Provincial Government nominate the others.

The National Council for Homeopathy is responsible for the education, examination and registration of homeopathic practitioners. Several hospitals, outpatient clinics and dispensaries are attached to homeopathic medical colleges. There are 21 members in the National Council for Homeopathy; some are elected through postal ballot and some are nominated by the Government.

There are 300-350 Herbal/Tibb-e-Unani manufacturing companies and around 300 companies manufacturing homeopathic medicines. Pakistan is amongst the leading exporters of medicinal plants; according to the Export Promotion Bureau, Pakistan exported 8500 tons of medicinal plants in 1999 and earned US$ 6 million from export, compared to US$ 31 million spent on import of herbal products. This is mainly because the technology is not yet developed to export the processed form of herbal products, which could be a major source of revenue.

There are around 5000 species of wild plants in Pakistan. According to the National Institute of Health of Pakistan, about 400 plant species are used in traditional medicine. Medicinal herbs and spices have great value in Pakistan. The ecosystem in which they are growing has intrinsic association with environmental values in conserving soil, water and providing a habitat for other species. The genetic diversity of traditional medicinal plants is continuously under the threat of extinction. The conservation of this biological diversity at the level of ecosystem, species and genetic sources is to be prioritized for sustainable medicinal resource management.

22.5. INFORMATION ON STRUCTURAL INDICATORS

22.5.1. Legislation and Regulation

The practice, education and registration of homeopathic doctors and Hakims are made under Unani, Ayurvedic and Homeopathic Act, 1965. A Bill to regulate Tibb-e-Unani, Ayurvedic, homeopathic, herbal and any other non-allopathic medicine has been recently approved by the Federal Cabinet of Islamic Republic of Pakistan and will be enacted very soon.

The National Drug Policy is an essential part of national health policy and traditional medicine is a component of the 2001 Policy, which advocates for special regulations and legislation and encourages the modern practitioners to conduct research on traditional medicine on scientific lines. It also calls for updating the inventory of traditional medicines used in Pakistan.

22.5.2. Endurance of Traditional Medicine in Pakistan

Advanced therapeutic and diagnostic devices, quick treatment and new drugs have encouraged the people, particularly the educated elite and those living in the urban areas, to seek treatment for their ailments in the allopathic sector. Despite the pressure from the modern system of medicine, traditional medicine has never completely disappeared from the lives of ordinary people especially those living in far-flung and least-developed areas of the country. The reasons for its endurance include:

- The continued existence of medicinal herbs and public demands for the herbs.

- The inability of the modern health care system to cure and curtail certain chronic diseases and ailments.

- The interest of the people in turning to their indigenous and national capabilities, knowledge and resources, and their desire to use natural products.

22.5.3. Education

There are 30 Tibbia colleges in the private sector and one college in the public sector offering four-year diploma courses in Tibb-e-Unani that follow the prescribed curriculum and conditions laid down in the regulations. Recently, a five-year degree programme has been launched by the Faculty of Eastern Medicine of Hamdard University, Karachi, and by Islamia University, Bahawalpur, and the curricula are revised and standardized by the Higher Education Commission.

There are 119 officially-recognized colleges of homeopathic medicine imparting education and offering programmes for a four-year diploma course. Islamia University, Bahawalpur, and three private colleges have recently started five-year degree programmes in homeopathy.

22.5.4. Research

The varied climatic conditions and diverse ecosystems in Pakistan have set the stage for the growth of over 5000 plant species. The Government, in consultation with the indigenous peoples and with the assistance of NGOs, is working hard to preserve this natural habitat.

The Plant Genetic Resources Programme (PGRP) of Pakistan Agricultural Research Council is involved in the collection, conservation, characterization and evaluation of germplasm of various crops including medicinal plants. During the last three years the PGRP, under a Ministry of Food and Agriculture funded project and Agricultural Linkage Programme, has collected more than

3000 accessions belonging to 60 medicinal plant species. The material collected has been put in ex situ conservation as an active and base collection for long-term preservation.

22.5.5. Traditional Medicine Providers

Table 22.4. Types of TRM practitioners

Practitioners	Number
Hakims/Tabbibs	39 584
Homeopathic Doctors	90 000
Vaids	455

Source: Unani Section, Ministry of Health, Government of Pakistan.

22.6. PROSPECTS FOR INTEGRATION OF TRADITIONAL MEDICINE AND ALLOPATHIC MEDICINE IN THE HEALTH-CARE SYSTEM

The practice of traditional and allopathic health care in Pakistan function in isolation and the practitioners of the two systems usually keep their distance. This is evident from one example: practitioners of allopathic medicine learned to use ispaghula husk only after it was fully accepted all over the world, despite the fact that it is indigenous to South-Asian traditional medicine and South Asia is the largest exporter to the rest of the world. Research in general, and traditional medicine in particular, has been the priority of the present Government. The Ministry of Science and Technology has recently announced the establishment of the Institute of Aromatic Plants with special mandate for the promotion and sustainable use of these indigenous resources. The Government is also making concrete efforts to promote research on traditional medicine and to regulate herbal products, an essential step to gain the faith of consumers as well as acceptance by allopathic physicians.

The Aga Khan University Medical College has introduced the concept of traditional and complementary medicine to its undergraduate (both medical and nursing) and postgraduate curricula. A Study Group on Traditional and Complementary medicine has been constituted, comprising professionals from different disciplines, such as basic health sciences, family medicine, community health sciences, medicine and psychiatry.

22.7. CONCLUSION

The majority of the people of Pakistan have perpetually inherited faith in traditional systems of medicines. The Government of Pakistan has, historically, allocated meagre funds for promotion of the traditional medicine sector. However, the Government has taken appropriate measures to upgrade the standard of education in traditional medicine and the sale and storage of traditional medicine products. The future course of action for traditional medicine in Pakistan will be steered by:

- Comprehensive national policy on traditional medicines as part of the national health policy.

- Patronage and promotion of traditional medicine at the primary health-care level.

- Establishment of a databank of traditional knowledge and essential traditional medicines.

References

1. *Population Growth and Its Implications.* Islamabad, National Institute of Population Studies, Pakistan, July 2003.

2. Hyder AA, Morrow HH. Applying Burden of Disease Methods to Developing Countries: Case Study of Pakistan. *American Journal of Public Health,* 2000, 90:1235–1240.

3. *Annual Report of the Director General Health.* Ministry of Health, Government of Pakistan, 2000–2001.

4. *Health and Nutrition. In: Economic Survey 2002–2003,* Chapter 12. Islamabad, Ministry of Finance, Government of Pakistan, 2003 (http://www.finance.gov.pk/).

5. *Report of the Inter-Provincial Health Ministers Conference,* 30–31 July 2003, Islamabad, Ministry of Health, Government of Pakistan.

CHAPTER 23

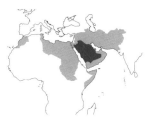

KINGDOM OF SAUDI ARABIA

Abdullah M.N. Al-Bedah

Supervisor, Alternative Medicine, Ministry of Health, Old Airport Road, Riyadh 11176, Saudi Arabia.
E-mail: aalbedah3@yahoo.com

23.1. INTRODUCTION

Traditional Arab medicine is often referred to, at least in part, as Unani Tibb or Greco-Arab medicine. Traditional medicine in general refers to indigenous knowledge, theories and practices for the maintenance of health as well as the prevention, diagnosis and treatment of various physical and mental illnesses. A large proportion of the population of the Kingdom of Saudi Arabia believes in some form of traditional medicine, such as Islamic and prophetic medicine, herbal medicine, bonesetting (al-tajbeer), cupping (al-hijamah), and cauterization (qai wasm), practised in different parts of the country.

The Arabian Peninsula, of which Saudi Arabia forms the major part, has historically been a major transit area for herbs, condiments and spices from the Indian sub-continent and countries of South-East Asia to Europe, North Africa and Eastern Mediterranean countries. Saudi Arabia, due to its holy places, Makkah and Madinah, receives millions of pilgrims every year from all over the world. These pilgrims bring with them their own traditional herbal remedies, whether for personal use or for sale and marketing. Accordingly, the holy cities of Makkah and Madinah have become centres for herbs and crude drugs.

23.2. BACKGROUND INDICATORS

National health-care agencies list the ten most common causes of morbidity in Saudi Arabia as upper respiratory tract infections; diseases of the digestive system; musculoskeletal diseases; skin diseases; dental problems; eye diseases; diabetes; chronic obstructive pulmonary diseases; urinary tract infections; and hypertension. Most morbidity is attributable to a high standard of living; rapid changes of lifestyle, including dietary habits and mass urbanization; the extreme weather conditions of the country; and the masses of international visitors during the pilgrimage season.

The ten most common causes of mortality in Saudi Arabia are cardiovascular diseases; accidents; complications of pregnancy and childbirth; neoplasm; haematological diseases; respiratory diseases; congenital deformities; endocrine diseases; infectious and parasitic diseases; and gastroenterological diseases.

In Saudi Arabia, only medical doctors are allowed to prescribe medicines. At present, the total number of doctors is 32 000 for a population of 22 million. However, over-the-counter drugs can be obtained without prescription.

Saudi Arabia is one of the few countries in the world in which most medical expenditure is borne by the Government. The total estimated expenditure in 1998 for the conventional medical-care sector was 27.4 billion Saudi riyals (US$ 7.3 billion); of this 30% is for primary health care and the remaining 70% is allocated to secondary and tertiary health care. The main health-care provider is the Ministry of Health with a yearly budget around 14 billion Saudi riyals (US$ 3.73 billion). The Ministry provides 65% of national health care, while the remaining 35% is provided by the Armed Forces, the National Guard and the Security Forces Hospitals mainly for secondary and tertiary care.

There are some qualified and trained health-care providers of traditional, complementary and alternative medicine (TCAM) present in various parts of Saudi Arabia but few are licensed to practise. As yet, only trained medical doctors have been licensed to provide acupuncture. Data on TCAM providers are not currently available. The size of the TCAM sector is difficult to estimate as no comprehensive national studies have been conducted on TCAM services, products, or utilization.

23.3. Information on Structural and Process Indicators

23.3.1. Policy and Legislation

The official national policy for TCAM is under development. The Government is currently considering its position with respect to TCAM, in response to public interest and concern. The Department of Alternative and Complementary Medicine at the Ministry of Health is dealing with matters related to recognition of TCAM, consumer education, licensing, and the implementation and integration of TCAM practices in Saudi Arabia. There are committees and sub-committees to review the strategies and recommendations for professionalization of TCAM practitioners.

Some regulatory activity has already taken place, including regulation of acupuncture practice and herbal medicine, and the licensing and registration of nutritional supplements and vitamins. The first protocol for selling herbs was issued as early as 1938. The first regulations on medicinal plants and preparations, issued in 1978, are entitled "Regulations for the registration of herbal preparations, health foods and supplementary foods, cosmetics and antiseptics that make medical claims". The regulation certificate covers 29 points.

Although the Ministry of Health has stated that there is no TCAM regulation of a general nature, a literature search has identified an Act Governing the Practice of Pharmacy and Trade in Medicines and Medical Products, issued by Royal Decree M/18, dated 26 February 1978. Articles 44 and 50 of this act prohibit the handling of locally-produced or imported products prior to their registration with the Ministry of Health. Paragraph 13A of the Special Provisions on Registration Regulations for Pharmaceutical Companies and their Products, which was amended by Ministerial Resolution 1214/30 dated 25 January 1989, requires the registration of medicines and all products having medical claims, including herbal preparations containing active ingredients that possess medicinal effects.

The Herbal, Health Food and Natural Products Licensing Committee, established under the Ministry of Health in 1993, is responsible for approving or disallowing products, primarily on the basis of safety and efficacy. Approval by this Committee is mandatory for products intended for public use. By late 2003, the Committee had approved only 630 out of 1950 herbal-based or natural products submitted for licensing. The Committee oversees the marketing and use of all herbal products, health food products and natural health products, including items for cosmetic and antiseptic use. The Ministry of Health has also established a central scientific committee to examine traditional healers' claims. Decisions are made through these two committees, and finally approved for implementation by the Minister of Health.

Following WHO guidelines, the Ministry of Health has restricted acupuncture licences to medically-qualified anaesthetists, rheumatologists and orthopaedists who have at least 200 hours of training, and comply with official standards of hygienic practice.

Regarding integration of services and professionalization of TCAM practitioners, no private institutions have, as yet, been established in Saudi Arabia.

23.3.2. Education

There are no dedicated TCAM educational institutions in Saudi Arabia. However, the College of Pharmacy at King Saud University, Riyadh, opened a specialized complementary and alternative medicine (CAM) unit in December 2003, with the aim of providing information regarding herbal and alternative medicines to governmental and private agencies, and also to the public. Recently, the Department of Pharmacognosy, at the College of Pharmacy, King Saud University, introduced a course on CAM for undergraduate students. Similarly, the colleges of medicine in Riyadh and Jeddah have also introduced a limited number of lectures on CAM for both undergraduate and postgraduate students.

23.3.3. Research

A major scientific study has been conducted on local medicinal plants to assess their potential biological activity (1). Research has included collection, identification, description of plant habitats and literature survey, as well as phytochemical, microbiological and pharmacological screening. The project was entitled "Phytochemical and Biological Evaluation of Saudi Plants" and took place during the period 1983–1986.

Another national project (1984–1990) was entitled "Scientific Evaluation of Merits and Demerits of Crude Drugs Used in Saudi Folk Medicine" (2). This study aimed to survey the prevalence of Saudi folk and/or traditional medicine practice in the country. The study focused on interviews with herbal medicine practitioners. Questionnaires were administered to both the general public and practitioners. Interviews were also conducted with the Attarine (sellers of herbs and crude drugs). Samples of crude drugs and poly-herbal formulations (compound drugs) were collected, and claims for them were recorded. The claimed activities of the collected material were then tested in laboratory animals at the College of Pharmacy, King Saud University. Both projects were funded by the King Abdulaziz City for Science and Technology (KACST), Riyadh.

23.3.4. Utilization

Traditional medicine remains widely utilized in rural areas. However, a considerable number of people, mostly highly-educated members of the professional community, remain hesitant about accepting and using TCAM. Accordingly, retail outlets selling modern herbal and health-food products offer well-presented packs of herbal or nutritional supplements, aiming to attract the young and educated community to try their products at least once. Public awareness is now growing, although this strategy is still in its infancy.

Saudi Television occasionally conducts national debates, lectures and specialized programmes related to TCAM, and in particular, the potential for integrating TCAM into the mainstream medical system. Participants in such debates represent all levels of society.

23.4. Discussion

Surveys and interviews of local populations, including herb sellers (attarins), folk and/or traditional medicine practitioners (practitioners of qai, hijamah, herbal medicine treatment using honey and recitation of Quranic verses), showed that large numbers of the general population are interested in using one or more TCAM modalities alone or in conjunction with modern health facilities. This trend is escalating even in the urban areas. Moreover, in Saudi Arabia, national and international conferences, symposia, annual meetings and seminars are being conducted from time to time by some institutions and societies and are sponsored by some commercial organizations dealing with natural herbal or nutraceutical products.

The present trend indicates that the future of TCAM in Saudi Arabia is bright and expected to take a leap forward with the support of the Ministry of Health and flexible legislation. On the other hand, recognition and easing of licensing policy may have an impact on the national economy by utilizing local natural resources and emerging indigenous human resources in health-care sector.

In view of the interest and mounting demands of local inhabitants and expatriates (who form more than 50% of the country's population), the authorities are reconsidering the official policy to develop a revision of the legislation on TCAM.

23.5. Conclusions and Summary

Official national policy regarding TCAM is under development in Saudi Arabia. Some regulatory activity has already taken place regarding acupuncture practice. Official policy and legislation are being formulated to cover the sale and marketing of herbal, nutritional and vitamin products; consumer awareness is being assessed; and there is research into selected traditional herbal practices. A national committee is being formed to regulate TCAM education, and a national voluntary self-regulatory system of TCAM practice is under study as a matter of priority. The Department of Alternative and Complementary Medicine in the Ministry of Health is now preparing guidelines and reviewing its strategies for issuing a mandate on the integration of TCAM into national health policy.

References

1. *Al-Yahya MA et al. Phytochemical and biological evaluation of Saudi plants. Periodical reports submitted to the King Abdulaziz City for Science and Technology (KACST).* Riyadh, 1983–1986.

2. *Ageel AM et al. Scientific evaluation of merits and demerits of crude drugs used in Saudi folk medicine. Periodical reports submitted to the King Abdulaziz City for Science and Technology (KACST).* Riyadh, 1984–1990.

CHAPTER 24

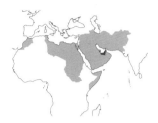

UNITED ARAB EMIRATES

Sassan Behjat

Coordinator, Office of Traditional, Complementary and Alternative Medicine, Federal Ministry of Health, P. O. Box 848, Abu Dhabi, United Arab Emirates. E-mail: sbehjat@moh.gov.ae

24.1. INTRODUCTION

The United Arab Emirates is an amazing combination of the traditional values of the East and the modern technologies of the West. It is a melting pot of various nationalities and cultures, and has a standard of living comparable to the world's most advanced nations. For centuries, due to its convenient location on the trade routes between Asia and Europe, the United Arab Emirates has gained a reputation as a host and trade partner for diverse peoples. Although 65% of its 85 000 km² area is desert, the country is characterized by rich microclimates and microecologies. There are hills, valleys, different kinds of dunes, plains, marshes and even mangrove forests. The desert extends from the westernmost tip of Abu Dhabi, on the borders of Saudi Arabia, towards the east to the land border with Oman and the Indian Ocean.

The United Arab Emirates had an estimated population of 2 407 460 in 2001, with a density of 29 persons per km². However, several aspects of its population are unusual. The population in 1995 was 15 times larger than it was 30 years previously, mainly due to the immigration of oil workers. Of the total population, 80% consists of foreign workers and their dependents. Due to the influx of young foreign workers, the cultural preference for large families and improvements in medical care, the United Arab Emirates also has a very young population.

The citizens have access to some of the world's best medical facilities, where provision of medical care is mostly free-of-charge. Life expectancy is increasing rapidly. Infant and perinatal mortality rates are the lowest in the region. The relative decrease in communicable diseases has exposed a pattern of disease and injury that is unique to the United Arab Emirates.

24.2. CURRENT SITUATION

Rapid social change during the past three decades has brought about increasing literacy rates, increasing empowerment and employment of women, and rapid economic development, leading to rising standards of living and high disposable incomes. As a consequence, there have been considerable changes in epidemiological trends, resulting in a sharp decline in mortality rates for all ages, and a decreased incidence of communicable diseases, prenatal, perinatal and maternal diseases, and nutritional disorders. At the same time there has been an increase in the incidence of noncommunicable and degenerative diseases, as well as accidents and injuries. Chronic diseases have become a significant cause of morbidity and mortality. Cardiovascular disorders, accidents and cancer are the major causes of mortality in the United Arab Emirates. In 2001, these three problems accounted for 61% of deaths in the country. The leading causes of deaths in 2001 were as follows: cardiovascular diseases, accidents, cancer, congenital anomalies, pneumonia and bronchitis, nephritis and nephrosis, diabetes mellitus, chronic liver disease and cirrhosis. National health strategies in the United Arab Emirates are being revised to accommodate these new trends according to their priority.

During 2001, total Government expenditure on health was 68 million UAE dirham (US$ 18.7 million) and total private expenditure on health was estimated to be 21.7 million UAE dirham (US$ 5.9 million). Therefore, total expenditure on health for 2001 was approximately US$ 24.5 million, which was 3.6% of gross domestic product for that year.

24.3. Development of Traditional Medicine in the United Arab Emirates

The Abu Dhabi Herbal Centre was established in July 1998 as an outpatient herbal treatment clinic, following the instructions of the President, HH Sheikh Zayed Bin Sultan Al Nahyan. Its subsequent development and expansion in 1996 to the Zayed Complex for Herbal Research and Traditional Medicine was an important milestone in the development of scientific research on medicinal herbs in the United Arab Emirates. Since its inception, the Zayed Complex has been actively involved in generating knowledge about new herbal treatments and verifying old traditions regarding the therapeutic properties of local medicinal herbs. These discoveries are made available for clinical use and further research for validation and documentation. Researchers from the Zayed Complex have been involved in many seminars on the advancement of the science of herbal and traditional medicine, and their cooperation has been sought by different international agencies active in research and development of medicinal herbs.

During the past decade, there has been an increased awareness by consumers, and subsequent rise in demand for natural and alternative therapies in the United Arab Emirates, as elsewhere in the world. Widespread public interest and reactions from both government and private health-care providers led to the creation of a legal mandate for the official recognition of alternative medicine practitioners and minimum standards for the quality of health care. In response to these challenges, and as a necessary function of its duty to protect the public interest, the Ministry of Health established a Complementary and Alternative Medicine Unit by Ministerial Decree on 25 June 2001.

Traditional, complementary and alternative medicine (TCAM) is regulated in the United Arab Emirates jointly by two departments at the Ministry of Health. The Drug Control Department regulates the registration of non-conventional medicines such as herbal, homeopathic, Ayurvedic, and Chinese, as well as natural products in drug stores and pharmacies, while the Complementary and Alternative Medicine Unit coordinates the licensing and regulation of TCAM practitioners.

By 1 July 2003, the Drug Control Department had registered 53 herbal medicines, with a further 120 in the process of registration, from 48 companies that have fulfilled criteria of the Ministerial Decree No. 3278 of 1997 regarding the 'rules and regulations for registration and re-registration of medicines and products derived from natural sources'. Food supplements and other natural and herbal medicines without any clinical claim are being registered under a general list.

Between January 2002 and December 2003, 132 TCAM practitioners – homeopaths, herbalists, Ayurveda and Unani practitioners, traditional Chinese medicine practitioners, acupuncturists and chiropractors – passed the TCAM qualifying examinations, which are held four times a year by the Ministry of Health. Many have started practising in clinics and private hospitals in the United Arab Emirates. These TCAM practitioners, like other primary health care physicians, can see patients without referral and prescribe non-allopathic medicines according to their specialization, as well as over-the-counter medicines that have been registered by the Pharmacy Department and sold through licensed pharmacies.

24.4. TCAM Licensing Procedure

In exercising its licensing authority, the Ministry of Health has the power to determine the qualifications that a TCAM licence applicant must possess. It may investigate educational credentials, professional competence and moral character. The applicant is responsible for proving that he or she fulfils all requirements for licensing.

No person is permitted to practise TCAM in the United Arab Emirates without first being licensed by the Ministry of Health. Successfully passing the TCAM qualifying examination is a precondition for evaluation and grant of a TCAM practice licence.

To be eligible to apply for the TCAM qualifying examination, the applicants should possess one of the following:

- A medical degree (e.g. MBBS, MBChB, MD) and a diploma or a postgraduate certificate in any of the TCAM specialities approved by the Ministry of Health, achieved after no less than six months or two semesters of full-time study.

- A diploma or bachelor degree, after full-time study in an accredited institute, college or university (e.g. doctor of chiropractic, bachelor or MD in homeopathy, bachelor or MD in Ayurvedic medicine, bachelor or masters in traditional Chinese medicine) in any of the TCAM specialities approved by the Ministry of Health. These courses should be of not less than three years for diplomas and not less than four and a half years for degrees.

In addition, allied health diploma or bachelor degree holders (e.g. nurses, dieticians, occupational therapists, physiotherapists) who have successfully completed a course in any branch of recognized alternative medicine of no less than two years' duration from recognized institutions, can also be considered on an individual basis to sit for the examinations.

Further to the above requirements, sufficient clinical experience in the field of speciality is required. For medical degree holders, it is a minimum of one year of TCAM experience, and for TCAM degree holders, it is a minimum of two years of work experience in an official clinic or hospital setting. The following TCAM specialties are recognized by the Ministry of Health:

- herbal medicine

- traditional Islamic medicine (Unani)

- traditional Chinese medicine

- traditional Indian medicine (Ayurveda and Siddha)

- homeopathic medicine

- naturopathy

- chiropractic medicine, and

- osteopathy.

Candidates who successfully pass the written examination based on clinical, diagnostic and public health sciences are called for interview in their field of speciality. An examination board consisting of professionals from different specialities conducts the interviews. If necessary, the examination board may invite TCAM professionals from the private sector to assist in conducting the interviews.

Successful candidates who have passed both written and oral/practical examinations are awarded a licence to practise in their field of speciality.

24.4.1. TCAM Licence Categories

The Ministry of Health awards TCAM practice licences in the following categories:

- TCAM Medical Specialist/Medical Category

- TCAM Therapist/Paramedic Category

- TCAM Assistants/Technician Category

TCAM Technician and Paramedic Categories are awarded to non-medically qualified TCAM applicants, while TCAM Medical Specialist licences are awarded to those having basic medical education in addition to a degree in TCAM from recognized institutions.

24.4.2. Practice Categories

The educational qualifications, depth and field of experience, and results of the TCAM examinations and recommendations from examination board are considered in evaluating the candidates and their category of practice. The evaluation committee may permit the following two categories of TCAM practice privileges on the licences:

Independent TCAM Practice Category: TCAM practitioners who have basic medical degrees or MD-level qualifications in TCAM specialities, or extensive proven experience, or others at the recommendation of the examination board, may be awarded licences for independent TCAM practice. These practitioners may start their own clinics or treatment centres and may employ other supporting staff such as nurses, technicians and even other TCAM specialists, as necessary.

Clinic Licence Category: These practitioners are permitted to work only in an established polyclinic or clinic where a licensed medical general practitioner is on duty. Based on the policy or decision of the management of the clinic, these TCAM practitioners may see patients directly or after referral from the resident medical general practitioner.

24.5. Good TCAM Practice and Care

TCAM care must include an adequate assessment of the patient's condition, based on history, clinical signs and symptoms and if necessary an appropriate physical examination and investigations.

24.5.1. Evaluation of Patients

TCAM practitioners in the United Arab Emirates must conduct an appropriate medical history and perform physical examination of the patient and review of the patient's medical records, before providing any treatment. TCAM practitioners may use allopathic diagnostic methods, in addition to other TCAM methods of diagnosis, provided that such diagnostic methods are based on currently-accepted safety standards. They are required to document all the investigations and findings in the patient's medical record. Medical records and patients' files should remain current and be maintained in an easily retrievable manner.

24.5.2. Treatment Plan

The TCAM practitioners are required to provide TCAM treatment according to a documented treatment plan based on the individual needs of the patient. Treatment plans help in evaluating the progress and success of a given treatment method, such as relief of pain and inflammation, improved physical and/or psychosocial function and attainment of a general state of well-being.

24.5.3. Consultations and Referral to General Practitioners and Specialists Licensed by the Ministry of Health

The TCAM practitioners may refer patients as necessary for additional evaluation and treatment in order to achieve treatment objectives.

24.6. Guidelines for TCAM Care

In providing TCAM therapies, practitioners must:

- recognize and work within the limits of their professional competence;
- be willing to consult allopathic and alternative medicine colleagues;
- be competent when making diagnoses and when giving or arranging treatment;
- keep clear, accurate and up-to-date patient records which report the relevant clinical findings, the decisions made, the information given to patients and any drugs, regimen or treatment prescribed;
- keep colleagues well informed when sharing the care of patients;
- pay due regard to efficacy and use of resources;
- prescribe only the treatment, drugs or appliances that serve the patient's needs.

TCAM practitioners are prohibited from:

- carrying out procedures not related to their speciality, including performing operations;
- administering injections, parenteral solutions and vaccinations;
- practising midwifery;
- withdrawing blood;
- claiming or offering to treat cancer;
- treating communicable diseases;

- performing internal examinations;

- prescribing controlled medicines or drugs such as prescription-only medications;

- selling medicines, goods, or health related products from their clinics or treatment centres;

- advertising that is false or misleading or that claims the cure of any condition or disease;

- preventing any person from being treated by an allopathic physician or improperly influencing any person to abstain from such treatment.

TCAM practitioners who do not possess a basic medical degree (e.g. MBBS, MD) or having a medical degree but not having yet passed the medical licensing examinations conducted for general medical practitioners, are prohibited from claiming to be, or leading people to understand that they are, an allopathic, or conventional medical doctor.

24.7. Discussion

During the past decade there has been evidence of an increase in consumers' awareness of natural and alternative therapies in the United Arab Emirates which has given rise to official recognition of the TCAM practice in the country. As well as an exclusive government research centre, alternative systems of medicine have started to become a part of existing private health-care institutions, providing individuals with an option for alternative or complementary medicine.

The past four years have seen continuing efforts to give legal status to most of the health-care traditions of the world, and to address the concerns of safety and efficacy. Both of these issues are critical to the licensing of the medicines and practice. To tackle the former issue, TCAM practitioners are being put through a very dynamic, yet systematic, method of evaluation by a multidisciplinary group of experts. Efforts to maintain the communication between TCAM providers through periodic continuing medical education are also being implemented.

As TCAM is being gradually introduced and integrated into the health-care delivery system, efforts to promote rational use and identification of safe and sound therapies will be crucial. To assure quality and proper use, natural medicines are put through a series of evaluations. Many recipes, especially the poly-herbal combinations, have yet to obtain registration due to the existing rules and regulations based on herbal medicine quality parameters. Further discussions are underway to address this issue. Research programmes in pharmacological and clinical studies, directed by the Government research centre, are periodically disseminated for clinical use and validation.

24.8. Conclusions

A review of the current approaches in evaluation and integration of TCAM has contributed to improvements in implementation of the integration system. An important role will, no doubt, be played by the TCAM sector as concerns about degenerative and chronic diseases grow with the increasing life expectancy. In the coming years the major thrust will be to emphasize improving the quality of the medicine and practice in the country.

Bibliography

Model guidelines for the use of complementary and alternative therapies in medical practice. Dallas, TX, Federation of State Medical Boards of the United States Inc., 2002.

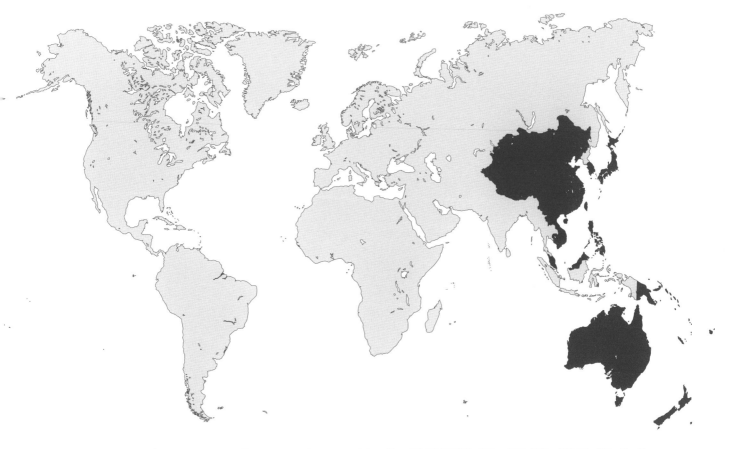

WHO WESTERN PACIFIC REGION

REGIONAL OVERVIEW AND
SELECTED COUNTRY CHAPTERS

CHAPTER 25

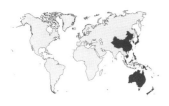

REGIONAL OVERVIEW: WESTERN PACIFIC REGION

Pyong-Ui Roh

Dean, School of Public Health, Daegu Haany University, 290, Yugok-dong, Gyeongsan-si, Gyeongsanbuk-do, 712-715 Republic of Korea. E-mail: puroh@dhu.ac.kr

25.1. Introduction

In the WHO Western Pacific Region (WPR), traditional medicine is practised in many countries, but is not always included as part of the health systems recognized by the respective governments. It is one of the many types of non-standard health care services, and national policy, legislation, administration, public financing, education and practice vary between countries (1).

After the introduction of allopathic medicine into the countries of the Region, traditional medicine was in most cases rejected by the formal health-care service systems. Nevertheless, traditional medicine still exists in all countries and areas in WPR. It provides an alternative to the formal health-care service for people living in developed countries, while for a large proportion of the population in many developing countries it is the only available, affordable and accessible health service.

Interest in traditional medicine has increased over the last decade and seems likely to continue to do so in the future (2). People now are more prepared to look for alternative approaches to maintain and promote their health. With the increase in public demand, governments have begun to pay more attention to traditional medicine and in most countries and areas in WPR they have shown a willingness to promote its proper use and to try to integrate it into formal health-care systems (2). The integration of traditional medicine into the mainstream health-care delivery system is a challenge for countries and areas where allopathic health care predominates.

25.2. Traditional Medicine Systems in WPR

Some traditional medicine systems are highly developed and well documented. They are based on systematized knowledge, a comprehensive methodology and rich clinical experience. Traditional Chinese medicine falls into this category. It originated in China and was later introduced into neighbouring countries such as Japan (see Chapter 27), the Republic of Korea, Viet Nam (see Chapter 29) and others, which then developed their own variations. Traditional Indian medicine (see Chapter 12) is another well-developed traditional system of medicine that is practised in parts of WPR, for example, Malaysia (1).

The Region contains a large number of simpler traditional practices that have been developed within small and isolated ethnic groups. Such practices are based largely on empirical experiences of treatment. Most of the knowledge has never been written down, and is transmitted orally from generation to generation. Most practitioners in this case do not obtain knowledge through an organized training process. The therapies used by healers from different communities and islands can be quite different. In these communities, psychological therapies tend to predominate, and often merge with magical and religious practices. The diversity of the people in WPR means that traditional medical practices differ widely from one country or area to another.

25.3. Structural indicators

25.3.1. National Policies

Eighteen countries and territories in WPR have already developed national policies in traditional and/or complementary medicine and in two other countries are currently under development (3).

The Australian Commonwealth Government has recently made funds available to traditional medicine practitioners to assist them in formalizing accreditation standards and developing appropriate participation. The Government of the State of Victoria, Australia, has passed legislation and implemented a regulatory system for practitioners of traditional Chinese medicine (4).

In China, there has been strong support for traditional medicine. The constitution of the People's Republic of China makes specific reference to the need to develop both allopathic medicine and traditional Chinese medicine and in 1997 the Government reiterated that it attached equal importance to both medical systems. In China, Hong Kong Special Administrative Region (SAR), article 138 of the Basic Law states that the Government shall formulate policies to develop allopathic and traditional medicine and provide medical and health services in both branches of medicine. The Chinese Medicine Ordinance enacted by the Legislative Council in 1999 makes provisions for the registration of practitioners in Chinese medicine, licensing of traders in Chinese medicine, the registration of proprietary Chinese medicines and other related matters.

Japan provides a good example of the integration of traditional medicine in mainstream health services in an industrial country. More than 140 herbal medicines are covered by the national health insurance system, and a large number of physicians use herbal medicine or acupuncture to supplement their practice of allopathic medicine (1).

Mongolian traditional medicine has been developed over centuries in accordance with Mongolia's geographical and climatic conditions and the lifestyles of her people. However, Mongolian traditional medicine was largely ignored from the 1930s until the end of the 1980s. In 1990, the Government made development of Mongolian traditional medicine a priority, and in 1996, announced its support for incorporation of traditional remedies into the mainstream health-care system (3).

In New Zealand, standards for traditional Maori healing were released by the Ministry of Health in June 1999. These emphasize the role of Rongoa Maori in New Zealand's health sector, and provide national standards of practice for traditional Maori healing. Recent legislation established an expert committee to evaluate, and provide information and advice on, complementary health care (5).

In the Philippines, a Traditional and Alternative Medicine Act was passed in 1997. It states that it is the policy of the state to improve the quality and delivery of health-care services to the people in the Philippines through the development of traditional and alternative health care and the integration of this into the national health-care delivery system. The Act also created the Philippine Institute of Traditional and Alternative Health Care to accelerate the development of traditional and alternative health care in the Philippines (1).

In the Republic of Korea, the National Medical Law was passed in 1952 and traditional medicine was formally recognized. Since 1987, the National Health Insurance has included traditional medicine. The Traditional Medicine Bureau was established in 1996 as one of the major bureaus of the Ministry of Health and Welfare (6).

In Singapore, the Ministry of Health appointed a committee headed by the Senior Minister of State for Health and Education to review the practice of traditional medicine, and to recommend measures to safeguard patients' interest and safety. The committee's report, published in 1995, recommended that the practice of traditional medicine in Singapore should be regulated and training standards should be upgraded. The Ministry of Health established a Traditional Medicine Unit in November 1995 to coordinate implementation of the committee's recommendations. A Traditional Medicine Practitioners Act was passed in 2000 (1).

In Viet Nam, Government policy on traditional medicine is based on a statement by President Ho Chi Minh in 1995 that Viet Nam should inherit valuable experiences from traditional medicine and at the same time study the possibility of integrated medicine. The Constitution of 1980 calls for the integration of traditional and allopathic medicine and traditional medicine is extensively integrated into secondary as well as primary heath care (1).

25.3.2. Public Financing Systems and Self-regulatory Associations

In some countries in WPR, such as China and Viet Nam, traditional medical treatments and drugs are covered by the national health system. In other countries, such as Japan and the Republic of Korea, some of the traditional medical practices are covered in part by public insurance systems. Generally speaking, insurance systems differ from country to country and many countries in WPR do not have any health insurance system for traditional medicine.

There are many professional bodies for traditional medicine and some are highly professional associations. For example, in Australia, there are many associations, but in the Republic of Korea, there is only one association whose members are exclusively traditional medicine practitioners (4, 6).

25.3.3. Education and Research

Generally speaking, there are four main categories of traditional health practitioners. The first includes those who have received training in both allopathic and traditional systems of medicine. The second covers those trained mainly in traditional medicine, although they often have elementary knowledge of allopathic medicine. They practise in both urban and rural areas, but many practise most extensively in rural areas. The third group practises only traditional medicine. They have no formal training, but possess diplomas in some traditional system. The fourth category includes those practitioners with neither institutional training nor qualifications, e.g. traditional birth attendants and herbalists but who practise after several years' apprenticeship with an established traditional health practitioner. The countries in the region which have formal education systems for traditional medicine are Australia, China (including Hong Kong SAR and Macao SAR), Japan, Malaysia, Mongolia, the Republic of Korea, Singapore and Viet Nam (2).

Many allopathic medical doctors have begun to use traditional remedies and techniques in their daily practice. Universities and medical schools in several countries offer full-time degree courses or short courses on traditional medicine. Scientists are trying to re-evaluate the safety and efficacy of traditional medicine, and some are involved in research to develop new drugs and other products derived from the plants used in traditional medicine (3).

25.4. Current Practices of Traditional Medicine

There may be great differences in approaches to traditional medicine and health care between countries, and even within a country. In many countries, there are several types of traditional health practitioners. There is a vast spectrum of traditional medicine practitioners including traditional birth attendants and traditional folk healers, spiritualists, diviners and numerous others. In the majority of cases, these people have no clear legal status, and there is a very limited amount of systematic information available about them and their practices (7).

25.5. Discussion

Some Member States have adopted the WPR regional strategy for traditional medicine (1). One part of this strategy calls for political support, and in WPR, 18 countries and areas have developed official government documents which recognize traditional medicine and its practice.

However, many Member States have not established solid national policies, while others have adopted advanced national policies. Some countries like China and the Republic of Korea have traditional medicine practitioners fully recognized by the law, and other countries like Japan, Malaysia and Singapore recognize only some traditional medical arts such as acupuncture and herbal medicine. In South Pacific areas, many kinds of traditional medical arts are practised but most of them are not legally recognized.

Medical costs have been increasing in this region and some Member States have adopted national health insurance systems to help the people who need medical services. The health insurance system in some countries covers traditional medical therapies.

Some countries in WPR have formal higher-education systems for traditional medical practitioners, while many others do not and the art of traditional medicine is passed down to the next generation by word-of-mouth (8). The WHO Regional Office for the Western Pacific held a meeting in Melbourne, Australia, in November 2003 and the experts drafted guidelines for traditional medicine education for the Member States in WPR.

Self-regulatory associations are organized in some Member States. For example, Mongolia recently established a traditional medical association. In the South Pacific area, voluntary associations have been organized.

Only limited numbers of studies on the use of traditional medicine have been conducted and few have been published in international journals. It is very difficult to estimate the cost-effectiveness and economic impact of traditional medicine. It is recommended that well-planned studies be conducted in these areas, and that the results should be published in international journals. A few studies have been carried out on the mechanisms of traditional medicine for treatment (*3*).

At the working group meeting of the WHO Regional Office for the Western Pacific held in Kyongju, Republic of Korea, in September 2003, the ways to improve traditional medicine by evidence were reviewed. Herbal medicine and acupuncture were the major areas for discussion.

The WHO Regional Office for the Western Pacific has produced a number of documents which are listed in the Regional Strategy for Traditional Medicine (*1*) and can be accessed through the web-site of the Regional Office of the Western Pacific (*9*). It is believed that these publications are very helpful for research and development of traditional medicine in WPR.

25.6. Conclusions

Traditional medicine is not standardized in WPR. Eighteen countries and areas have already developed national policies on traditional medicine but some Member States are not yet ready to adopt national policies. Some Member States have government bodies to take care of traditional medical affairs.

A small number of countries have self-regulatory associations to regulate traditional medical affairs. Public financing systems for traditional medicine are available in only a few countries. The funds for research and development are limited.

Surveys on the use of traditional medicine in countries in WPR are limited and the results of only a few have been published in international journals. Many studies were not well planned in advance and it is difficult to estimate the use of traditional medicine by the people.

References

1. *Regional strategy for traditional medicine in the Western Pacific.* Manila, WHO Regional Office for the Western Pacific, 2002.

2. *Traditional and modern medicine: harmonizing the two approaches.* Manila, WHO Regional Office for the Western Pacific, 2000.

3. *Legal status of traditional medicine and complementary/alternative medicine: a worldwide review.* Geneva, World Health Organization, 2001 (WHO/EDM/TRM/2001.2).

4. Bensoussan A, Myers SP. *Towards a safer choice. The practice of traditional Chinese medicine in Australia.* Sydney, MacArthur, University of Western Sydney, 1996.

5. *Standards for traditional Maori healing.* Wellington, Ministry of Health, Manatu Hauora, New Zealand, 1999 (http://www.moh.govt.nz/moh.nsf/0/93c2f1462ab854154c2568230074bf0f/$FILE/ MaoriHealing.pdf, accessed 23 April 2004).

6. *Traditional Korean medicine service.* Seoul, Ministry of Health and Welfare, Republic of Korea, 2000.

7. Bannerman RH, Burton J, Wen-Chieh C. *Traditional medicine and health care coverage.* Geneva, World Health Organization, 1983.

8. Roh PU, et al. Traditional medicine education system and integration of traditional medicine into health care delivery system. *Journal, Institute for Culture Studies.* Kyungsan University, Republic of Korea, Vol. 5, 2001.

9. WHO Regional Office for the Western Pacific (http://www.wpro.who.int/themes_focuses/ theme3/focus1/trm_pub.asp, accessed 28 October 2004)

CHAPTER 26

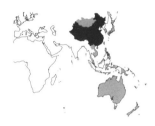

PEOPLE'S REPUBLIC OF CHINA

Liu Baoyan[1],
Wang Xiaopin[2],
Ren Dequan[3]
and Zhu Jiaqing[4]

[1] Vice President, China Academy of Traditional Chinese Medicine, 16 Nanxiaojie, Dongzhimen Nei Street, Beijing 100700, China. E-mail: liuby@mail.cintcm.ac.cn

[2] Division Director, Department of International Cooperation, State Administration of Traditional Chinese Medicine, No. 13 Baijiazhuang Dongli, Chaoyang District, Beijing 100026, China. E-mail: Wangxiaopin@natcm.gov.cn

[3] Deputy Director-General, State Food and Drug Administration, A 38 Beilishilu, Beijing 100810, China. E-mail: ren.dq@sda.gov.cn

[4] Institution of Chinese Medicine Information, China Academy of Traditional Chinese Medicine, 16 Nanxiaojie, Dongzhimen Nei Street, Beijing 100700, China. E-mail: puszzzx@sohu.com

26.1. HISTORICAL OVERVIEW OF THE REGULATION OF TRADITIONAL CHINESE MEDICINE

Traditional Chinese Medicine (TCM) is the summation of the experiences and theories gained by the Chinese people through many years of fighting diseases. TCM has its own unique theory and methods of diagnosis which are different from allopathic (Western) medical philosophy and modalities. The forms of treatment are usually considered to include the following: acupuncture and moxibustion; TCM medication consisting of Chinese herbal medicines, animal and mineral materials; massage (Tui-na); dietary regulation; therapeutic exercise (Qi-qong); and others (1). The medications can be classified into Chinese crude drugs, processed TCM preparations based on drug formulas, marketed products such as raw Chinese medicinal materials and Chinese proprietary medicines.

The Government of China has paid significant attention to the development of TCM since the founding of the People's Republic of China in 1949. The TCM Division of the Ministry of Public Health was established in 1951 and became the Department of TCM in 1954.

The Chinese Constitution stipulates that "both modern medicine and traditional Chinese medicine must be developed" thereby giving both equal emphasis and taking into account a principal area of work for health in China (1). A programme of Integrated TCM and Modern Medicine (MM) was established in 1957 within the Ministry of Health. The TCM Department was revamped in 1978 and the State Administration of TCM (SATCM) was established in 1986, under the Ministry of Health.

In 1988, the State Council established SATCM as an independent administrative body in its own right. Since then, more than 200 statutes and policies have been promulgated to promote the development of TCM and these have been the basis for developing an organizational framework for TCM. They include institutional development, health care, education, science and technical research, production and management of herbal medicines, and international exchange and cooperation in the field of TCM.

26.1.1. TCM Legal Framework

TCM is now protected by law in China. The Government's commitment to "develop modern medicine and Traditional Chinese Medicine" has been written into Article No. 21 of the Constitution of People's Republic of China (1982) (2). This is the first time in the world that the promotion and development of traditional medicine has been included in a national constitution. On 7 April 2003, the State Council promulgated the Regulations of Traditional Chinese Medicine of the People's Republic of China and these came into effect on 1 October 2003. This has had the effect of giving significant support to the continuous development of TCM.

26.1.2. TCM Central Framework and Administration

SATCM is a relatively independent government agency under the Ministry of Health and has the overall responsibility to develop and regulate TCM activities in China. It comprises five major departments (3):

- General Office (Department of Financial Affairs)
- Department of Personnel and Policy (Department of Personnel)
- Department of Medical Administration
- Department of Science, Technology and Education, and
- Department of International Cooperation

SATCM's major responsibilities are to:

- provide guidelines and policy for the development of TCM, and the integration of TCM with allopathic medicine and other ethnic medicines in China;
- establish and enforce standards and regulations for technicians and organizations for procedures involved in TCM;
- coordinate the distribution of TCM resources to hospitals, research and development centres, and universities;
- organize major research and development projects;
- plan education programmes for TCM training;
- guide and coordinate international cooperation (including Hong Kong Special Administrative Region, Macao Special Administrative Region and China (Province of Taiwan) and to promote globalization of TCM.

26.2. GENERAL OVERVIEW OF TCM SITUATION

26.2.1. Practice of TCM

As at December 2002, there were 4 808 640 people working in 85 705 medical organizations in China. Of these, 3801 are TCM organizations (approximately 4.4%) with 435 082 TCM staff (9.1%). At present, there are 213 919 TCM doctors and 18 304 TCM pharmacists in China. There are 2864 government TCM hospitals with a total of 272 861 ward beds (4). Approximately 200 million outpatients receive treatment in TCM hospitals annually.

In the rural areas, TCM takes care of one third of outpatient services and approximately a quarter of inpatient services. In 95% of hospitals providing allopathic medicine, there are also Chinese medicine departments. Over 50% of the 1 330 000 rural doctors use both types of medicines.

26.2.2. Science and Research in TCM

There are approximately 15 000 professionals involved in scientific research on TCM in China, working either in research institutes or in colleges and universities. TCM systems in China have more than 2000 hospitals, about 30 specified research institutes at provincial, municipal and county levels, and about 30 colleges (5). Some scholars from large universities also participate in the studies related to TCM. Research on Chinese materia medica has been listed as one of the country's key scientific projects.

In recent years, the main directions of research on Chinese materia medica have been in:

- survey of Chinese materia medica resources;

- standardization and quality control of commonly-used raw materials;

- research on adventitious herbs, cultivation of herbs and non-polluted green raw materials;

- biotechnology, preparation and processing methods of herbal drugs, new drug studies, new excipients, technological studies and quality control of Chinese patented medicines.

In order to enable more people in the world to understand and use TCM, practitioners have emphasized research on the standardization of quality control including the establishment of appropriate methods of analysis.

Emphasis is also placed on systematic research on complex prescriptions, research on the indications for use of Chinese medicines, pharmacodynamics, pharmacology, quality control and evaluation of safety. Many related government bodies and financial organizations are involved in important research projects at different levels. The national strategy for "Modernization of Chinese Medicine" was promulgated in 2003 (2).

Since the 1990s, enormous changes have been achieved in the TCM industry in China, with the promotion of efficient modes of production in place of the traditional methods of mass production. Notably, integration of farming, industry and commerce for supply and marketing has been taking place in the form of joint operations.

26.2.3. TCM Education and Licensing Practices

There are 27 TCM universities and colleges with an enrolment of over 40 000 students in China. These are postgraduate students for doctoral and master degrees, undergraduate students, and specialized students with no degrees. There are 51 secondary schools of TCM. The curriculum includes some modern sciences such as in allopathic medicine, as well as courses on TCM. Graduates are assigned to work in TCM hospitals, drug manufacturing facilities and general hospitals. In addition, about 3000 overseas students are studying in TCM universities and colleges in China.

Besides those who have finished their undergraduate studies and have received a diploma at a recognized TCM educational institute, qualified doctors, nurses and pharmacists, who meet the necessary requirements, can apply for the TCM examination organized by the Ministry of Health (2, 6). On passing the examination, they can obtain a license to open their own practice.

At present, there are 70 000 registered TCM doctors who have opened their own private clinics. The same numbers of doctors are employed in public TCM hospitals in China. Hence, the public-sector to private-sector ratio of TCM doctors is 1:1. The number of doctors who have their own clinics is steadily increasing.

26.2.4. The Market and Industry of TCM

Since the beginning of the reform in China and the opening of the country to the outside world, the national TCM industry has been developing continuously. The TCM industry has been seen as strategic for development and the growing global market is important in the developing economy and society of China.

In 2000, export of TCM products increased by 8.9% (7). In 2002, Asia was the largest TCM market for China, followed by North America which had the highest rate of growth – above 40% during the previous year. The total output of the TCM industry reached 71.7 billion renminbi (c.US$ 8.64 billion), 16.63% higher than the previous year; the income from sales reached 67.9 billion renminbi (c.US$ 8.18 billion), 15.87% higher than the previous year; and the profits were 7.394 billion renminbi (c.US$ 0.89 billion), 15.9% higher than in 2001.

TCM has become more properly classified and controlled. TCM offers around 2000 kinds of herbal medicine and 3300 other traditional remedies; products include injections, intravenous bolus preparations and aerosols. The production of TCM medicines has reached 370 000 tonnes per year, making continuous double-digit growth in terms of value of the TCM pharmaceutical industry since the mid-1980s (8).

China has just 5% of the global market of traditional medicine in 2004. However, this market growth has been expanding solidly at the rate of 2% in 1998 (7) and 3% in 2001(9).

All TCM manufacturers and commercial enterprises must be certified and registered by the local drug regulatory authorities. After years of planning and implementation of new standards for the TCM industry, all manufacturers must now comply with the Good Manufacturing Practices (GMP) established in 1995 and Good Supply Practices (GSP) promulgated in 2000. Farms producing raw medicinal materials and ingredients will have to meet Good Agricultural Practices (GAP) by 2007. Improvement in the preparation of TCM in China by GAP, GMP and GSP is to be followed by the introduction of Good Laboratory Practices (GLP) and Good Clinical Practices (GCP), in accordance with the guidelines relating to chemistry, manufacturing and control (10).

26.2.5. Regulation of TCM Medicines and Products

TCM is widely used in China to fight diseases and promote health and quality of life. For example, the current role of TCM is shown in the national Essential Drugs List with 1249 items of TCM medicine, in comparison with 770 items of allopathic medicine. The sales of TCM products in 2003 amounted to about US$ 10.3 billion (10). There are national standards for marketed TCM medicines, including the Chinese Pharmacopoeia and Pro-pharmacopoeia in which the progress and achievements in respect to quality control are reflected. All TCM products must meet these national standards and if revealed unqualified by government market sampling, product distribution is suspended and sanctions imposed on the manufacturer.

Under the Drug Administration Law enacted in 1985, marketing authorization is required for all drugs. Under the provisions for the approval of new TCM drugs issued in 1985, products marketed before 1986 can remain on the market if no adverse drug reaction (ADR) events have been reported. In 1988, an ADR monitoring protocol was initiated in China under the supervision of the Bureau of Drug Administration, Ministry of Health. The Centre for ADR Surveillance and Inspection was established officially in 1989 by the Ministry of Health, renamed the National Centre for ADR Monitoring in 1999, and was affiliated to the Drug Re-evaluation Centre, State Drug Administration.

Since 1986, the application for approval of new TCM products consists of two steps; application for clinical trial, and for marketing. Products can only be launched after approval (10). To obtain TCM product registration, applications for new products require: general data, pharmaceutical data, pharmacological and toxicological data and clinical data. The administration of research, production and distribution of TCM products has adopted the international practices of modern drug administration. In this connection, GLP and GCP are formulated and implemented based on the characteristics of TCM. The efficacy of TCM should be evaluated not only with the quantification indices of allopathic medical systems, but also with the indices of TCM systems in order to carry forward the characteristics of traditional medical theory and provide complementary functions to allopathic medicines (10).

26.2.6. Utilization of TCM

During 2001-2002, SATCM conducted a survey on the requirements and quality of service of TCM in 10 provinces and cities of China. The sample sites in the study were: Beijing, Guangdong, Hebei and Jiangsu provinces in eastern China; Heilongjiang, Henan and Hubei, in central China; and Ningxia, Shanxi and Sichuan hui municipalities in western China. The sites were located around the cities or districts that had been included in a study of national health services in 1998. The total sample included 10 provinces, 30 counties or districts, more than 60 towns, 180 rural villages or committees and 10 880 families, with a total of 38 880 people.

Medical organizations surveyed included 30 TCM hospitals, 30 general hospitals, 60 urban and rural clinics or community health centres, 180 clinics, 3 integrated TCM-MM hospitals, 21 employee hospitals, 8 specialist TCM hospitals, 10 specialist MM hospitals and 257 individual clinics.

In a population of almost 1.3 billion, it is estimated that there are 3.1 billion outpatient visits per year. Integrated TCM and MM treatment accounts for 1.03 billion cases, or 33.4% of the total outpatient visits. Most outpatient services are provided by village health centres, which care for 38.9% of patients, followed by rural TCM hospitals, which provide care to 27% of the outpatient population. Town health centres provide 16% of care, general hospitals 9.7%, and individual clinics 6.2% of care.

26.3. Discussion

Sound TCM production and promotion in China is critical to evolve and maximize the opportunities offered in the new century. With full GAP, GMP and GSP certification schemes in place, progress is being achieved in quality assurance with regulated and centralized product quality control.

The Government's support to improve the safety of TCM products needs to be further encouraged by monitoring production and introducing standards that compare to international practices, and by explaining the sound use and practices of TCM to MM practitioners who are confused by complicated traditional systems of diagnoses and prescriptions (11). Simultaneously, comprehensive efforts to empower the industrial structure of TCM manufacturers should be enhanced in China, in order to redress the lack of resources to drive the research and sustainable development efforts in modernizing TCM production.

26.4. Conclusions

TCM has been used in China for more than 2000 years and it still plays an important role in the health care of the population. Since it is being introduced to other countries, the experience of the Chinese government in the areas of policy, regulation, education, and research in the field of TCM can help facilitate its proper use worldwide.

References

1. Dong H, Zhang X. An overview of traditional Chinese medicine. In: *Traditional Medicine in Asia*. New Delhi, World Health Organization Regional Office for South-East Asia, 2002 (SEARO Regional Publications No. 39):17-29.

2. *Anthology of policies, laws and regulations of the People's Republic of China on Traditional Chinese Medicine*. Beijing, The State Administration of Traditional Chinese Medicine of the People's Republic of China, 1997.

3. State Administration of Traditional Chinese Medicine, Beijing, People's Republic of China, (http://www.satcm.gov.cn/english_satcm/eindex.htm/, accessed 25 May 2004).

4. *China Statistical Yearbook*. Beijing, China Statistics Press, National Bureau of Statistics of the People's Republic of China (published annually).

5. *A Report on China's Hospital System and Medical Equipment Market* (http://www.chinavista.com/database/cides/hospital.html, accessed 28 June 2004).

6. Information available at: http://www.satcm.gov.cn/english_satcm/jiaoyu.htm/ (Education) (accessed 25 May 2004).

7. *Overview of Chinese Pharmaceutical Market in 1999 and 2000*, Chinese Medical News, issue 107. Beijing, Beijing Consultech, 2001.

8. National Statistic Bureau, People's Republic of China, Rapid Growth of Pharmaceuticals, Trend Report: China's Pharmaceutical Industry, *ACHEMA Worldwide News*, 23 February 2004, 10-12.

9. *Traditional Chinese Medicine, China Wishes to Modernize Traditional Medicine*. Beijing, The State Food Administration and the Ministry of Commerce of the People's Republic of China. (http://www.english. mofcom.gov.cn/article/200211/20021100051361_1.xml, accessed 28 June 2004). National Library Board 2003, Issue 1, No.1, June 2003.

10. Dequan, R. *Current status of TCM in China*. State Drug Administration, People's Republic of China, for the International Conference of Drug Regulatory Authorities (ICDRA), Geneva, World Health Organization, 2004.

11. The Chinese Economy in a New Era: Reform and Innovation. In: *China Business Summit 2001 Report*, 2001:35-36.

Useful Link

Traditional Chinese Medicine Database System, Institute of Information on Traditional Chinese Medicine, China Academy of Traditional Medicine, (http://www.gfmer/ch/TMCAM/TNCAM_database_system.htm/, accessed on 28 June 2004).

CHAPTER 27

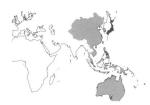

JAPAN

Haruki Yamada

Director, WHO Collaborating Centre for Traditional Medicine, Oriental Medicine Research Center, the Kitasato Institute and Professor, Kitasato Institute for Life Sciences, Kitasato University, 5-9-1, Shirokane, Minato-ku, Tokyo 108-8642, Japan. E-mail: yamada@lisci.kitasato-u.ac.jp

27.1. INTRODUCTION

Japan has a history of selection and integration of medical traditions, and has developed specifically intra-complementary medical systems to provide traditional medicine practice. Medical practice coverage in Japan has been provided by registered medical doctors since the 19th century within the legal framework of its historically-established medical policy. In this manner, in contrast to many other countries that maintain their own indigenous and imported traditional medical systems quite independently, the Japanese medical system has integrated its TCAM systems.

In this context, there have been lots of segments of traditional medicine systems in Japan, including indigenous medicine which may vary in respect to local climes and cultures. In addition, a range of TCAM systems have been introduced from outside Japan.

In this chapter, only officially-certified Japanese traditional medicine systems are discussed. These are classified into two groups: herbal medicines and physical (manual) therapies. Herbal medicines include Kampo medicine and indigenous Japanese medicine; and physical therapies include acupuncture, moxibustion, Japanese traditional massage (An-ma), finger pressure (Shiatsu), and Judo-seifuku therapy (judotherapy). Kampo medicine is considered to be Japan's mainstream herbal medicine system.

27.2. KAMPO MEDICINE

27.2.1. History and Social Background

Chinese traditional medicine was introduced into Japan through cultural exchanges beginning in the 6th century. Chinese medicine continued to grow and was further developed in Japan, and by the 18th century, Kampo, a modified version of Chinese medicine, was established as Japan's herbal medicine system. When Japan opened its door to the West in the 19th century, Kampo medicine was discarded by the Government in favour of contemporary Dutch and German medicine. Despite this unfavourable trend, Kampo continued to thrive through the efforts of a few medical leaders. Today, Kampo and allopathic medicines are used together throughout Japan (*1*).

The use of Kampo medicine as a complementary therapy was spurred by the fact that, while antibiotics and other allopathic medical approaches continue to fight many of the world's epidemics, the latter half of the 20th century saw a marked increase in chronic, endogenous metabolic disorders. There has also been an increase in non-specific, constitutional or psychosomatic diseases. Some severe adverse effects associated with some natural and synthetic compounds have also resulted in occasional disillusionment with allopathic medicine. As a result, Kampo medicine is now very popular in Japanese society and plays an important role in modern therapy. The 2002 production value of Kampo medicine was 1.7% of the total medicine production in Japan (*2*) including crude drug materials and ready-made prescriptions of Kampo preparations for clinical and over-the-counter use and for household distribution (*3*). Among these uses, pharmaceutical Kampo extract preparations for clinical use accounted for 84.3% (*2*).

27.2.2. Clinical Applications

Kampo medicines are most commonly used by patients who have problems concerning physical functions, fitness to undergo surgery, side-effects of allopathic medicine, persistent symptoms, psychosomatic disorders, geriatric conditions and declining physical strength, and those patients seeking improvements in their overall health. Kampo medicines are commonly used to treat many disorders including hepatitis, menopausal disorders such as autonomic nervous and hormonal manifestations, autonomic imbalances, bronchial asthma, cold syndrome, digestive disorders, atopy, dermatitis, eczema, hypersensitivity to low temperatures, allergic rhinitis, general malaise, nephritis, constipation, chronic articular rheumatism, irritable bowel syndrome, hypertension, psychogenic pharyngeal symptoms, weak constitution, dermatitis, chronic bronchitis, diabetes, lumbago, neurosis, chronic paranasal sinusitis, neuralgia, sterility, degenerative joint disease and psychosomatic disorders.

Many of these conditions are difficult to treat with allopathic medicine. Yet, because Kampo medicine addresses imbalances in the whole body, it is reported to be effective in many cases. This can be seen particularly in the elderly where diseases are caused by problems occurring simultaneously in several organs. Allopathic therapy treats these diseases with a variety of medicines. Kampo, however, prescribes one individualized formula to treat the whole body, and eventually restore a normal physiological environment. In general, Kampo medicines also have fewer adverse effects than allopathic medicines. Recently, some Kampo medicines have been recognized as effective for the prevention of the progression of dementia such as Alzheimer's disease and cerebrovascular disorders in Japan. Therefore, Kampo medicine seems to be a very suitable treatment for elderly patients.

The action of allopathic medicine relates specifically to the causes and functions of disease, whereas Kampo medicines function to harmonize the disturbed pathophysiological conditions of the patient (so-called sho) as a whole, to eventually equilibrate a normal physiological environment in the system.

27.2.3. Characteristics of Kampo Medicines

Kampo medicines traditionally consist of a formulation of five to ten different herbs. In contrast, Japanese folk medicine generally uses a single herb for each treatment (1). Kampo medicines are mainly administered as decoctions, but may also be made in the form of powders, pills and ointments. In 1972, the Ministry of Health and Welfare (predecessor of the current Ministry of Health, Labour and Welfare) of Japan designated 210 Kampo formulae as over-the-counter drugs. This selection was based on Kampo practitioners' experiences. Preparations were adapted to the modern clinical setting by spray-drying decoctions into granule or powder forms. Their acceptance took place through traditional clinical experience, but without clinical validation studies. As these pharmaceutical preparations are convenient and highly portable, they have become popular and widely used throughout Japan.

Traditional Kampo decoctions provide very useful "made-to-order" medicines, as the ratio of components can be modified to best fit the patient's physiological condition. In Japan, more than 70% of physicians of allopathic medicine have experience in the use of Kampo medicines (3).

Since 1976, the Ministry of Health and Welfare has approved 148 Kampo formulations, as well as their individual herbal components, to be covered by the national health insurance system in Japan. The Pharmacopoeia of Japan (4) lists 165 raw herbs used in Kampo prescriptions and the Japanese Herbal Medicine Codex (5) lists an additional 83 items. For each herbal material listed in these two documents, the plant origin, physical properties and criteria for identification with respective testing methods are rigorously specified.

27.2.4. Education and Licensing

Several countries in Asia, such as China and the Republic of Korea, license two types of medical doctors – allopathic doctors and traditional medicine doctors, whereas Japan licenses only allopathic doctors. Therefore, in Japan, Kampo extract pharmaceutical preparations may only be prescribed by allopathic physicians holding a medical licence.

Kampo medicine was not included in formal medical education in Japan, with the exception of a few specific schools, until 2001. Since then, Kampo medicine has been formally introduced into the model core curriculum for medical education and, by 2002, Kampo medicine had been included in the curriculum of 88.8% of Japan's medical schools (6), although the content and extent varies depending on the medical school.

For many years, pharmaceutical schools and faculties have provided lectures in pharmacognosy, but have included in their thematic curriculum only a few issues about Kampo medicines, mainly from viewpoint of resource development of isolated or synthesized active components in allopathic use. In 2002, the Pharmaceutical Society of Japan also proposed a model core curriculum for pharmaceutical education which officially employs the agenda of orthodox Kampo medicine. Kampo medicine is now taught in 89.1% of pharmaceutical schools and faculties in Japan (6), but the content and extent vary.

27.3. Acupuncture and Moxibustion

27.3.1. History in Japan

Due to improved transportation and communication, Chinese medicine, together with acupuncture and moxibustion, was introduced into Japan, along with Buddhism, in the 6th century. In the 16th century, Japanese acupuncture began to develop independently of China. In the 17th century, needles were made using iron, and eventually using silver and gold. During this era, the "hammer" insertion method was also developed. In search of a simple and speedy insertion method, the insertion tube, which is a small cylindrical tube through which the needle is inserted, was developed. This insertion method is still used in Japan by over 90% of acupuncturists.

With the introduction in the 19th century of allopathic medicine as a new medical system in Japan, acupuncture and moxibustion were excluded. Today, however, acupuncture is widely accepted and used in medical treatments throughout Japanese health-care systems.

27.3.2. Clinical Applications

According to the WHO guidelines (7, 8), acupuncture has clinical applications in the treatment of lower back pain, hemiplegia, disc herniation, spondylosis deformans, rheumatoid arthritis, whiplash injury, arthrosis deformans of knee joint, cervical syndrome, cold syndrome, asthma, and other conditions. However, adoption of such guidelines may lead to some misconceptions, particularly in Japan, about "officially authorized clinical application" of systems of acupuncture for the disorders stated. Therefore, it is important that there is a proper conceptual understanding during the development of guidelines or standards and appropriate translation by the national experts concerned or academic societies providing ethical information (9).

27.3.3. Education and Licensing

Acupuncture is performed by licensed acupuncturists in Japan. These practitioners are graduates of technical schools and universities of acupuncture and moxibustion, and all have passed national qualifying examinations for licensure set by the Minister of Health, Labour and Welfare, with revisions in the acupuncture and moxibustion practitioner's law enacted in 1998 (10).

There are 113 000 registered practitioners of acupuncture and moxibustion as of 2001. According to the estimate in 2000, around 70 000 are engaged in clinical practice of acupuncture and moxibustion (11). By the end of 2000, 94 colleges and vocational schools had been established in Japan for sighted students and the blind; 63 schools for the blind provided the training curriculum as of 2002. Three-year programmes in vocational schools are most common.

27.4. An-ma and Shiatsu

27.4.1. History and Social Background

An-ma is Japanese traditional massage derived from the therapeutic touch with the hand; an ancient way to treat people's discomfort. People cast their hands instinctively to relieve pain and the traditional hand-casting method of treatment, developed in China, was introduced into Japan 1200 years ago and integrated into original Japanese practices. It was not until 1964 that Shiatsu was recognized as distinct and independent from An-ma.

27.4.2. Clinical Applications and Present Situation

An-ma techniques involve stimulating vital energy points (acupoints) along meridians in order to release muscular tension, promote circulation of blood and ultimately self-healing. They do not use oil, in contrast to most of other "western" massage systems.

Shiatsu is a technique of finger-pressure massage, as is one of the an-ma techniques, the pressure method. An-ma employs various techniques including kneading, which combine with several different applications to compose a round of therapy.

27.4.3. Education and Licensing

To practice as a provider of An-ma and Shiatsu requires training and education at the certified schools authorized by the Ministry of Health, Labour and Welfare or the Ministry of Education, Culture, Sports, Science and Technology under the School Education Law in Japan (*10*). Trainees pursue a three-year curriculum of practical training and basic medical knowledge. After graduation, they need to pass the national board examination for registration by the Ministry of Health, Labour and Welfare.

27.5. JUDOTHERAPY

27.5.1. History

Judo-seifuku therapy (judotherapy) is a unique medical technique that originated in the Japanese martial arts and the history of judotherapy can be traced back to jujutsu (a prototype of judo). The kappo methods of physical damage control, including the emergency resuscitation technique of jujutsu, Japanese folk remedies transmitted from the past, and ideas of Buddhism and Confucianism that emphasize maintaining one's body bestowed from heaven intact to the end of one's life, have been integrated and developed as folk remedies. These remedies preserve medical techniques which promote natural healing without blood-shedding and have contributed to the present-day judotherapy, which combines oriental medicine dating back before the 10th century and western medicine of the 18th century. The name of Judo-seifuku is recognized by law, together with the other names of Sekkotsu (bone-setting) and Honetsugi (setting-bone). Seikotsu (bone-adjusting) is also a method that is increasingly popular.

27.5.2. Clinical Use and Present Situation

Judotherapy is regarded as a therapeutic method under the national health insurance policy in Japan. Judotherapies include treatment of the membrane parts of the body such as sinews, tendons and ligaments, in patients with broken bones, dislocation of joints, contusions and sprains. In the case of broken bones and dislocation of joints, allopathic physicians must be consulted.

27.5.3. Education and Licensing

In 1999, there were approximately 29 000 accredited judotherapists in Japan. Accreditation in judotherapy requires a high-school diploma or a certificate to enter university; a degree from an accredited judotherapy institute; and successful completion of a national examination, which leads to licensure by the Ministry of Health, Labour and Welfare (*10*). Generally, judotherapists start their own clinics after two to five years of clinical training at a bone-setting or orthopaedic clinic.

Of manual therapies practised in the field of TCAM, only the services provided as acupuncture and moxibustion, An-ma, Shiastu and judotherapy are officially recognized under respective laws. In addition to each specific law, the Medical Practitioners Law applies overall to Japanese TCAM practices, covering those medical practices linked with hospitals/clinics regulation. Those traditional manual therapies are categorized as "practices similar to medicine", distinguished from allopathic systems, and national insurance coverage is provided only when such therapies are approved in writing by registered medical doctors.

27.6. LEGAL ASPECTS OF TCAM IN JAPAN

In general, legislative and control systems for TCAM practitioners, medical doctors, pharmacists, acupuncturists and moxicauterists, An-ma and Shiatsu practitioners and judotherapists are regulated under the Medical Practitioners Law, the Pharmacists Law, the Law for Practitioners of Massage, Finger Pressure, Acupuncture and Moxibustion, and the Judotherapists Law, respectively (*10, 12*).

Practices, facilities for treatment, and quality of medicines of Japanese TCAM are regulated comprehensively by the Medicine Law and the Pharmaceutical Affairs Law, which form the nucleus of the control of pharmaceuticals in Japan.

27.7. DISCUSSION

Japan has maintained a variety of traditional cultures and systems of medicine, in spite of various political pressures over time. Nevertheless, treatment based on consumer preference, be it traditional or allopathic, is a growing trend in Japan, as in other industrialized countries.

It is becoming crucial for the Japanese traditional medical systems to respond effectively to issues such as the high dependency on medicinal raw materials imported from abroad. The cost of traditional remedies is affected by globalization of the crude drugs market. The recent implications of intellectual property rights, along with environmental conservation issues, have compounded the problem.

Proper education and training systems in traditional medicine need to be well established. The political will to give proper recognition to TCAM is justified. Practical communications among traditional and conventional (allopathic) medicine practitioners should be strongly encouraged to promote rational use. Safety and efficacy are issues that are common to TCAM and conventional medicine and must be addressed in order to improve the use of these remedies and realize the full potential of TCAM in Japan.

27.8. CONCLUSIONS

In order to encourage policy development for whatever modality of TCAM, proper information about traditional remedies, their uses and practices is vital for TCAM in Japan. Under the present circumstances with insufficient information available for rational use, development of education systems associated with safety and efficacy, and proper access to TCAM in Japan, the following issues need to be discussed further:

1. The unbiased knowledge and experiences from both the public and private sectors need to be accurately and promptly exchanged to enable information networking systems to cover the broad range of areas of TCAM for future health policy development in Japan.

2. There is a need for evaluation of the current status of information-sharing in the area of TCAM, both within and outside the policy framework.

3. There is a need also to improve the understanding of information systems by policy-makers, experts and those in the private sector dealing with trade and commerce.

References

1. Yamada H. Modern scientific approaches to Kampo medicine. *Asia Pacific Journal of Pharmacology.* 1994, 9:209–217.

2. *Situation Update on Domestic Production of Kampo Prescriptions and Herbal Medicines in Japan, Japan Kampo Medicine Manufactures Association (from Annual Report of current survey of Pharmaceutical Industrial Production).* In Japanese. Japan Kampo Medicine Manufacturers Association, 2003 (http://www.nikkankyo.org/frame.html, accessed 13 May 2004).

3. *Pharmaceutical Affairs.* Japan Self-Medication Industries (JSMI) (http://www.jsmi.jp/english/pharma/index.html, accessed 10 May 2004).

4. *Japanese Pharmacopoeia Fourteenth Edition (JP14), English version.* Ministry of Health, Labour and Welfare, Government of Japan, 2002 (http://jpdb.nihs.go.jp/jp14e/, accessed 13 May 2004).

5. *Japanese Herbal Medicine Codex, Augmented Edition of 1989.* Tokyo, Yakujinippou-sya, 1997. In Japanese.

6. Kampo Medical Symposium 2003. *Nikkei Medical.* 2003, Suppl. 5:12–21. In Japanese.

7. *Guidelines for Clinical Research on Acupuncture* (ISBN 92 9061 1146), WHO Regional Publications, Western Pacific Series No. 15. Manila WHO Regional Office for the Western Pacific, 1995.

8. Acupuncture: Review and analysis of reports on controlled clinical trials (ISBN 92 4 1545437). Geneva, World Health Organization, 2002.

9. *Consensus Development Conference on Acupuncture. Issues from the NIH Consensus Development Conference in 1997 to Invited Speech by Dr. Ferguson in 1999.* Tokyo, The Japan Society of Acupuncture and Moxibustion, 2004 (in press).

10. *Medical Laws and Regulation Database System, the Ministry of Health, Labour and Welfare.* Ministry of Health, Labour and Welfare, Government of Japan, 2004 (http://wwwhourei.mhlw.go.jp/hourei/, accessed 10 May 2004) (in Japanese).

11. *Introduction of the Japan Society of Acupuncture and Moxibusion (JSAM).* Tokyo, the Japan Society of Acupuncture and Moxibusion, 2003 (http://www.jsam.jp/english/, accessed 10 May 2004).

12. Mitsuhashi H et al. A study on Judo and Judo-seifukushi (no surgery) techniques. Judo-seifuku. *Sekkotsu-Igaku [Japanese Journal of Judo Therapy].* 2000, 8:103–110.

Useful Links

Pharmaceutical Administration and Regulations in Japan. Japan Pharmaceutical Manufacturers Association (http://www.jpma.or.jp/12english/parj/index.html, accessed 28 October 2004).

CHAPTER 28

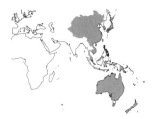

REPUBLIC OF THE PHILIPPINES

Alfonso T. Lagaya

Director General, Philippines Institute of Traditional and Alternative Health Care, Department of Health, Philippines. E-mail: lagaya_md_ac@yahoo.com

28.1. INTRODUCTION

The practice of traditional medicine in the Republic of the Philippines is thought to have existed for hundreds of years, even before colonization by the Spaniards. The roots of traditional medicine appear to have originated from the practices of ethnic and indigenous groups of Filipinos. The assumption is that the spectrum of traditional medicine in the Philippines has been brought about by the influences mainly of ethnic Chinese traditional medicine systems, local folklore and experiments with the use of medicinal resources. Thus the Philippines, due to the long influence from Spanish colonization, has merged its ancestral beliefs with the formal Christian influence. The use of amulets to ward off sickness, to protect from natural disasters and even from man-made aggression, is combined with prayers adapted from the churches.

One of the most interesting forms of traditional medicine, which has become a worldwide phenomenon, is Philippine faith healing with its fantastic and controversial bare-handed, painless operations ("psychic surgery"). The healers claim to operate on the body of the patient, resulting in the diseased blood and entrails being removed, but no sign of a wound is visible after the procedure. Sceptics have challenged such phenomena as simply the sleight of a magician's hands, but local research claims otherwise (1). Psychic surgery belongs to an order of reality not fully understood nor accepted by present-day science, but this is not to say that such a reality does not exist. Another Filipino-based healing practice is the understanding of energies emanating from the patient's body; once these are swept away by the hands, pain relief, and even cure, may result (2).

The above local healing practices are generally tolerated by the Philippine Government since they are primarily non-invasive and do not compromise the patient's safety, and most especially because of their long cultural heritage that goes well with primary health care.

In the Philippines, traditional, complementary and alternative medicine (TCAM) may be divided broadly into two categories based upon the types of personnel who provide the treatment and care, i.e., TCAM used by popular folklore practitioners, and TCAM-trained allopathic health professionals.

28.1.1. TCAM used by Popular Folklore Practitioners

In the TCAM used by popular folklore practitioners, both rural and urban populations rely on time-honoured practices and remedies such as local herbal decoctions, oils and poultices, massage, bone-setting, cupping and prayers. For diagnosis, the folklore practitioners use palpation, pulse diagnosis, or methods of determining heat and cold imbalance in the body. Most of the healers rely on local devices and insights to aid them in determining the cause of the patient's illness, such as pouring candle wax on water and analyzing the shapes formed; examining the entrails of a young chicken lightly passed around the patient's body; examining the contents of a raw egg placed on a saucer after lightly passing it around the patient's body, and others.

For most healers, locally known as herbolarios, the practice of alternative healing is usually a combination of physical, energetic and spiritual (magico-religious) methods of therapy. Some ethnic Chinese and Indian healers use their healing skills within their own community. Another minority group uses knifeless psychic surgery to extract diseased tissues and organs (see above).

The Philippines Government has generally accepted such folklore practices, including spiritual, divine, faith and energy healing, as long as they are within the context of primary health care, and where such practices may be performed without any invasive techniques, thereby ensuring public safety even if the issue of efficacy is still under study.

28.1.2. TCAM provided by TCAM-trained Allopathic Health Professionals

Only registered physicians, including trained acupuncturists, are allowed to provide legally-recognized TCAM therapies (3). In the TCAM used by formally-certified allopathic health professionals, a handful of physicians have applied traditional Chinese acupuncture, homeopathy, chelation, naturopathy and anthroposophy, together with conventional therapies, as part of their medical practice. Most physicians are trained by foreign and local medical institutions, and their practice of TCAM is accepted, as they have an official licence to practice medicine and assure the public of competence to access medicine with safety.

Further specific regulation for TCAM use and practitioners has been in the process of development since 2003, aiming at formulation of qualified standards of practice, accreditation procedures, and licensing and training of practitioners.

28.2. Background Indicators

28.2.1. Morbidity

For the past years, most of the ten leading causes of morbidity have been communicable diseases. Between 1987 and 1997, these included diarrhoea, pneumonia, bronchitis, influenza, tuberculosis, malaria and chicken-pox. Sometimes measles and dengue are among the top ten, due to outbreaks. Leading non-communicable causes of morbidity are diseases of the heart, hypertension, accidents and neoplasm (4).

The prevalence of communicable diseases is still very high, while that of non-communicable diseases is increasing. This double burden of disease places a great toll on the health and economy of the people and the nation as a whole. As the Philippines becomes more urbanized and industrialized, and with the increase in life expectancy and improvement in the control of communicable diseases, the disease burden is expected to shift further towards non-communicable diseases. Strategies must be in place to address current and future situations with regard to the disease burden.

28.2.2. Mortality

Unlike the leading causes of morbidity, deaths are mainly due to non-communicable diseases, and this trend is increasing. Diseases of the heart and the vascular system are the two most common causes of death, and comprised 39.6% of the ten leading causes of death. Cancer deaths ranked fifth in 1975–1990 and moved to fourth in 1995. Pneumonia, tuberculosis and diarrhoeal diseases remain consistently among the ten leading causes of death, but deaths due to diarrhoea have significantly lessened. Deaths due to accidents and injuries are increasing and must be addressed aggressively. Diabetes mellitus is emerging as one of the leading causes of death. Meanwhile, deaths due to kidney diseases, avitaminosis and other nutritional disorders, although no longer in the top ten causes of death, are still of serious concern. Deaths from measles have decreased significantly (4).

28.2.3. Total Number of Prescribers

The Philippines has a large health workforce with more than 120 doctors and 450 nurses for every 100 000 population according to the National Statistics (5). In the period 1990–1995, there were reported to be 82 494 doctors, 259 629 nurses, and 102 878 midwives (5).

28.2.4. Total Number of TCAM Providers

There has been no national survey to determine the number of TCAM providers outside the conventional health system. As of 2003, there were approximately 250 physicians who had been trained in acupuncture by the Department of Health, and had integrated it into their professional practice (3).

28.2.5. Total Health Expenditure for the Conventional Health Care Sector

In 1997, 88 billion pesos were spent on health care, which represented 3.5% of gross national product. There is no breakdown of expenditure for primary, secondary and tertiary care. However, the share spent on public health, which may represent primary health care, grew from 8% in 1991 to 14% in 1997. On the other hand, the share spent on personal health care declined from 76% in 1991 to 72% in 1997. The continued dominance of family out-of-pocket spending would suggest that a large portion of health expenditures are likely to be spent on personal health-care services.

A 1994 survey of family out-of-pocket health expenditure showed that 2% of the health expenditure of Filipinos is spent on TCAM. The balance was spent at government hospitals (35%); at retail outlets for drugs and other non-durable purchases for self-care (27%); at non-hospital medical facilities (20%); private hospitals (11%); dental facilities (3%); other professional facilities (1%); and retail outlets for vision products and other medical durables for self-care (1%) (6).

28.3. STRUCTURAL INDICATORS

28.3.1. Legislation

The Philippines Government officially recognized TCAM in 1993, when the Traditional Medicine Programme was established in the Department of Health. The Programme was elevated into a Government-Owned and Controlled Corporation when the Philippine Institute of Traditional and Alternative Health Care (PITAHC) (3) was established in 1997 by Presidential and Congressional approval of Republic Act No. 8423 (also known as " Traditional and Alternative Medicine Act (TAMA) of 1997). Its guiding principles are that the policy of the State is to improve the quality and delivery of health-care services to the Filipino people through the development of traditional and alternative health care and its integration into the national health-care delivery system. It is also the policy of the State to seek a legally workable basis by which indigenous societies can own their knowledge of traditional medicine (7). The law also guaranteed permanent legislation and a budget for the development of TCAM in the country (7).

Objectives for PITAHC initially focused on herbal medicines, therapeutic massage and energy healing in the context of primary health care approaches, as well as acupuncture provided by officially-certified physicians. After the initial establishment phase of PITAHC from 1997-2000, the Institute began to reach out to the un-served and underserved Filipino populations. This was done through advocacy, and by introducing training in TCAM skills development; this is consistent with the concepts of primary health care, as recommended by the local scientific community and WHO.

With respect to general medical legislation, the general law applies to the practice of medicine, which may include the practice of TCAM by duly registered and licensed physicians. Indeed, only physicians are explicitly authorized to practise. The use of TCAM by non-physicians within the context of primary health care is generally tolerated within the bounds of safe practices as accepted by local health authorities. Licensed nurses, physiotherapists and midwives, with or without TCAM training, are also allowed to practise TCAM therapies as long as these are non-invasive, e.g. therapeutic massage or herbal food supplementation.

At present, the following TCAM providers are not legally recognised: herbalists; spiritual or faith healers; traditional birth attendants/midwives; traditional bone-setters/orthopaedists; Unani practitioners; Ayurvedic practitioners; osteopaths; chiropractors; homeopaths; acupuncturists/practitioners of Chinese medicine; others including energy healers (Pranic healing, qi-gong, Reiki, etc.). However, spiritual, divine, faith, and energy healing are generally accepted as long as they are performed without any accompanying invasive techniques, in order to ensure public safety. Traditional birth attendants/midwives are not legally recognized nor licensed, unlike the midwives who are licensed and regulated. However a number of trained traditional birth attendant/midwives who are usually TCAM practitioners, have been assisting the government as health-care volunteers to augment the human resources available for primary health-care delivery in the country.

The Philippines Government is mandated to regulate quality assurance, testing and accreditation of TCAM practices provided by physicians in the future. Pharmacists are allowed to recommend herbal medicines based upon ethical procedures. These prescriptions are now legally marketed nationwide either as herbal medicines or herbal food supplements, upon registration with the Bureau of Food and Drugs. Other herbal proprietary materials are also registered as cosmetics.

A database of TCAM practitioners is being developed, which will eventually lead to the formulation of standards of practice, procedures for the accreditation and licensing of practitioners, and for the establishment and operation of clinical and training facilities.

28.3.2. Education and Research

In 2001–2002, the WHO Regional Office for the Western Pacific provided financial assistance to PITAHC to conduct a consultative workshop for the formulation of the national curriculum to guide the integration of TCAM into courses in medicine, dentistry, pharmacy, physical therapy, nursing, nutrition/dietetics and midwifery. At present, PITAHC is advocating the integration of TCAM into health colleges and universities. PITAHC is also training the general public in the safe and effective use of massage therapy and herbal medicines within the context of primary health care.

National agencies including the Ministry of Health, the Ministry of Education, and the National Institute of Health, have varying responsibilities for TCAM control, information, education and/or research within their mandates. Currently, a National Expert Committee for TCAM is being established, along with a National TCAM Advisory Board. Other related national institutions dedicated to TCAM development are in the process of establishment.

Information and advisory services relating to TCAM are now being offered by most TCAM-related colleges and universities, which are providing outreach activities to inform the general public on the safe and efficacious use of TCAM.

28.3.3. Professional Organizations

Concerning the existence of professional organizations of TCAM practitioners, at present the Philippines have registered such non-government organizations as the Philippine Academy of Medical Acupuncturists, Inc.; the Philippine College for the Advancement of Medicine; the Philippine Scientific Acupuncture Association, The Philippine Institute of Acupuncture; the Integrative Medicine for Alternative Health Systems (INAM), Inc.; etc. There is an emerging trend for some of these to act as voluntary self-regulatory bodies, with membership restricted to qualified and licensed practitioners, developing codes of practice and ethical guidelines.

28.3.4. Financing Systems

Financing systems for TCAM are emerging. The Philippine Health Insurance Corporation is in the process of accrediting acupuncture performed by licensed physicians. Most government hospitals with trained physician-acupuncturists have been offering free acupuncture services. In these hospitals, herbal medicines are also offered free-of-charge, as are the herbal teas, ointments and soaps used in primary health care. Some government hospitals have initiated regular pranic healing treatment for patients.

Apart from the Philippine Health Insurance Corporation, no other financing systems are being developed. However, four widely-marketed herbal medicines in the Philippines have been included in the Philippine National Drug Formulary, thus qualifying inpatients for reimbursement of such purchases from the Philippine Health Insurance Corporation.

28.4. RESEARCH ON TCAM UTILIZATION

A major national survey was conducted by the Department of Health in 1998, in conjunction with data collection on maternal and child health. Other small-scale surveys have been conducted by colleges and universities. However, to date there have been no patient surveys which provide information on the utilization of specific TCAM therapies or reasons for use, satisfaction, perceived outcomes or out-of-pocket expenditure. There is a survey in progress on TCAM practitioners, which will generate a listing of practitioners (see section *28.3.1*).

A national study of TCAM was conducted from 1995–2001 by a partnership formed by the University of the Philippines (UP) Manila Research Group, the De La Salle Research Group, and the UP Mass Communications Research Group. This was a survey of the general population, including the ethnic groups of Ifugao, Mangyans, natives of Palawan, and others. Data were collected by a combination of methods, including focus group discussions and questionnaires. TCAM use over the previous 12 months and lifetime use were studied. The findings are summarized below and in Table 28.1.

Herbal medicines and massage, with or without any accompanying religious ceremonies, are considered to be the most frequent TCAM usage due to their accessibility and availability, especially in the remote rural areas. The knowledge of safety and efficacy is derived from the long years of utilization, passed down from one generation to another. In the more densely populated urban areas, herbal medicines and massage are considered as a cost-effective health-care modality in contrast to the more expensive pharmaceutical preparations. However, other more educated and economically affluent sectors of the population have been patronizing such herbal medicine modalities because of their use of natural resources rather than artificial chemical drugs.

Table 28.1. Estimated percentage of the general population using any form of TCAM, and the five most popular individual TCAM therapies

Therapy	Visiting a TCAM provider (%)	Self-medication (%)
Any form of TCAM	20	35
Herbal medicines/foods as a primary health care modality	15	25
Massage (traditional Filipino, other Oriental and/ or Swedish)	15	25
Acupuncture, homeopathy, naturopathy	1	1
Spiritual/divine healing (including psychic healing or surgery)	2	1
Energy healing (Pranic healing, Qigong, Reiki, Tetada Kalimasada, etc.)	1	1

Acupuncture is mainly practised by ethnic Chinese and has been sought by Filipinos, but since needles are generally invasive, causing repulsion for many, its popularity remains low. The Philippines Government supports the recommendation of WHO on the safety and efficacy of acupuncture, and around 200 physicians have been trained to integrate acupuncture in their allopathic-based clinical practice.

The most common medical determinants of TCAM use and of visits to TCAM providers were found to be pain and stress-related conditions, virility (men), fertility (both men and women); and chronic degenerative disorders and other health conditions, such as malignant neoplasm, in which allopathic medicine fails to cure the patient. Treatment of virility and fertility problems usually involved the use of herbs. Treatment for pain and stress complaints, and chronic degenerative disorders, were all associated with herbs, massage and acupuncture, while treatment of malignant neoplasm was associated with prayer as well as herbs, massage and acupuncture.

Reasons given for TCAM use were affordability, availability, safety, effectiveness, and the use of TCAM as a last resort after the failure of allopathic medical care. Seventy percent of respondents were satisfied with their TCAM treatment.

There are no official data available on sociodemographic characteristics of consumers, such as age, economic status or gender, associated with TCAM use. The quality of the survey is low, as is the quality of data on process indicators.

28.5. DISCUSSION

At present, the Philippines Government has established the master-key for the development of TCAM, through the passage into law of Republic Act No. 8423, the Traditional and Alternative Medicine Act of 1997. However, the realities of organizational change in a developing country constitute a major challenge for the officials directly involved. At present there are only two policies directly related to TCAM modalities. The first of these is the Bureau of Food and Drugs regulation for herbal medicines, food and cosmetics, which adopts only the biomedical (allopathic) approach to standards of quality assurance. The other is the licensing of massage therapists, simply to ensure hygienic practice.

If TCAM is to boost the health-care delivery system of the country, professionalization of practitioners and the legal practice of TCAM by both physicians and non-physicians are warranted. Such a move is now under way, focused initially on herbal medicine, massage therapy and acupuncture, where priority is being given to training, research, standards and accreditation. The other TCAM modalities will follow, once acceptance of TCAM in general has been accomplished. The strategic approach is based on organizational change, social marketing and an operational approach to quality assurance. These approaches are being applied to training and formal education; research and development; financing and legalization of TCAM practice and its practitioners. There is also a need to focus strategically on a win-win relationship with established health-care professionals and product manufacturers.

The remaining challenges are to reach out to marginalized populations, assuring safe, effective and qualified medicinal products and services, and to carry out further research and development on other TCAM modalities that could be appropriate and beneficial to Filipinos (*8*).

28.6. CONCLUSIONS

Networking with countries supportive of TCAM is one of the most important ways in which the future development of TCAM can be improved. The compilation of this worldwide atlas on TCAM will help to guide the Philippine health authorities to determine which among the other countries are at par with each other and may share information on their successes and failures that have led to the present state of TCAM development. Through this sharing of important information between countries, we shall hand-in-hand attain maximum but wise utilization of our natural health resources and indigenous knowledge. The Philippines will benefit from the expertise of those countries with more advanced levels of government recognition and technical expertise on TCAM. Likewise, the Philippines may share its humble accomplishments with the other countries with similar socioeconomic development but with zero or minimal government recognition.

References
1. Licauco JT. *The Truth Behind Faith Healing in the Philippine.* Manila, National Bookstore Inc., 1981.

2. Sui CK. *Miracles through Pranic Healing.* India, Sterling Publishers Pvt. Ltd., 2001.

3. Philippine Institute of Traditional and Alternative Health Care, (http://www.doh.gov.ph/pitah, accessed 1 June 2004).

4. *Philippine Health Statistics 1995.* Manila, Department of Health, Republic of the Philippines.

5. *Country Health Information Profile.* Manila, WHO Office for the Western Pacific (2002), (http://www.wpro.who.int/chips/, accessed 1 June 2004).

6. National Objectives for Health, Philippines 1994–2004 & 1999–2004. Department of Health, Philippines, 2004.

7. Republic Act No. 8423 (S. No. 1471, H. No. 10070), Congress of the Philippines, Republic of the Philippines, Approved: December 9, 1997.

8. *Medicine Research in the Philippines, Herbal Medicine Research in the Philippines: Current status,* Philippine Council for Health Research and Development, Department of Science and Technology, (http://www.pchrd.dost.gov.ph/philmedplants/whatsnew08012001_01page_02.html, accessed 1 June 2004).

CHAPTER 29

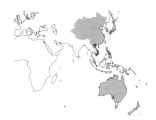

SOCIALIST REPUBLIC OF VIET NAM

Tran Van Hien[1]
and Chu Quoc Truong[2]

[1] Head of Laboratory of Research in Traditional Medicine, the National Hospital of Traditional Medicine, 29 Nguyen Binh Khiem, Hanoi, Viet Nam. Email: tranvanhien@fpt.vn

[2] Director, The National Hospital of Traditional Medicine, 29 Nguyen Binh Khiem, Hanoi, Viet Nam. Email: truongcq@yahoo.com

29.1. Introduction

The Socialist Republic of Viet Nam has a rich diversity of local medicines for the whole range of human diseases. Located in one of the richest biodiversity regions Viet Nam is considered the sixteenth most biodiverse country in the world. With one quarter of its area being rain forest, it has an estimated 12 000 plant species, of which 350 species are listed as endangered. Viet Nam has been a meeting-point for traditional systems of medicine for millennia, including classical Chinese medicine from the north, Hindu and Islamic influences from the west, and Austronesian practices from the islands of the South Pacific.

Vietnamese traditional medicine is a combination of modified classical Chinese medicine (as a result of a millennium of Chinese domination until the 12th century) and the indigenous practices of the diverse ethnic minorities making up Viet Nam. Practices based in Chinese medicine, including acupuncture, are more common among lowland groups and urban populations. The Vietnamese modification of Chinese medicine, although influenced by the indigenous population, may be more akin to the Chinese practices of some centuries ago. Furthermore, differences in the patterns of disease and in the plant species found in warmer and more humid Viet Nam necessitated different emphases in diagnosis and treatment. Traditional medicine practice is further influenced by the medicines of the ethnic minorities in Viet Nam, who number about 7 million in a national population of about 80 million. The minorities may be divided into 54 ethnic groups from several language groups.

29.2. Background Indicators

Viet Nam has made impressive gains in its health indicators during the last decades. It has achieved what few low-income countries have been able to achieve— a reduction of infant, child and maternal mortality to levels that are typically observed in countries that have two or three times the per capita income of Viet Nam. This has been done, for the most part, without much external assistance. Viet Nam has significantly reduced morbidity and mortality from communicable diseases, but finds itself facing a new generation of health problems associated with economic development, increasing affluence and ageing of the population. Diseases, such as diabetes, cancer and heart ailments are beginning to appear, especially in the urban areas, in part due to high rates of smoking and changes in diet. HIV/AIDS has the potential to become a major cause of morbidity and mortality in the future.

The ten most common causes of morbidity noted in the *Health Statistics Yearbook* of the Ministry of Health in 2000 (*1*) were:

1. Pneumonia
2. Acute pharyngitis and tonsillitis
3. Acute bronchitis and bronchiolitis
4. Diarrhoea and gastroenteritis
5. Influenza

6. Injuries

7. Respiratory tuberculosis

8. Traffic accidents

9. Hypertension

10. Complications of pregnancy and delivery.

The ten most common causes of mortality (*1*) were:

1. Pneumonia

2. Intracerebral haemorrhage

3. Intracranial injury

4. Heart failure

5. Respiratory tuberculosis

6. Transport accidents

7. Stroke, not specified as haemorrhage or infarction

8. Slow foetal growth, foetal malnutrition, low birth weight

9. Acute myocardial infarction

10. Other respiratory disorders originating in the prenatal period.

Total health expenditure for the allopathic health-care sector in 1999 was 27.7 billion Vietnamese Dong (VND), equivalent to approximately US$ 2.1 million (*2*), which included the state budget, health insurance and out-of-pocket spending. There has been a substantial increase in public spending on health over the last decades. Both total and per capita public spending on health increased about threefold in real terms, representing an annual rate of growth of around 20%. However, per capita public health spending in Viet Nam is still low, only VND 72 688 or US$ 5.62 in 1997, while total health spending is US$ 27.95 per capita. At 9.4% of gross domestic product, this places Viet Nam among those countries in Asia that spend the most on health care. Data on primary, secondary and tertiary health care spending are not available.

29.3. DEVELOPMENT OF TRADITIONAL MEDICINE IN THE HEALTH SYSTEM

In Viet Nam, traditional and allopathic medical systems are combined to bring traditional medicine into nationwide public health care. There are explicit government policies for traditional and complementary medicine (TCAM), dedicated agencies, regulation of practice and herbal medicines, research, formal coursework and associations of practitioners. There is a legal and regulatory infrastructure, with updated legislation on registration and inspection of herbal medicines and a licensing system to control the activities of traditional medicine practices. Most recently, the official national policy document in traditional medicine has been approved by the Government (*3*).

As a result of the Government's orientation in the development of the health sector, TCAM is extensively integrated into both primary and secondary health care. Viet Nam is one of only four countries (the others are China, Democratic People's Republic of Korea and the Republic of Korea) which WHO considers to have fully integrated TCAM into the formal health-care system. With this integrated national health-care system, there is a life expectancy of 69 years (in 1999) (*4*) despite a national per capita income that year of only US$ 390. This is substantially better than other countries with similar levels of economic development.

Regulated TCAM provision is available in two main sectors. The first of these is the government sector, including institutes of traditional medicine, hospitals of traditional medicine, and departments of traditional medicine in general hospitals, town and village centres. The second is the nongovernmental sector, including private traditional medicine clinics, companies and traditional medicine services. In addition to these two main sectors, professional traditional medicine associations, such as acupuncture associations, are also regulated.

Only certain TCAM providers are legally recognized. They are traditional doctors, traditional medicine practitioners, assistant doctors of traditional medicine, and those having remedies handed down from ancestors. All of these providers must have a license to practise medicine granted by the relevant bodies and based on conditions stipulated in Ministry of Health circulars.

These four categories of providers are entitled to provide the TCAM therapies which are commonly used. These include: (a) procedure-based therapies such as acupuncture, chiropractic, Qigong, energy methods and osteopathy; (b) body-work therapy including massage and reflexology; and (c) herbal medicine, including Chinese and Vietnamese herbal medicine.

29.3.1. Coordination Structure for TCAM Activities

There is a centralized management system for the TCAM sector. At the level of the Ministry of Health, there is a department of traditional medicine. At the central level, there are TCAM institutes, such as Institutes of Traditional Medicine and the Institute of Acupuncture. At the local levels there are many hospitals of traditional medicine. General activities include:

- recording, conveying and studying the heritage of traditional Vietnamese medicine, and combining it with allopathic medicine;

- training medical staff specialized in traditional medicine, from central to local levels;

- building-up a strong network of traditional medicine throughout the country;

- promoting traditional methods of disease prevention and health promotion;

- developing international cooperation.

29.3.2. Education and Training

With respect to education, there are TCAM faculties, TCAM departments in medical colleges, traditional hospitals, and institutes to train medical staff, as required by the Ministry of Health and according to the requirement of each locality. There are also public and private schools which offer training in TCAM.

Most TCAM training for health personnel is organized by the government system and concentrates on training medical doctors, secondary medical doctors and pharmacists in traditional medicine. This training is provided by:

- the Faculty of Traditional Medicine within the Hanoi University of Medicine;

- the Faculty of Traditional Medicine within the Ho Chi Minh City University of Medicine and Pharmacy;

- Departments of Traditional Medicine within a college of medicine in each of the following four provinces: Thai Binh, Thai Nguyen, Can Tho and Hai Phong;

- the Department of Traditional Medicine within the Military Academy of Medicine;

- three secondary schools in traditional medicine, namely Tue Tinh One and Tue Tinh Two belonging to the Ministry of Health and a private school belonging to the Hanoi Education and Training Bureau;

- the Viet Nam Institute of Traditional Medicine in Hanoi.

The Viet Nam Institute of Traditional Medicine is in charge of traditional medicine training for allopathic doctors and for continuing medical education. The Institute also provides certified TCAM training for overseas students. There is no school specialized in herbal medicines and acupuncture. All the above medical education institutions use a common curriculum, which includes a basic knowledge of traditional medicine; herbal medicine; acupuncture, massage, and vitality preservation; and other procedure-based therapies. The difference in training between colleges and schools lies in the length and level of the training course. There is also a separate training system organized by associations of traditional medicine at different administrative levels. Graduates who are successful in the examinations receive a certificate from provincial medical bureaux.

A team of medical professionals specialized in traditional medicine has been officially trained in traditional methods for treatment of diseases. About 19% among them are working in the government health sector and the remainder in the private sector. Training and refresher courses in TCAM are offered by various institutions of higher education and universities. Around 1500 physicians have graduated from traditional medicine departments of medical colleges. Of these graduates, 17% have undergone postgraduate training in a combination of traditional and allopathic medicine; 200 have Masters degrees with a specialization in traditional medicine; and approximately 20 have doctorates in traditional medicine.

29.3.3. Research

Research is conducted at various levels, including state-level projects, projects within the central Ministry, and studies at institutes of traditional medicine. This research aims to evaluate the safety and efficacy of herbal medicines; to improve the quality and form of final products; to combine traditional medicine with allopathic medicine; and to facilitate the modernization of traditional medicine in diagnosis and treatment of disease.

In scientific research, attention is paid to combining allopathic and traditional medicine by comparing the advantages and disadvantages of the two systems. Clinical research, research into basic theory, experimental investigations, diagnostic and therapeutic evaluations, as well as studies to develop new remedies and new forms of herbal medicine products, are all carried out.

Scientific research in traditional medicine is of interest not only to scientists in TCAM institutions, but also to others aiming to:

- develop sources of medicinal plants in Viet Nam;

- promote the inheritance of experiences of traditional medicine utilization among people in different areas of the country;

- promote the potential of traditional medicine in community health care;

- integrate traditional and allopathic medicine for the treatment of culture-bound syndromes (social diseases) and chronic diseases;

- improve the quality of herbal medicine products.

29.3.4. Regulatory Control

Hospital codes of ethics and statutes are enacted by the Ministry of Health to control examination and treatment of patients. A formal National Drug Policy governs the use of herbal medicines. There is a list of 186 herbal medicines identified as essential medicines, of which 40 herbal preparations are for use by the community and 60 herbal medicines are for use in the treatment of common diseases in village health centres. The Ministry of Health has issued guidelines for the study and evaluation of Viet Nam traditional medicines in the context of a Cabinet Statute on traditional medicine and an accompanying circular (5).

29.3.5. Funding

The Government provides funding mainly for the activities of the national traditional medicine network. At the central level, there are three research institutes with beds for inpatients. In the provinces, there are 52 provincial hospitals of TCAM, and about 254 departments of TCAM in general hospitals. District, inter-district and communal health centres have staff responsible for TCAM.

In general, hospital budgets are provided from the national health budget, depending on hospital classification. At the central level, the budget is allocated at the rate of VND 20–23 million (c. US$ 1546–1778) per bed. At the provincial level, the rate is between VND 8–13 million (c. US$ 618–1005) per bed, depending on the type of hospital. The annual budget for the hospital includes salaries for staff. The Government funds health stations at different administrative levels. Traditional therapies are covered under the health insurance system.

The national budget for TCAM is approximately 2.7% of the national health budget. Health expenses for TCAM therapies are about VND 614 (c. US$ 0.05) per capita per year. This is equivalent to 1.28% of national per capita health expenditure.

29.4. Utilization Surveys

There have been at least three TCAM user surveys conducted in Viet Nam during recent years:

1. A survey of the need for provision of primary health care with traditional medicine, carried out from 1994 to 1996 by the Department of Traditional Medicine, Ministry of Health.

2. A study on the situation of human resources for traditional medicine and utilization of traditional medicine in Viet Nam. This study was designed at the request of Ministry of Health, aiming to draw a picture of TCAM development at the moment before the implementation of the Viet Nam National Drug Policy. The implementation unit was the Viet Nam Institute of Traditional Medicine. The head of the research group was the Institute's Director, Professor Tran Thuy. The study was sponsored by the Swedish International Development Agency, conducted in 1997, and Dr Tran Van Hien wrote the report in 1998 (6).

3. A survey on the utilization of traditional medicine and perceptions of users of traditional medicine in Viet Nam. The implementation unit for this study was the Viet Nam Institute of Traditional Medicine. The World Bank sponsored the study and the report was written by Dr Tran Van Hien in 1999 (7), in consultation with Global Initiative for Traditional Systems of Health, Oxford University. The objectives of the study were:

   - to outline the current situation in terms of human resources for traditional medicine (amount, quality, structure and distribution);

   - to investigate the utilization of herbal medicines for common illnesses;

   - to recommend solutions for inequalities in human resources and utilization of traditional medicine.

29.4.1. Utilization of Traditional Medicine

The survey conducted in 1997 by the Viet Nam Institute of Traditional Medicine showed that 50% of the population preferred to be treated by traditional rather than allopathic medicine. In 1995, herbal medicines represented 31% of registered drugs in Viet Nam. Traditional medicine is practised not only at the primary level of health care, but also in hospitals providing secondary and tertiary care. In Viet Nam, traditional medicine is not expensive, it is locally available and it is the system most utilized and preferred by the poor.

By tradition, Vietnamese people have some knowledge of herbal medicine. In the survey conducted in 1999 by the Viet Nam Institute of Traditional Medicine, 85.2% of respondents could name at least 10 plants and describe their use for common diseases. In community health care, herbal medicine is used to treat 15 different kinds of diseases and symptoms: common cold, digestive disorders, stomach ache, insomnia and headache, asthenia, arthritis, jaundice, urinary problems, poor lactation, menstrual disorders, skin problems, burns and wounds, and dengue fever.

29.4.2. Attitudes of Traditional Medicine Users

Rural people, of whom 80% are peasant farmers, prefer traditional treatment for new and common diseases in the community, due to the low cost of these therapeutic methods. This is particularly the case in remote and mountainous areas, where traditional medicine is almost the only choice available for health care. In the majority of cases, people do not have to spend any money, since they collect medicinal plants in their local area. The cost of curing chronic diseases at medical stations at the grass-roots level is acceptable, and the effectiveness is equivalent to that obtained by conventional therapeutic methods.

Traditional medicine is commonly chosen by people to treat common diseases and chronic diseases. A survey done by the Viet Nam Institute of Traditional Medicine in 1997–1998, investigated the treatment of diseases in traditional hospitals. The study looked at 85 different medical conditions from 3351 clinical records. The ten most common conditions treated were: weakness, rheumatism, sciatica, haemorrhoids, hypertension, the sequelae of cerebral accidents, neurasthenia, lumbago, gastro-duodenal syndrome, pain in the shoulder area.

29.5. Discussion

Traditional medicine is part of the cultural heritage of Viet Nam. Vietnamese traditional medicine is a combination of modified classical Chinese medicine and indigenous medicine. Vietnamese traditional medicine has been documented by honourable Vietnamese practitioners in many valuable medical masterpieces covering different specialties.

Vietnamese traditional medicine forms an integral part of the national health care system in Viet Nam and has an important role in promoting the health of the Vietnamese people, particularly in difficult cases, geriatric diseases and primary health care at the commune level. In Viet Nam, the government supports public-sector facilities for traditional medicine and encourages people to mobilize resources for the development of traditional medicine. A number of official documents indicate clear support for traditional medicine; the most recent being the national policy on traditional medicine. According to Ministry of Health statistics, about 30% of patients receive treatment with traditional medicines, provided by both government and private traditional medicine systems. Traditional medicine is practised not only at the primary health care level, but also in hospitals providing secondary and tertiary care. In Viet Nam, traditional medicine is not expensive, is locally available and is the system most utilized and preferred by the poor. As the result of research in traditional medicine, many herbal medicine products derived from classical formulae or new formulae have been developed and modernized. This has made a great contribution to solving the problems of epidemic, viral and social diseases.

29.6. Conclusions

Traditional medicine in Viet Nam is formally and effectively integrated into national health care. Regulation is designed to ensure quality of services and products. Education and training are conducted according to a standardized curriculum, and produce practitioners and researchers from the level of provincial institutions to national level institutes. Research plays an important role in the modernization of traditional medicine practice in Viet Nam, making it more efficient, effective and safe.

References

1. *Health statistics yearbook.* Hanoi, Ministry of Health, Viet Nam, 2000.

2. *Vietnam health sector review.* Hanoi, World Bank, 1999.

3. *National policy in traditional medicine.* (No. 222/2003/QD-TTg), 3 November 2003. Hanoi, Government of Viet Nam, 2003.

4. *Health statistics yearbook.* Hanoi, Ministry of Health, Viet Nam, 1999.

5. *Guidelines issued for the study and evaluation of Viet Nam traditional medicines in the context of a Cabinet Statute on traditional medicine and an accompanying circular (MOH circular No. 371).* Hanoi, Ministry of Health, Viet Nam, 1996.

6. *A survey on the situation of human resources for traditional medicine and utilization of traditional medicine in Viet Nam. Hanoi, Viet Nam.* Institute of Traditional Medicine, 1998.

7. *The utilization of traditional medicine and perceptions of users of traditional medicine in Viet Nam.* Hanoi, Viet Nam Institute of Traditional Medicine, 1999.

INDEX